Bodies of Knowledge

Bodies of Knowledge

The Medicalization
of Reproduction in Greece

Eugenia Georges

Vanderbilt University Press
Nashville

© 2008 by Vanderbilt University Press
Nashville, Tennessee 37235

12 11 10 09 08 1 2 3 4 5

This book is the recipient of the 2006 Norman L. and Roselea J.
Goldberg Prize from Vanderbilt University Press for the best project
in the area of medicine.

Designed by Dariel Mayer

Library of Congress Cataloging-in-Publication Data

Georges, Eugenia.
Bodies of knowledge : the medicalization of reproduction in Greece /
Eugenia Georges.
p. ; cm.
Includes bibliographical references and index.
ISBN 978-0-8265-1598-8 (cloth : alk. paper)
ISBN 978-0-8265-1599-5 (pbk. : alk. paper)
1. Human reproduction—Greece—Rhodes (Island)—History—
20th century. 2. Childbirth—Greece—Rhodes (Island)—History—
20th century. 3. Birth control—Greece—Rhodes (Island)—History—
20th century. 4. Women—Health and hygiene—Greece—Rhodes
(Island)—History—20th century. 5. Ethnology—Greece—Rhodes
(Island)—History—20th century. I. Title.
[DNLM: 1. Reproductive Behavior—history—Greece.
2. Anthropology, Cultural—methods—Greece. 3. Family Planning
Policy—history—Greece. 4. History, 20th Century—Greece. 5. Social
Conditions—Greece. 6. Women's Health—history—Greece. HQ 766
G8 G351b 2008]
QP251.G357 2008
612.609495—dc22
2008028081

For my mother, Nafsica,
and my daughter, Christa

Contents

Acknowledgments

Returning year after year to do fieldwork on a Greek island sometimes conjures skeptical, even cynical, reactions from people. I am therefore especially grateful to all those friends, colleagues, family members, and funding agencies who, despite such preconceptions, supported me in this research over the years.

Like every anthropologist, I owe an irredeemable debt to the many people who shared their lives and stories with me, and without whose generosity and goodwill this book would never have been possible. Most must remain anonymous, but it is a pleasure to personally thank my friends in Rhodes: Debbie Hadzidiakou, Maria Karagianni, Vasilia Kazoulli, Ghianis Kazoullis, Vangelis Pavilides, Evmorphia Stratis, Stathis Stratis, the late and greatly missed Evi Triandafilou, Georgia Vitsilaki, and Dimitris Zanetoulis. Because of their friendship and hospitality, Rhodes genuinely came to feel like home for me and my daughter, Christa. Heartfelt thanks go to Evmorphia Stratis for allowing me to use her painting for the cover of this book, as well as for teaching Christa how to draw. Ana Maria Kazdagli taught me much about medieval Rhodes and pointed me to resources that I would have never found on my own. I am especially grateful to Dr. Chrisy Vitsilaki, not only for over a decade of friendship, but also for making her office at the University of the Aegean in Rhodes available to me whenever I needed it. The research assistance provided by Christina Karagianni, Anthoula Hadzipetrou, and Penny Papakosta was critical to this project, and I thank them all for their friendship as well.

I am also deeply grateful for the guidance and hospitality I received from colleagues in Greece as I began to formulate this project and then throughout the ensuing years. Dimitra Gefou-Madianou welcomed me into her home and into her department at Pantion University. Deanna Trakas literally led me to Rhodes, where she had conducted her own research, and personally introduced me to the staff of the hospital, as well as to other Rhodians who would eventually become good friends. I am additionally grateful for the affiliation she arranged with the Institute of Child Health in Athens, which provided important institutional support at an early phase of this project. Eleni Papagaroufali, together with her husband, Kostas, and son, Ghiorghos, offered me and my daughter endless warmth, laughter, and hospitality whenever we were in Athens. Deanna, Dimitra, and Eleni have also provided invaluable insight and guidance over the course of my research, and have read and commented on various versions of the project as it progressed. My friendship with Dr. Lida Triantafillidou, formed during the three years she was my Greek teacher in Houston, continued when she moved back to Athens. I thank her and her husband, Dr. Fivos Verdelis, for the many delicious dinners and stimulating conversations we've shared over the years.

For the selfless act of reading and commenting on the entire manuscript, my heartfelt thanks to Lambros Comitas, Robbie Davis-Floyd, James Faubion, Dimitra Gefou-Madianou, Eleni Papagaroufali, Deanna Trakas, and the unsung anonymous reviewers for Vanderbilt University Press.

Many colleagues at Rice University's Department of Anthropology, my academic home for nearly two decades, have provided assistance and advice on this project. George Marcus, my chair for most of this time, grumbled only slightly when I asked for research leaves and encouraged this project in his own inimitable style. In particular, I remain grateful for his invitation to contribute a piece to the *Late Editions* project, which showed his confidence in the research at a very early stage (and led to one of the most enjoyable collaborative experiences of my academic career). Over the years, I have benefited in many ways from conversations with Sharon Traweek, Julie Taylor, Kathryn Milun, and the unstinting Jim Faubion. Many colleagues elsewhere have offered valuable advice and commentary on various aspects of this research as well. Thanks to Athena Athanasiou, Carole Browner, Michael Herzfeld, Werner Kelber, Ann Millard, Lisa Mitchell, Lynn Morgan, Barbara Rylko-Bauer, and Lida Triantafillidou. I owe a special and immeasurable debt of gratitude to Robbie-Davis Floyd, friend and reader extraordinaire.

Financial support from the American Council of Learned Societies, the National Science Foundation, the Foundation for Hellenic Studies, and the Center for the Study of Institutions and Values at Rice University has supported this project over the years. A Faculty Fellowship from the Center for the Study of Culture at Rice University helped launch the writing of this book, and I thank its director, Werner Kelber, for his support and encouragement. I owe special thanks to the RISM–Ruth Landes Foundation and its director at the time, Lambros Comitas, for awarding me an individual faculty fellowship as well as a generous developmental grant that allowed me to take four Rice students to the field with me each summer for three years. The projects undertaken by Aimee Placas, Lindsay Smith, Erkan Saka, and Sophia Roosth produced fascinating original research on cross-cultural romance and marriage and on Rhodes's Muslim and Sephardi communities that helped deepen and extend my understanding of Rhodian society.

My heartfelt thanks go to Michael Ames, my editor at Vanderbilt University Press, for his faith in this book, and the enthusiasm and patience with which he has supported its publication. I also appreciate the quick responses that Jessie Hunnicutt and Dariel Mayer always provided to my queries and uncertainties. I am particularly grateful to Bobbe Needham for her extraordinarily careful and skillful copyediting.

I also wish to acknowledge the University of Wisconsin Press for permission to use portions from a chapter previously published in the volume *Body Talk: Rhetoric, Technology, and Reproduction*, edited by Mary Lay, Laura J. Gurak, Clare Gravon, and Cynthia Myntti (2000); the University of California Press for permission to adapt portions of an article originally published as "Fetal Ultrasound Imaging and the Production of Authoritative Knowledge in Greece" in *Medical Anthropology Quarterly* 10(2): 157–75 (1996), © Society for Medical Anthropology; and Elsevier Science, Ltd., for permission to include portions of an article originally published as "Abortion Policy and Practice in Greece" in *Social Science and Medicine* 42(2): 509–19 (1996).

From the start, my husband, Bob Etnyre, has been the linchpin of this project. He has given me the unconditional support year after year without which the undertaking and completion of this book would have simply not have been possible. He also read and commented on the entire manuscript. For all of this and for so much more, no thanks are enough.

Note on Transliteration

Because no universally accepted standard of transliteration exists for modern Greek, each of us who attempt to render the language readable to an English-speaking audience must decide on a system that more or less satisfactorily suits our purposes. I have opted for a mix of phonological and orthographic representation, not least because some of the Greek I render is local Rhodian dialect for which no standard orthography exists. I use *dh* for the Greek delta, *kh* for the Greek chi, and *gh* for the Greek gamma. For place names, I have retained the forms most familiar to English speakers, but I have used my own system when transliterating proper names, including those of Greek authors not published in English.

Chapter 1

Introduction

This book is about the recent shifts in knowledge and power that have profoundly transformed how women on the island of Rhodes perceive, make sense of, and manage their reproductive bodies and experiences. These shifts, which began soon after the end of World War II and took roughly a generation to complete, can be summed up in the term "medicalization." Medicalization refers to the increasingly global process by which biomedicine has achieved the authority to redefine and treat an expanding array of individual life events and social problems as medical problems and ultimately to make exclusive claims over the body. Well into the middle of the twentieth century, the full range of Rhodian women's reproductive concerns remained largely outside the purview of biomedical experts. Women relied on the long-standing body of knowledge and practices known as the *iatrosophia*, literally, "medical wisdom," on the one hand, and on rituals improvised from the Greek Orthodox religious tradition on the other, to enhance and control their fertility, protect their pregnancies, successfully birth their babies, and navigate the hazards of the postpartum period. Every village on the island and every neighborhood in the capital city of Rhodes had at least one local midwife to whom women could turn for expert assistance in these matters. In the early 1990s, when I began this study, all the midwives had died or long since stopped practicing. By then, the specialized knowledge of the recent past, of which young women usually knew little or nothing, could be spliced together only from the recollections of their mothers and grandmothers. Such practices as women in their twenties and thirties might be aware of—the obligation of pregnant women to sample any food they happened to smell to prevent miscarriage and birthmarks, for instance—were liable to be dismissed as *vlakies*, "stupidities." Or, less harshly but equally revealingly, they might be referred to by the loan words *tabou* and *folklor*. Either way, young women unmistakably signaled their distance from practices that, now hopelessly undermined, had come to be either seen as the irrational traces of an earlier, benighted time or, at best, objectified and relegated to the realm of anthropology and folklore.

As also hinted by the use of these terms, medicalization has succeeded not just by changing women's behavior, but more fundamentally, by demoting and disallowing existing knowledge of the body and replacing it with new discourses based in biology and medicine (Duden 1991). Official efforts to eradicate local midwives and other practical healers, and along with them, the iatrosophia medical tradition in general, began almost as soon as the Greek nation achieved independence from Ottoman rule in 1828. Just six years later, a new regulatory institution, the Iatrosynedrio, was established to organize public health and administer medical examinations, issuing licenses only to those who succeeded in passing them (Korasidou 2002, 157–58). Rhodes, and the Dodecanese Island chain of which it is the major hub, remained part of the Ottoman Empire into the early twentieth century, passing through Italian hands before finally joining the Greek nation in 1947. Under the banner of its own modernizing mission, the Italian colonial government that ruled Rhodes between 1911 and 1944 waged a remarkably similar campaign to suppress local practitioners and replace them with certified, preferably Italian-trained, biomedical professionals. Still, on Rhodes as on the Greek mainland, such attempts at medical reform rarely reached beyond more than a sliver of the elite echelons of the population. Throughout Greece, the medicalization of reproduction and the realization of biomedical hegemony in general had to await fundamental changes in both institutional structures and the broader cultural logic of Greek society. Until then, women relied heavily—and in rural areas, almost exclusively—on what I refer to in this book as ethnogynecology and ethno-obstetrics and its specialist practitioners, the local midwives, to address a host of reproductive concerns, from the inability to conceive a child to breech presentations in childbirth. In the first half of this book, I offer the first comprehensive ethnographic description of this richly elaborated body of reproductive knowledge, which, as I will show, comprises a remarkably smooth braiding of three distinct strands: a secular ethnogynecology replete with parallels to humoral medicine as codified by Galen and the countless other medical theorists who followed his lead through the early modern period; an ethno-obstetrics with numerous parallels to the equally durable and influential obstetrical treatise of Soranus of Ephesus, who self-consciously distinguished his approach from that of humoral medicine; and, finally, though not least, a host of salient idioms and rituals rooted in the Greek Orthodox Church. In doing so, I bring into focus the neglected figure of the practical midwife, a unique female specialist whose practice also seamlessly embodied ritual and secular answers to the pressing health concerns of the women who depended on her care.

The exponential increase in literacy and education and the explosive growth in the medical profession after the Second World War provided the institutional moorings for the unraveling of much of this body of knowledge—and along with it, the demise of its specialized practitioners—and paved the way for the ascent of Greek biomedicine that I describe in the second half of this book. But, by its very nature, the achievement of biomedical hegemony, like any hegemony, depends also on the active desire and demand of the larger population. It depends, in short, on transforming subjectivity—the ways people experience, know, and feel. Because such transformations are always conditioned and shaped by local configurations of power and contingencies of history and culture, however, the specific features of medicalization, like the processes of modernization and globalization of which it has formed an integral part, are inevitably stamped by the society in which they develop. Furthermore, because these transformations are always ongoing and never totally realized, women and their families, both as consumers of medical knowledge and practices and as producers of new self-knowledge, have also inevitably helped shape the process. As a result of the interplay of these and other factors that will be examined in the course of this ethnography, the medicalization of reproduction in Greece has assumed its own distinctive signature, a mosaic of responses that, depending on the specific reproductive technology, range from ebullient embrace, through qualified acceptance, to adamant refusal. The specific ways in which women have helped shape the contours of this medicalization process across an array of reproductive concerns, and amid the particular circumstances of their lives, is the theme of the second half of this book.

Conceptualizing the Medicalization of Reproduction

It is a basic insight of medical anthropology that all medical knowledge, whether ethno- or bio-, is implicated in the maintenance of social control. Biomedicine as it developed in Europe in the eighteenth and nineteenth centuries, and spread globally in the twentieth, is distinguished moreover by its intimate alliance with *institutional* apparatuses of power concerned with the rational regulation of both the individual and the social body (B. Turner 1995). Because of this tight linkage, even as new medical definitions and categories based on developments in anatomy and pathology advanced the understanding and treatment of disease, they also did much more. Most significantly for my purposes, they made available a distinctive and authoritative mode of discourse that performed a significant role in the process that Foucault termed "biopower." On Foucault's view, biopower comprises a "great bipolar technology" of modernity that has increasingly displaced the use of repressive force as a form of social control. Drawing on a variety of discourses and practices, biopower at one level directs the performance of the individual body—attempting to shape its everyday movements and dispositions and innermost motivations and desires. Biopower also operates at the social level through a series of institutions and technologies, from clinics and hospitals to censuses and statistics, to supervise and intervene in and regulate the life of national populations (Foucault 1978 [1990], 139–40).

Although not explicitly discussed in these terms by Foucault, biopower has historically been a profoundly gendered process. The obsession with national population that developed among an array of elites over the course of the nineteenth century had divergent implications and consequences for men and women. Representing a major departure from older Malthusian fears of *over*population, the new demographic discourse was concerned with both increasing the number of national citizens and improving their overall "quality" in terms of health, productivity, and reproductivity. Within this discourse, men's citizenship came to be defined largely in terms of their contributions as disciplined and conscientious soldiers and productive and compliant workers. Women, on the other hand, were assigned the primary responsibility for reproducing and ensuring the health and vigor of these "stalwart sons" of the nation (Cole 2000; de Grazia 1996; Ram and Jolly 1998). Over time, the ideological bond between women and motherhood, and between women's citizenship and the quality of their reproductive contribution to the national body, became increasingly tight.

The new concern with the quantity and quality of national populations was accompanied by the "discovery" of children and their migration from the ideological margins to the center of concern in family life (Aries 1962; Donzelot 1979). Statistics emerged at this time as "the major technical factor, or one of the major technical factors," deployed by the state to effect the governmentality of the national population (Foucault 1991, 99). By the latter part of the nineteenth century, these newly devised statistical and survey techniques were revealing declining fertility and alarmingly high rates of infant and child mortality in nation after nation across Europe and North America (Blum 1999; Cole 2000; Korasidou 2002). Prominent Athenian physicians of the day, like their counterparts in France and elsewhere, turned to records newly gathered by the police in an attempt to identify the factors responsible for these deaths.

By means such as these, they were able to conclude, for example, that the diarrheal diseases claiming so many children's lives at the time were caused primarily by their mothers' "wrong-headed" feeding practices (Korasidou 2002, 195). More generally, the high rates of infant and child death, as well as the declining birth rates, uncovered by the new methods of statistical analysis were widely read as an abdication on the part of women to do their duty as citizens, either by not reproducing in sufficiently large numbers, or by contributing to the premature death of their children through ignorance and the pursuit of irrational childbirth and child-rearing practices (Korasidou 2002). In either case, the stage was set for a series of interventions whose objective it was to medicalize motherhood, that is, to replace existing maternal understandings and practices with novel ones based in science and medicine. This was a project in which medicine and its auxiliary professions, as well as education, the law, and later on, the mass media, all played pivotal roles (Apple 1995; Donzelot 1979, xx). The process of medicalization inevitably took different forms and routes in bourgeois, poor, and later, colonial families (Donzelot 1979, xxi; Ram and Jolly 1998; Ross 1993). Yet across the board, it was women who were assigned the core responsibility for learning and following the canons of scientific hygiene and medicine to ensure the successful birth, survival, and health of their children (Apple 1987). "Good mothers" were those who did so, "bad mothers" those who did not. And since all women were now expected to reproduce, their contributions to society increasingly came to be gauged by their "successes and failures as mothers" (Cole 2000, 15). Medicalized definitions and categories thus had a potent role to play in reconfiguring gender roles and meanings in the nineteenth and twentieth centuries. Ultimately, however, rather than unifying women in a common project of scientific reproduction, they offered a new (and constantly mutating) set of tools for dividing, condemning, and regulating them (Litt 2000).

Authoritative Knowledge, Rationality, and Power

The perspective on the medicalization of reproduction I have just outlined contrasts dramatically with most popular accounts. On the popular view, the ascent of biomedicine tends to be cast as part of a larger celebratory story of progress, modernization, and continual improvement of the conditions of life achieved through the application of science and technology. However, the aura of rationality and inevitability that hovers over this widespread modernist narrative—its "halo of disinterestedness," in Benedict Anderson's evocative phrase—obscures the play of powerful interests and their vital stake in the narrative itself. Historically, the global triumph of biomedicine has relied on alliances with the state and other sources of structural power that have frequently had as their objective the repression of competing approaches, as the example of the passage of laws outlawing midwifery and other nonbiomedical specialties in North America and elsewhere attests (Baer 1989; Leavitt 1986; Wertz and Wertz 1989). It is for this reason, as Davis-Floyd, Pigg, and Cosminky caution, that biomedicine is best conceptualized "not so much as a free-floating system of knowledge and techniques as a nationally and internationally authorized project often linked to state efforts of modernization" (2001, 114).

Perhaps even more fundamental has been biomedicine's ideological success in pushing alternative perspectives "to the margins of reasoned discourse" (Young 1982, 275). Vested with the structural and cultural authority to define an experience or event as legitimately medical or not medical, biomedical knowledge has become, in Brigitte Jordan's influential term, *the* authoritative knowledge of the body. Ultimately, this cultural authority endows biomedicine with a dominant voice in the ongoing negotiation of consensus regarding what is thinkable and what is unthinkable, imaginable and unimaginable, rational and irrational (Williams 1980; Jordan [1978] 1993). In short, biomedicine becomes hegemonic.

Thus, eclipsed behind the halo of celebratory narratives of medical progress there is usually a shadow story of how competing ways of understanding and approaching reproduction and the body have been displaced along the way. At the same time, repressed alternatives return from the margins of reasoned discourse to be rhetorically recast as quackery, traditional ignorance, and irrational superstition, or, in the more polite Rhodian locution, as taboos and folklore. Against the foil of this now delegitimated body of knowledge, biomedicine is represented, and often experienced, not as hegemonic and coercive, but as another freedom from the traditional constraints and, even worse, mortal dangers of the past that modern women and men are privileged to enjoy (D. Miller 1994, 72).

Despite their fundamental differences, popular and sociological perspectives on the medicalization of reproduction share embedded teleologies that in the end shortchange the ways in which women themselves actively engage with and help shape the process. Whether as the instrument of a (patriarchal) medical profession surreptitiously wielded in the service of expanding social control or, alternatively, as the beneficent outcome of a disinterested quest for scientific knowledge and progress, the medicalization of reproduction tends to be conceptualized as a monolithic process unremittingly imposed on women from the outside (Lock and Kaufert 1998; Lock 2004; Lupton 1994; Rapp

1999). Either way, their reactions and responses as users, consumers, and, above all, as subjects of medical discourse and practice are barely audible. A rapidly growing number of feminist-informed ethnographic studies, however, persuasively argues for the inadequacy of such approaches and underscores both the scholarly and practical benefits of paying close attention to women's embodied experiences as they attempt to interpret and assign meaning to an ever-expanding array of reproductive technologies and practices (Becker 2000; Inhorn 1994, 2003; Lock and Kaufert 1998; Rapp 1999; Saetnan 2000).

As these studies accumulate, it has become apparent that women's responses to medicalization are often surprisingly selective and culturally specific. Which reproductive technologies and procedures are embraced and how tightly and which rejected or ignored varies, often markedly, from context to context (Lock and Kaufert 1998). In other words, women do not receive and accept new technologies, procedures, and knowledge in a docile or unreflective manner; rather, they actively and flexibly interpret and assess their meanings and implications for their everyday lives. In doing so, they may draw on a variety of disparate and not always mutually compatible discourses. Even so, it is important to underscore that, given the uneven distribution of power and authority that underpins most biomedical systems, women's creativity and interpretive scope are never fully free or unconstrained. Rather, within the intersecting grids of powerful discourses and practices, they generally "make do" in the sense elaborated by de Certeau: although women may continually improvise meanings and deploy tactics to serve their own pragmatic ends, inevitably they do so bounded by "the space of the other" (de Certeau 1984, 37). Their ability to flexibly interpret and recode the meanings of technologies and procedures is thus usually limited. How precisely limited, however, varies with the kinds of power relations in which women find themselves entangled. The techniques of biopower are heterogeneous and the degrees to which they allow for deviance from a set of norms has implications for the extent to which women are able to flexibly interpret the array of biomedical technologies and procedures they encounter in the course of dealing with their reproductive concerns. As a result, women may often exhibit the seemingly paradoxical and fragmented stance of simultaneously consenting and dissenting to various features of the medicalization process (Fisher and Davis 1993; Lupton 1999). Since ethnographic studies often tend to focus on a single reproductive technology (in vitro fertilization, amniocentesis, medical contraception), it can be difficult to follow the complex logic by which women discriminate among, and selectively respond to, the array of technologies that most now face across their reproductive lives. Comparing Rhodian women's responses to different technologies thus offers a unique opportunity for understanding how and why diverse discourses and pragmatic concerns recede or come to the fore as women deal with a range of reproductive concerns and, ultimately, of the roles they have played in shaping the process of medicalization.

Studying Medicalization in Context: Interpretive Ambiguity and Divergent Knowledge

In the contemporary world, a number of different discourses exist alongside biomedicine, opening up its technologies and procedures to a variety of meanings and posing the possibility of alternative interpretations. As a result, and notwithstanding the continuing appeal of the modernist narrative just described, medicalization today is rarely received as a story of undiluted triumph (S. Williams 1997). Fed by a steady stream of information and images in the mass media, public concern over the undesirable by-products of science and technology and the potential hazards they pose to health and well-being has grown and intensified. By now, awareness of the iatrogenic risks of biomedicine is widespread, while the dystopic possibilities of the new genetics create novel apprehensions and uncertainties. Beginning in the 1960s, critiques articulated by a variety of grass-roots social movements such as environmentalism, feminism, and consumer health advocacy groups have helped shape and give political direction to sometimes inchoate anxieties and fears. Consumer concern and dissatisfaction with biomedical risks and side effects have helped fuel the impressive expansion and (re)legitimation of complementary and alternative medicine in Europe, the United States, Japan, and elsewhere (Baer 2002; Micozzi 2002; Ohnuki-Tierney 1986). Health and consumer activists have also helped devise influential critiques that have even succeeded in partially demedicalizing such specialties as psychiatry and obstetrics, two historically classic loci of the medicalization process. As a result, if until fairly recently medical scientific expertise was regarded as the "guarantor" or "arbiter" of truth (Nelkin 2003, xii; Rabinow 1989, 14) about health, illness, and the body, in the contemporary late or postmodern world, this is no longer unqualifiedly the case. Instead, science, medicine, and technology have come to be regarded as sources of a proliferating array of "manufactured risks" that potentially threaten human health and well-being (Giddens 1991). In short, disparate and diverse discourses now intersect the authority of science and medicine, creating new knowledge and offering novel possibilities for competing interpretive perspectives.

Among these, the pervasive discourse of risk has been especially influential in generating compelling critiques of science and medicine. In his influential "risk society" thesis, Ulrich Beck (1992a) has argued that a heightened awareness of an overwhelming volume of contemporary risks is a distinctive feature of the late modern sensibility. The hallmark of this sensibility, according to Beck, Giddens, and others, is reflexivity, a disposition of thought that most crucially entails the habitual questioning of science and medicine through alternative sources of expert knowledge (Lash and Urry 1994, 36). Increasingly, this disposition has also come to entail the expectation that nonexperts, including consumers themselves, should acquire the appropriate knowledge necessary to make responsible decisions about their own future. From this perspective, the notion of risk may be understood as an increasingly global technology "for assembling populations through expert knowledge so that these populations may become 'experts of themselves'" (Phillips and Ilcan 2007, 108). Critics of the risk society thesis have dissected its shortcomings on a number of fronts: its propensity to sweeping generalizations, its neglect of cultural difference, and the relatively unrefined implicit typologies (premodern-modern-late modern) on which it rests (e.g., Mallaby 2002; Nichter 2003; Tulloch and Lupton 2003). Without losing sight of these important qualifications, one may still appreciate the basic insight that anxiety over, and responsibility for, acquiring knowledge about an ever-expanding array of manufactured risks represents a significant dimension of health management throughout the contemporary world (Lupton 1999; Stacey 2001, 134; Tulloch and Lupton 2003).

Beck, however, would ethnocentrically, and quite erroneously, exclude Greeks from participation in this late modern disposition. Writing of the pervasive contemporary sense of nuclear risk and fear of radiation, for instance, Beck asserts that "everyone between the Alpine cottages and the North Sea mudflats now understands and speaks the language of the nuclear critics" (1992b, 115). In locutions such as these, Greeks (along with many others) periodically find themselves relegated to the margins of influential discussions of modernity, a rhetorical move with which they have long been acquainted, as I discuss later. *Pace* Beck, however, concern and anxiety over the harmful effects of radiation, as well as a host of other manufactured risks—hormones, dioxins in the food supply, and genetically modified foods, to mention some of the most salient—are in fact commonplace in contemporary Greek life. The local responses to Chernobyl, a global emblem of scientific and technological development gone horribly awry, offered one early and unmistakable manifestation of such concerns. As Adriana Petryna (2002, 3–4) has observed in her recent ethnography of the site: "Chernobyl was an 'anthropological shock' for Western Europe, bringing the efficacy of everyday knowledge to a state of collapse and underscoring how much the conditions for secure living in what have been termed risk societies lie in the hands of experts of all kinds." In Greece, anxiety and fears produced by the "shock" of Chernobyl and its radioactive aftermath were dramatically expressed in the unprecedented 10 percent drop in the birth rate that followed the accident, a decline that took two years to fully rebound (Emke-Poulopoulou 1994, 23–24). Almost twenty years later, Chernobyl still reverberated in the minds of Rhodian women I spoke with. When Evangelia, a twenty-eight-year-old civil servant expecting her first child, learned from an ultrasound examination that her fetus had a serious kidney problem, she searched for some explanation to help her make sense of this devastating news. Her thoughts kept returning to Chernobyl, she told me, and she wondered: Was it the contaminated rains that drenched her as she walked home from middle school that winter and sent her rushing to the shower for a thorough scrubbing the moment she got in the door? Since Chernobyl, Greece has continued to be rocked by exposure to new risks manufactured elsewhere that migrate unimpeded across its borders.[1] In 1999, anxiety over the effects of radiation was rekindled by the news, widely reported in Greece (but not in the United States) that U.S. troops fighting in Kosovo were using weapons containing depleted but still radioactive uranium. Women I spoke with that summer were once again worried about the effects of radiation on their pregnancies, and many Rhodians also voiced fears of a future spike in the incidence of cancer, as well as other health problems.

As a consequence of the global circulation of information and the increased awareness of a dizzying array of manufactured risks, biomedicine in Greece, as elsewhere, has acquired a "dilemmatic" complexion (S. Williams 1997). Increasingly, it is perceived both as source of "goods" as well as "bads"; as symptom at the same time as solution; vehicle of hope, optimism, and a sense of control on the one hand and of hidden risks, potential disease, and injury on the other (Beck 1992a; Tulloch and Lupton 2003; S. Williams 1997). New developments in medicine, science, and technology are still actively desired and embraced, to be sure, but in the context of a pervasive discourse of risk, often not without some measure of ambivalence.

This dilemmatic quality of biomedicine and the ambivalence it can provoke, I argue, are reflected in the signature unevenness that characterizes the medicalization of reproduction in Greece today. Certain domains, such as pregnancy, birth and abortion are indeed intensely medicalized while others, such as birth control, have resisted medicalization almost entirely. Whereas up until the end of World War II, nearly all women who lived outside the major cities birthed at home with the help of local midwives, today nearly all women give birth in the hospital attended by obstetricians. As I describe in Chapter 5, in the span of a single generation, Greek obstetrical care has acquired one of the most technologically intensive profiles found anywhere in the world. A study comparing a dozen nations in the early 1990s, for instance, found that Greek maternity care was marked by the heaviest reliance on technical interventions (Stephenson et al. 1993). The use of fetal ultrasonography in prenatal care offers one particularly arresting example of this technological intensification. When I began my research in 1990, Rhodian women underwent an already high average of three to four scans over the course of a routine pregnancy. Ten years later, monthly ultrasounds had become the norm. By far the most invasive and dangerous obstetrical intervention is, of course, the caesarean section. Up from about 15 percent in the late 1980s to an average of around 40 percent today (and reaching 50–60 percent in Athenian hospitals), the rate of caesarean births in Greece is now the highest in the European Union and among the highest in the world (Mossialos et al. 2005; Skalkidis et al. 1996). When caesareans are added to the other commonly performed obstetrical interventions, nearly all Greek women today experience what are medically classified as "operative deliveries" (Skalkidis et al. 1996).

In contrast to the intensively technological profile of pregnancy and birth, birth control remains largely unmedicalized in Greece. Barely 10 percent of Greek women use any form of medical contraception. More intriguing still, this percentage has hardly budged over the last couple of decades, a period otherwise characterized by stunningly rapid change in the fabric of Greek life. Greece's birth rate of 1.27 children per woman, one of the lowest in the world, has been attained largely through the use of coitus interruptus (withdrawal) and condoms, techniques conventionally coded by demographers as "traditional" and "nonmedical." Abortion, on the other hand, heavily relied upon by Greek women, was fully medicalized decades before becoming officially legal in 1986. Overall, as I describe in this book, Greek women display an intriguing mosaic of refusal, acceptance (both qualified and enthusiastic), and indifference to the medicalization of their reproductive experiences. Distinctive though this Greek signature may be, such selective responses are by no means unique, as the cross-cultural studies collected in Lock and Kaufert (1998) amply demonstrate. In providing an ethnographic portrait of the social, political, and cultural context of Greek women's responses to an array of reproductive technologies, *Bodies of Knowledge* seeks to contribute an anthropological perspective on what might perhaps best be thought of as the cross-cultural study of medicalization.

Comparative Medicalization, Biopower, and the Politics of Numbers

To this point, I have been referring to medicalization as if it were a uniform or universal process. Since the mid-1980s, however, scholars examining biomedicine as a cultural system have increasingly challenged overly rationalist interpretations of biomedicine as singular and value free, immune to the effects of the social, cultural, and political forces of the particular societies in which it is found. Medical anthropologists long ago recognized the role of these forces in shaping the ethnomedicine of others. It is only more recently, though, that the boundary between biomedicine's inside and the messy outside world was discovered to be equally permeable and continually traversed (Berg and Mol 1998, 8). This realization has led many scholars to recast biomedicine as a species of ethnomedicine—although one with unique properties, to be sure. Over the last two decades or so, ethnographic studies have demonstrated that, whether ethno- or bio-, all medical traditions contain implicit meta- medical components that simultaneously reflect and reproduce cultural values, interests, and conflicts (see, e.g., Baer 1989; Gaines and Davis-Floyd 2004; Hahn and Gaines 1985; Hahn and Kleinman 1983; Lock 1993a; Lock and Gordon 1988; Rhodes 1996; Worsley 1982).

While this is undoubtedly true across medical specialties, recent scholarship also suggests that, in actual practice, obstetrics and gynecology may well display the greatest range of cross-cultural variability. In a unique study comparing several countries in North America and Europe, DeVries et al. found wide variation in regimes of maternity care, ranging from Holland at one end, where one-third of births take place at home and all normal births are attended by midwives, to the United States at the other, where nearly all births, whether normal or high risk, occur in the hospital and are subject to a broad array of technological interventions. The discovery of these notable cross-national differences led the authors to conclude that "more than any other area of medical practice, . . . the organization and provision of maternity care is a highly charged mix of medical science, cultural ideas and structural forces" (2001, xii). A similar claim could be made for gynecology: wildly divergent patterns of contraceptive use across nations, for example, point to considerable variability in the preferences and practices of gynecologists and other providers of contraceptive services (Norgren 2001; J. Potter 1999).

The pronounced cross-cultural variation often found in the clinical practice of obstetrics and gynecology can be traced to several factors. In the first place, these are specialties distinguished by their intimate association with sexuality, gender, family, and kinship. It would indeed be surprising if historically and culturally specific understandings of these highly charged and often hotly contested domains of social life did not inflect both medical knowledge and clinical practice, at least to some extent (Davis-Floyd 1992; Martin 1987). A second, related factor pertains to the salient role that obstetrics and gynecology (along with pediatrics) perform in the exercise of biopower. Deeply implicated in the nineteenth-century European obsession with population and the ensuing "discovery of the child" that I outlined earlier, these specialties have been intimately tied to national biopolitical projects ever since (Armstrong 1983; Arney 1982). As a consequence, whether implicitly or explicitly, their discourses and practices often reflect and transmit historically and culturally specific visions of what it means to be a proper citizen—and, what's more, a properly gendered citizen—of a particular nation. Finally, obstetrics and gynecology, along with pediatrics, are central sites in the production of politically charged signs and symbols that powerfully index a nation's location within a hierarchical global order. Rates of infant and maternal mortality, for example, are routinely used as proxies to measure a nation's level of economic development and pinpoint its rank among nations. Average life expectancy is another such highly symbolic statistic in the global "politics of numbers" that is itself heavily influenced by the survival of infants and children (Declerq and Viisainen 2001; Jenkins 2001; Stillwagon 1998).

A glance at these recent statistics for Greece reveals that, across the board, the nation's health has in fact posted stunning improvements in the postwar period. When compared to the United States, for example, Greece's rates of infant mortality, maternal mortality, and life expectancy are all consistently superior—an accomplishment all the more impressive given that Greek per capita GNP is roughly one-third that of the United States. However, the usual frame of reference for Greece is the other nations of the European Union (to which Greece acceded as a full member in 1981). In widely reported statistical comparisons issuing from Brussels, with which Greeks are routinely barraged by the media, Greece usually finds itself at or near the bottom rung of the (admittedly impressive) EU ladder. In a similar vein, statistics on birth rates, abortion ratios, and the use of medical contraception among women are often deployed as importantly gendered signifiers of a nation's modernity (Chatterjee and Riley 2001; Kanaaneh 2002). Within this discourse, women's knowledge and practices carry an especially heavy symbolic load, as critical signs and signifiers of national progress toward the highly desired project of modernization and, in the case of Greece, its close relative Europeanization (Herzfeld 1986a; Jolly 1998, 3). Greece's high abortion rate, for example, has been debated and decried in Parliament and periodically deployed by journalists, politicians, and religious leaders, as well as doctors, to publicly critique Greek women's "backwardness" and "immaturity" on a number of counts (Athanasiou 2001; Halkias 2004; Paxson 2004; Skilogianis 2001). Given their ostensible objectivity, statistics are more difficult to talk back to than negative news stories that can be attributed to the self-interest of powerful others. Because of their intimate association with these highly charged statistics, obstetrics and gynecology inevitably become embroiled in issues central to national identity. As a result, they attract political attention and interference in ways that other specialties infrequently do.

Medicalization, (Belated) Modernity, and the Reproduction of National Identity

If statistics are "part of the ways subjectivity is constituted in the modern world" (Urla 1993, 837), then stories in the press and on television constantly comparing members of the European Union and reminding them of their numerical rank become another way that Greeks come to learn their place among nations. This is by no means a new phenomenon, however intensified by the mass media today. Historically, comparison has served as an essential technique in the creation of modern national identities. For Greece and a host of other "belated" modernizers, as Gregory Jusdanis (2001) has argued, forging a national identity has in fact entailed a process of "perennial comparison" with those (few) Western European nations that modernized early—essentially, England, Holland, and France. The "belated" dimension of Greek modernity has thus meant that the meanings of the modern have evolved in continual reference to definitions always already devised by more powerful outsiders (Faubion 1993, 143). The experiences of, and responses to, the cultural hegemony of the early modernizers ("the West") are themes that have been richly explored in the more recent anthropology of Greece and Cyprus (Argyrou 1996; Bakalaki 1994; Herzfeld 1987, 1992, 1995, 1997; Moutsatsos 2001). At the same time, forging a national identity under conditions of belated modernity is always an "intensely syncretic" process (Jusdanis 2001, 132). Defining cultural difference—what a nation was and was *not*—was an equally significant dimension of nineteenth-century projects of nationalism (McDonald 1993, 226). That is to say, even as belated modernizers assimilate "the drafts of others into their own national blueprints," the ideology of nationalism prescribes that they also assert their own cultural uniqueness and difference from those powerful others (Jusdanis 2001, 132). Modern national identities are thus shaped by broader patterns of power and hegemony, but only as these are refracted through specific cultural and historical contexts (Knauft 2002, 22).

Among the pillars of national cultural difference that have influenced the profile of medicalization and biopolitics more generally in Greece, the Greek Orthodox Church deserves special mention. Since the founding of the Greek nation, the close, if not always harmonious, relationship between Orthodoxy and the state has given the Church an influential hand in shaping the meanings of reproduction, children, and the family (Just 1989; Kokosalakis 1987; Paxson 2004; Sant Cassia with Bada 1992). Church and state have never been separate, and Greek Orthodoxy remains the official religion of the nation today. Although its intimate ties with the state have deeply politicized the Greek Orthodox Church and have consequently restrained its scope to function as an autonomous institution—it is part of the Ministry of National Education and Religion—in exchange it has been able to maintain religious hegemony over Greek society. All Greek students, for example, are obligated to take religion classes from elementary through high school. The Church has thus been able to play an influential hand "in the symbolization and mediation of power" in Greek society (Kokosalakis 1987, 225) and as a consequence, it retains a degree of authority over the body, health, and illness that is seemingly at odds with the otherwise relentless ascent of biomedicine and its institutions and the steady secularization of Greek society. In contrast to the secular strands of ethnogynecology and ethno-obstetrics, which have all but disappeared, religious healing (at least those elements that have been appropriated by the Church) continues to offer alternative therapeutic modalities and options that many women regard as valued complements to biomedicine when seeking answers to their reproductive concerns. Furthermore, as I show in Chapter 6, Rhodian women typically remain in dialogue with the central idioms and tenets of their Church when making their reproductive decisions—even when they repeatedly violate these tenets, as so many do by having abortions.

Belated Modernity and the Consumption of Technology

"Belated" and "advanced" represent just one pair in a concatenated set of binaries that today continue to be used as "paradigms of analysis of the modern Greek condition" (Panourgia 1995, 29). Others include: traditional/modern, backward/progressive, East/West, Third World (or the playful coinage *bananeo*, as in banana republic)/First World, Mediterranean or Balkan/Europe. Within this set of oppositions, fraught with implicit hierarchies that usually (though not always) privilege the second term of each pair, "Europe" and "European" are tropes that arguably carry particular rhetorical force.

Today, as in the preceding century, the idea of "Europe" is closely related to what has been called a "perennial crisis" in Greeks' sense of identity, to wit: Is Greece part of the East/Orient or of the West/Europe (Papagaroufali and Georges 1993)? In the nineteenth century, Greece's independence from Ottoman rule was contingent on the interests of the then-powerful nations of the West, the so-called Great Powers: England, France, and Russia. Support for the nascent project of Greek nationhood was also grounded in the European conceit that located the origins of European civilization in the genius of Greek antiquity. This crucial support was courted by the Greek elite who actively sought to align themselves and their emergent national identity with the Great Powers of the day and against the "Oriental" realities of everyday experience, the lamentable heritage of four centuries of Ottoman rule (Gefou-Madianou 1999; Gourgouris 1996; Herzfeld 1982a, 1995; Jusdanis 1992). These strategic appeals to the Hellenism of Western Europeans set the Greek struggle apart, and succeeded in eliciting a passionate level of support for independence denied other nationalist revolts against the Ottomans (Jusdanis 1992, 14).

Still, the conundrums of national identity that ensued are not peculiar to Greece; rather, they haunt the so-called margins of Europe. Thus, Spaniards, to take but one example, have grappled for at least two hundred years with the question of whether Spain was part of "Europe" or whether, as Alexandre Dumas put it in the early nineteenth century, "Africa begins on the other side of the Pyrenees" (cited in Douglass 1992, 69). In the end, persistent binaries such as Europe/Africa and Europe/Orient are perhaps most usefully conceived as contested symbols in a "dialogue about world view and the quality of life" (ibid.).

In Greece today, this perennial identity crisis has arguably deepened as a consequence of full membership in the European Union. The Greek public has generally embraced EU membership, with polls revealing the highest level of popular support among all the member states for the Europeanization process (Pettifer 1996, 17). Today, "Europeanization" is in fact commonly conflated with the highly desired national project of "modernization" (Featherstone 1998, 24). In practice, however, the more powerful EU states have often skeptically regarded Greece as an unruly and semi-Oriental junior partner, whose capability of applying such Western values and institutions as rationality and efficiency remains an open question (Papagaroufali and Georges 1993). Thus, within the paternalistic European "family of nations," Greece in recent years has been stereotyped as the disobedient "bad child" for its pursuit of foreign and domestic policies at odds with general EU trends (Borneman and Fowler 1997, 494; Michas 2002). Old binaries have an annoying habit of recurring in the scoldings that sometimes issue from the EU core, as when a reporter writing in London's *Spectator* of Greece's support for Serbia in the Balkan conflict of the early 1990s concludes with the pronouncement, apparently intended to be scathing, that "Greece, from being one of *us* since the war, has become one of *them* (*Balkans*)" (Nicholson 1992, quoted in Michas 2002, 140, my emphasis). Such dividing practices ("us" v. "them") can keep identities perennially teetering on an ideological seesaw from which it is relatively easy to tumble or, as in this example, be pushed off.

The persistent conundrum of national identity within a context of belated modernity, I submit, provides an important backdrop against which to study the medicalization of reproduction and the particular technological profile it has taken in Greece. This is so because biomedicine, science, and technology—over and above their pragmatic value in terms of technical efficacy and medical outcomes—also wield considerable power as signs and vehicles of the modern. Under conditions of belated modernity, as described by Jusdanis, notions of time, progress, modernity, and technological innovation were early on closely entwined:

> What enabled the conceptual separation between advanced and belated
> societies was not just the political and economic innovations themselves
> but the very notion of progress. Certain societies could be characterized
> as pioneering and others as backward only when time was understood as
> moving linearly forward. The ideology of ongoing development placed
> a premium on being modern, equating power and well-being with ever
> changing technological sophistication. No other epoch had so sacralized
> novelty, self-propelling change, and time itself. (2001, 106, my emphasis)

Once time was thus understood as a line "that ties past, present and future, and yet insists on their distinctiveness," individual and social actors inevitably became positioned along that line (Trouillot 2002, 225). Given their crucial role in indexing one's location along the rolling continuum of progress and modernity, it should not be surprising that technologies and technical procedures may be adopted or rejected for reasons that may have little to do with their efficacy as conventionally defined. This, of course, is universally true, as attested by clamorous and proliferating calls for "evidence-based medicine" in the United States and the United Kingdom in recent years. Over the last two decades, the undesirable effects of a large number of commonly used birth technologies and procedures have been repeatedly confirmed. Caesarean sections, episiotomies (incisions made into the perineum to enlarge the vaginal opening), the lithotomy (supine) position, electronic fetal monitoring, and fetal ultrasound imaging, among other practices, have all been shown to be unnecessary, overused, or downright harmful. WHO guidelines now advise the elimination of such procedures as episiotomies, pubic shaves, and enemas, and the reduction of caesarean rates to between 5 and 15 percent of births. Nonetheless, these guidelines and the by now voluminous body of scientific evidence have had curiously little impact on most regimes of maternity care. Indeed, the global diffusion and adoption of highly technological interventions have accelerated and intensified, especially in those nations of "the South," such as Brazil, Mexico, and India, that have experienced rapid economic growth and improvement in living standards (Davis-Floyd 2003; De Mello e Souza 1994; DeVries et al. 2001; Donner 2004). Similarly, within the European Union, the most intense levels of medicalization, and the highest rates of caesareans in particular, are now found in Greece, closely followed by Spain, Italy, and Portugal (Johanson, Newburn, and Macfarlane 2002; Whitaker 2000).

Although many forces have a hand in shaping national regimes of maternity care, attending to the cultural politics of technological activities helps reveal important, if sometimes overlooked, dimensions that help promote their diffusion and intensification (Jordan 1978 [1993]). As I will argue, in contexts of belated modernity, medicalization and its attendant technologies and procedures may also acquire important redressive dimensions (Pfaffenberger 1992). That is, the social actors or groups adversely affected by meanings and definitions devised by more powerful others may embrace technologies as means "to mute or counter the invidious status implications" of such domination (Pfaffenberger 1992, 505). From this perspective, the consumption of particular technologies can articulate an implicit negation or counterstatement to the dividing practices of those Westerners (or national elites) that would consign one's identity to the category of less developed, backward, or "the South." In this book, I use this analytical perspective, derived from cultural studies of science, medicine, and technology, in my attempt to understand how particular obstetrical and gynecological discourses and technologies work along a number of dimensions that may have little to do with their intended or professed medical outcomes. In particular, I am concerned to examine how, within the uneven symbolic and political context of belated modernity, they work to assist actors in constituting the modern gendered identities they desire to ascribe to themselves (D. Miller 1987, 215).

Studying Reproduction on Rhodes: An Evolving Project

Most of the research for this book was conducted in Rhodes Town, a small city of some fifty thousand inhabitants that I describe in detail in the following chapter. Rhodes Town is the capital as well as the regional medical center of the Dodecanese province, the string of islands that marks Greece's easternmost boundary in the southern Aegean Sea. Its General Hospital, the only one in the province, is the site of some thousand births each year out of a national total of about a hundred thousand. Due to its size, its history, and its robust tourist-based economy, Rhodes today is an island scored by numerous intersecting dimensions of social difference. This complexity afforded me opportunities to speak to women and men from a broad variety of backgrounds—from the wealthy hotel owners at the top of the local socioeconomic hierarchy to the women who cleaned their rooms. Its excellent road and transportation system made it easy for me to visit many of the island's twenty-two villages to interview the old women and men who formed their permanent core, and to select one, Ermia, for more intensive study of the medical knowledge and practices of the recent past.[2] Not least, Rhodes's well-developed tourist amenities made it possible for me to quickly settle in for the recurring episodic bouts of fieldwork dictated by the constraints of family and work on my time and mobility. For these reasons and many others, I found Rhodes an ideal place for this research. Rhodians themselves, however, sometimes begged to differ. I'd made a mistake in my choice of field site, I was told on more than one occasion when people learned I was an anthropologist. I should pack up my things, they advised me, and go study the island of Karpathos instead. Karpathos, which in fact has received more attention from anthropologists than has Rhodes, is a small rocky outpost of the Dodecanese archipelago with a regional reputation for proud (and stubborn) adherence to local tradition. For example, while no Rhodian woman, no matter how old, dressed in traditional island costume, Karpathian women as young as their forties or fifties still wore their distinctively full-skirted white cotton dresses with black aprons and embroidered headscarves, even when visiting Rhodes Town. (But challenging the Rhodian stereotype of Karpathian backwardness, I later discovered from a provincial survey that on a per capita basis, Karpathians own twice as many personal computers as Rhodians [Dhimos Rodhion 2002].) Rhodes, in contrast to Karpathos, was cosmopolitan and urbane. For a glimpse of traditional Rhodian culture, I was directed to the many village museums that had sprouted up throughout the countryside in the 1990s. Or I might be handed a copy of a book or pamphlet written by an educated native son or daughter that chronicled the now-vanished customs of the village in which they'd spent their childhood, a proliferating genre I came to think of as "local ethnography."

Despite the culturally salient contrast between Rhodes and the islands of its hinterland, the most significant differences in medical knowledge and reproductive experiences, I eventually discovered, were to be found among Rhodian women of adjacent generations. As I describe in this book, Greek society in the postwar period has been marked by significant reconfigurations of gender ideologies, of reproductive desires and imagined futures, and of the meanings attributed to children, motherhood, and fatherhood, among a host of other changes generally glossed and subsumed by the term "modernization." On Rhodes, conventional sociological dimensions of difference such as rural versus urban residence are today blurred by the intense traffic among the island's villages, Rhodes Town, Athens, and locations much farther afield.[3] "Class" was often an equally complex and slippery notion in the fluid postwar Rhodian context of rapid economic transformation and social mobility. Certainly, both place and relative socioeconomic position shaped the texture and quality of the life of each woman I came to know during the course of my study. However important, though, these dimensions seemed to pale in comparison with the shifts in knowledge and experience I found between the generations.

My research on Rhodes began in 1990 with the relatively modest aim of understanding how the contemporary experience of pregnancy and birth had been affected by the intensive use of one specific obstetrical technology, fetal ultrasound imaging. As I talked with the oldest women I met to gather background information on the past, a rich body of humoral medical knowledge unexpectedly came into focus, much of it, moreover, uncannily familiar from my earlier ethnographic familiarity with Latin America, particularly with the work of Carole Browner (1980, 1985) on menstrual regulation and early pregnancy and George Foster (1994) on popular medicine. Anthropologists have occasionally made note of the humoral flavor of Greek ethnomedicine (e.g., Beyene 1989; D. Sutton 1998b). Systematic ethnographic studies of the topic, however, do not exist. Indeed, until recently, attention to the subjects of health and medicine in general was sporadic or secondary to other areas of research in Greek ethnography (e.g., Danforth 1989; Dubisch 1995a; Herzfeld 1986b; Stewart 1991).

The relative paucity of medical anthropological research may be in part the case because Greek ethnography, like ethnography in many other locales, has been until recently tightly defined—and confined—by certain disciplinary gatekeeping concepts. For Greece, as Appadurai (1986, 357) has elaborated this notion, "the quintessential and dominant questions of interest in the region" have been family and kinship. Appadurai goes on to wonder whether gatekeeping concepts "really reflect something significant about the place in question, or whether they reveal a relatively arbitrary imposition of the whims of anthropological fashion on particular places" (357–58). Certainly, as Roger Just (2000, 5–6) writes of his attempt to escape this conceptual corral and study economics and politics on the Ionian island of Meganisi, understanding kinship and family still remains foundational to any anthropological study of Greece, including this one. Yet, the close association of Greek culture with these gatekeeping concepts arguably discouraged anthropologists from attending to other domains of inquiry. Nonetheless, the few studies of health and reproduction in rural areas undertaken in the 1980s and early 1990s proved to be of great help in situating the present study within the broader Greek context. These included studies of reproductive knowledge and practices and other health-related topics conducted by Arnold (1985) in Crete, Beyene (1989) in Evia, Gefou-Madianou (1992) in Attica, and Lefkarities (1992) and Trakas (1981) on Rhodes.[4]

More recently, intense ethnographic attention has been focused on the interrelated issues of demography, contraception, and abortion (Athanasiou 2001; Halkias 2004; Paxson 2004; Skilogianis 2001). Aside from certain differences of interpretation, *Bodies of Knowledge* complements this burst of scholarly interest in Greek demographic discourse and practices in at least two major ways. First, it provides a detailed and uniquely diachronic account of Rhodian ethnogynecology and ethno-obstetrics that strives to situate these local bodies of knowledge within broader intellectual currents of medical history. Second, by pursuing this diachronic approach through to the present, it also brings to light the various political, social, and cultural mechanisms that propelled the rapid demise of this body of women's ethnomedicine and theorizes how these mechanisms also helped shape the distinctive features of the medical system that replaced it. Thus, *Bodies of Knowledge* adds to the recent ethnographic focus on contemporary Greek women's reproductive practices through the scope of the reproductive themes it encompasses, as well as through its concern with the mechanisms of change over time.

Stumbling onto the body of reproductive ethnomedical knowledge late in my initial study, I decided to embark on additional research to document it in detail and attempt to understand the processes by which it had been so quickly displaced. So, in 1994, having completed my study of ultrasound use, I adopted a generational approach and deliberately began to seek out my interlocutors by broad age group. With the help of my research assistants, I eventually conducted a total of 157 formal interviews roughly divided among three cohorts of women. When my initial attempt to sample randomly met with numerous obstacles (not least being women's almost universal reluctance to be interviewed by someone with whom they could trace no connections), I turned to the time-honored snowball method. By this means, I was able to include many mother-daughter pairs in the study, as daughters referred me to their mothers (and sometimes their grandmothers) and vice versa. I demarcated three cohorts by significant historical events that, at some risk of simplifying, I have treated as watersheds in the shifting terrain of reproductive knowledge and practices. (1) What I call simply the "oldest generation" comprises all the women I interviewed who were born before the Second World War, and who thus married and had their children before most aspects of reproduction became medicalized. Most of these women were born between 1930 and 1940, but I also interviewed several who were born before 1920 and a few born as early as 1906. The great majority came of age under the agrarian way of life that all but disappeared on Rhodes after the war. Although this generation had the widest age range (from sixty to ninety-two), their medical knowledge and practices hewed closely and consistently to the humoral logic that I describe in detail in Chapters 3 and 4. (2) The "transitional generation" comprises women born between 1940 and 1955. These women came of age and began to form their families in the two decades following the war, a time of rapid transition from the humoral body of knowledge to the biomedical. This generation experienced the greatest degree of medical pluralism (the availability of more than one medical system within which to make sense of and manage their reproduction, as well as their health in general), and women in this cohort sometimes moved back and forth between the two systems. (3) The "youngest generation" comprises women born between 1955 and 1970. This was the generation that came of age during and after the *metapolitefsi*, the heady years of often exuberant social and political transformation that followed the fall of the repressive military junta that had ruled Greece from 1967 to 1974, an event widely regarded by Greeks themselves as the "end of an era" (Papagaroufali and Georges 1993). This was also the first generation to reach maturity after Greece had acceded to the European Union, another watershed for the nation, and it is its members who have borne the brunt of the influential discourses and practices clustered around the notion of Europeanization. By the 1980s, when these women began to marry and form their families, the hegemony of biomedicine was almost complete. This generation usually had only fragmentary awareness of the ethnogynecological and ethno-obstetrical knowledge and practices that had shaped their mothers' and grandmothers' reproductive experiences. In addition to my interviews with these three cohorts of women, I spoke informally with many men about reproductive issues; more formally, I managed to interview a total of fifteen married men on the subjects of birth control and fatherhood. Ideally, men's voices and experiences on the topic of reproduction should have figured more prominently in this project. For many reasons, this was not feasible, and this remains an area of research in which much remains to be done.

In addition to participant observation and interviews with these three generations of Rhodian women, I also studied the biomedical professionals on whom they relied for their health care. For more than four months between 1990 and 1992, I observed clinical visits and conducted interviews with doctors and patients in the Department of Obstetrics and Gynecology at the Rhodes Public Hospital. Over the course of this earlier study, I interviewed a total of twenty-six women (aged eighteen to thirty-nine) who had just given birth. At the hospital, I was allowed to observe on a daily basis the regimes of prenatal care and a variety of other clinical encounters; shadow obstetricians as they performed fetal ultrasound scans; and observe births and postnatal visits. I conducted numerous informal conversations with medical staff as they went about their daily work, and formally interviewed fourteen doctors and seven professional midwives. To learn something about how obstetrical regimes of care were taught to fledgling obstetricians, I spent an additional two months in a large Athens hospital observing the training of medical students in fetal ultrasound and prenatal diagnosis and interviewing professors and medical residents. In the late 1990s, I interviewed several Athenian activists who were helping organize the Greek alternative childbirth movement.

I also visited and conducted interviews in many of the island's villages, whose permanent core is today composed largely of old pensioners and retirees. For over four months, I lived in the village of Ermia, located on the southern end of the island, which I describe in Chapters 2 through 4. I also traveled to some of the smaller and more remote Dodecanese islands to collect comparative information (though regretfully, I never did manage to visit Karpathos).

My approach to fieldwork was in certain ways unorthodox and requires some commentary. From the very beginning, professional and personal concerns braided together to shape and give texture to both the conceptual and pragmatic aspects of this project. Like so many women anthropologists of my generation (baby-boomer) who study biomedicine and technology, my interest in the subject was inspired by my own reproductive trajectory (Traweek 1993). My story is fairly mundane compared to others who faced involuntary infertility, pregnancy loss, a diagnosis of genetic anomaly, or a traumatic delivery and went on to define the field of the anthropology of reproduction in the 1990s (see, e.g., G. Becker 2000; Davis-Floyd 1992; Inhorn 1994; Layne 2003; Rapp 1999). I became pregnant with my only daughter fairly late, both in terms of age and career. Like so many women of my class and educational background, I "took pregnancy as a reading assignment" (Rothman 1986). But, being an anthropologist, my syllabus included not only the usual pregnancy guides and advice literature, but also any ethnographic study of reproduction I could find. At that time, in 1988, it was still possible to read a great deal, if not most, of the existing literature. Today, this would represent a monumental task, as the anthropological study of nearly every aspect of reproduction has grown explosively over the last decade (for reviews see, e.g., Browner and Sargent 1996; Davis-Floyd and Franklin 2005; Davis-Floyd and Sargent 1997; Ginsburg and Rapp 1991, 1995). When my pregnancy shifted categories from "normal" to "high risk" because of a diagnosis of placenta previa, my plans for a midwife-assisted home birth were abruptly waylaid. And so, from my early ideal of a "natural" birth, for which I had been training "like a marathon" as advised by my midwife, I found myself undergoing (and anxiously fretting over the risks of) multiple ultrasounds, amniocentesis, and ultimately, a caesarean section. I recount this not as a complaint (How could I? Placenta previa unquestionably merits the "high-risk" label), but to offer a glimpse of my trajectory and personal experience with divergent ideologies of birth, as well as with a variety of obstetrical technologies. Of all the interventions I underwent, though, none provoked the deep emotional response I felt as I first glimpsed my daughter's shadowy image on the ultrasound monitor. When my doctor pointed out her spinal column, which shimmered up from the gray wash of the screen to remind me, oddly enough, of a string of luminous pop-beads I used to wear in junior high school, I surprised myself (and my doctor) by bursting into tears. Why did I have this intense reaction? Studies beginning to appear around that time (in particular, Petchesky 1987) offered provocative insights into the peculiarly potent impact of ultrasonography on North American women's experiences of pregnancy. How did women undergoing fetal ultrasound in other cultural and political contexts respond, I wondered? The initial germ of the project that would ultimately grow into this book was in place.

The boundaries between the personal and professional were also thoroughly blurred in the practical decisions involved in how to go about the extensive fieldwork this project required. For many American baby-boomer anthropologists in midlife and midcareer like myself, our decisions to undertake major second projects (after the dissertation) often bump up against the constraints of work and/or family. Trying to find a way to accommodate my desire to do cross-cultural research outside the Anglo-American context (at that time, almost all research on new reproductive technologies was being done in North America or the United Kingdom) with my personal and professional obligations, I decided to take my daughter, Christa, along with me each time I went to the field, even though my husband would have to remain at home in Houston because of his work. So, unlike the doctoral fieldwork that I'd done in my twenties, when I lived an uninterrupted and unencumbered year and a half in a village in the Sierra Mountains of the Dominican Republic, this project was conducted in fits and starts as professional and familial obligations permitted, mostly in the summers and during the occasional academic leave if it could be coordinated with my daughter's school calendar. The result was some twenty-two months of fieldwork stretched over more than a dozen trips, beginning in 1990 and lasting over a decade. My project thus unexpectedly became, at least in part, diachronic, as the practices and technologies that were the object of study sometimes changed over the course of the fieldwork. The disadvantage of this turn of events is that my object of study is destabilized to some extent and this inevitably complicates my effort to describe any particular moment. The obvious advantage is that I have been able to follow and describe processes of change over time.

Being Greek American, the granddaughter of four Greek immigrants, and the mother of a "halfie" daughter colored my fieldwork in many other ways. My ethnic background influenced my decision to work in Greece; but I soon discovered, as Michael Fischer (1986, 196) has cautioned, that being Greek American (or Chinese American, etc.) is decidedly not the same thing as being Greek (or Chinese, etc.) in America. Like many offspring of diaspora and exile, I derived my understanding of Greek culture mostly from my grandparents' stories of their youth, permanently fixed in the turn-of-the-century freeze-frame of their memories. While these stories enriched my childhood with alternative visions and meanings, they left me completely unprepared for my first encounters with Greek culture and society in the 1990s. My first task, then, was to unlearn many of the ingrained images of Greek life that I had acquired from my grandparents, images that ironically were reinforced by much of the ethnography of Greece up to that time (the late 1980s), focused as it was largely on remote villages. Even the language—the kitchen Greek—I'd learned as a child was often comically at odds with contemporary Greek reality. At first, I used antique terms that either puzzled my interlocutors or raised eyebrows. I unwittingly called the bathroom the "outhouse" (*apokhoritirio*), for example, or as my grandmother euphemistically put it, *piso* (behind), as I imagine most outhouses in her native town of Kalamata a century ago were located behind the house. Then I had to unlearn all the Greek Americanisms (Greenglish) that immigrants had devised for referents that didn't exist when they left the homeland (and that were a source of amusement for many educated Greeks). Ironically, this sometimes entailed substituting one unassimilated English loan word for another, assimilated one: for example, Greek

Americans say *barra* for "bar," and *groceria* for "grocery store," while Greeks today simply say *bar* and *super-market*.

Taking my daughter with me to the field also colored this study in a variety of ways and overall, I am convinced, greatly enhanced my research. For one thing, her presence helped many Rhodians make sense of me within a generally positive framework of meaning. Bringing Christa back year after year was often read approvingly (and correctly) as an indication that I valued my Greekness, and that I was taking pains to preserve and extend my heritage to the next generation. For another, as many anthropologists have also found, taking a child to the field opens up research in unanticipated ways that may offer a windfall of cross-cultural learning experiences (Cassell 1987; Sutton and Fernandez 1998). One of the best examples of this occurred in the fall of 1997 when Christa attended second grade in our neighborhood school in Rhodes Town. Each weekday I walked her to the schoolyard, stayed through the morning assembly, endured the principal's hortatory speeches, and often lingered afterward to chat or have coffee with another mother. Attending parent-teacher meetings and other school events, reading her school texts to help her with homework, and enrolling her in after-school lessons inserted me in an unexpectedly intimate way into the everyday world of Rhodian mothers with school-aged children. Finally, I believe that having my daughter almost constantly by my side helped legitimate me (to some extent, in any case) in the face of the common perception, discussed in the next chapter, that foreign women typically visit Rhodes looking for sexual liaisons with local men (see Dubisch 1995b; Smith 2002).

The fact that I had only *one* child, on the other hand, sometimes drew comments that were decidedly less approving. As I describe in Chapter 6, there is a widespread perception in Greece today that the nation's exceptionally low birth rate represents a major national problem. Even though the one- to two-child family is now the norm, many women, especially women my age and older, still held to an ideal of larger families and often challenged me to explain my singleton family: "Your only child? Why?" (cf. Anagnost 1995 for the flip side of this experience as a mother of two in one-child China). These were queries to which I soon grew accustomed. If my answers were judged unsatisfactory, I might be offered a range of advice, from how to make a vow at one of the island's several miraculous shrines to the names of fertility specialists in Athens and beyond. When, by the end of this study, I began to plead menopause, one woman reminded me of the doctor in Italy who'd just helped a woman in her sixties give birth.

Guide to the Chapters

The first half of this book focuses largely on women's procreative knowledge and practices in the prewar period. Chapter 2 provides the reader with a historical and social overview of the island of Rhodes and, in particular, of its capital, Rhodes Town. I have devoted considerable space to describing my field site in part because of my own fascination with the place and its history, but also, as Cowan (1990) has pointed out, because anthropologists studying Greece have paid little attention to such medium-sized, provincial centers. Most of the first wave of ethnographic research in Greece concentrated on villages and the countryside; over the last decade, a new wave, seeking to correct this rural bias and to bring Greek ethnography into conversation with contemporary theoretical concerns, has tended to focus primarily on Athens, where, after all, nearly half of all Greeks reside. Smaller cities like Rhodes have thus remained neglected (for exceptions, in addition to Cowan 1990, see Herzfeld 1991; Kirtsoglou 2004; D. Sutton 1998a).

Chapter 3 is devoted to a description of Rhodian ethnogynecology, the system of knowledge and practices that women of the oldest generation used to enhance and control their fertility and protect their reproductive health. This chapter also strives to situate this local body of medical knowledge within the broader history of Old World medicine by tracing its many intriguing parallels with the Galeno-Hippocratic model that dominated learned medicine in the Byzantine Empire and, later on, Arab and Islamicate medical scholarship, as well as that of the Latin West.

In Chapter 4, I go on to describe the ethno-obstetrical knowledge and practices that the oldest women and their midwives relied on to protect their pregnancies, successfully birth their babies, and manage the many dangers inherent in the postpartum period. The midwifery tradition I describe in this chapter has been extinct for some three decades, and the information on midwives and midwifery practices was pieced together from interviews with the few remaining midwives and their daughters, and from the birth narratives of older women who had been assisted by practical midwives well into the 1960s. Together, Chapters 3 and 4 present the argument that local medicine on Rhodes is best understood in conversation with far more widely broadcast bodies of medical knowledge and practice.

The remainder of *Bodies of Knowledge* examines the processes by which biomedicine became hegemonic in the postwar period and describes in detail younger women's interpretations of, and responses to, the new biomedical model of reproduction and its attendant technologies. Chapter 5 focuses on

the processes contributing to the intensification and routinization of technological interventions in pregnancy and childbirth and showcases one reproductive technology in particular, fetal ultrasound imaging, for a more detailed case
study. It also offers a close analysis of a significant but often neglected adjunct
to the medicalization of reproduction: the process of self-education through
the reading of popular guides intended to tutor pregnant women in how to become scientifically literate and biomedically prepared "experts of themselves."
Chapter 6 returns to the subject of fertility control and examines the distinctive contours of contemporary Greek contraceptive culture. In this chapter,
the dynamic and diverse ways in which Rhodian women make sense of and
respond to the process of medicalization amid the competing discourses that
shape their everyday lives emerge in sharpest relief. Alongside the preceding
chapters, it demonstrates the full range of women's reflexivity in dealing with
a diverse array of new reproductive technologies. In the conclusion, I discuss
the implications of this study for understanding the globalization of medical
knowledge as both a deep historical process and a fact of contemporary life.

Chapter 2

Transnational Rhodes

On Rhodes today, the global interconnections that are a hallmark of contemporary transnationalism are everywhere in evidence. They are literally embodied in the island's population, a fluid and constantly shifting mix of natives and the international tourists that seasonally outnumber them ten-to-one; of thousands of bilingual and bicultural offspring produced by the many unions that have taken place between native and tourist over the last several decades; of mounting numbers of migrants, both Greek and international, drawn to the island's vibrant tourist industry; and of diaspora Greeks returned from their sojourns in nearly every corner of the world to rebuild their lives on the island. The familiar logos of contemporary globalization are also hard to miss. McDonald's anchors a central venue in downtown Rhodes, and there are no less than three Body Shops from which to choose. With the deepening economic integration of the European Union, regional department store chains such as Marks & Spencer, British Home Store, and Zara now offer a much larger selection of goods than the smaller Rhodian shops and boutiques ever could.

Yet, however intense and accelerated the current Rhodian experience of transnationalism and globalization may be, it is not entirely new. For much of its history, Rhodes could be aptly characterized, borrowing Appadurai's term, as a "translocality" (1996, 192). Cross-cultural trade, religious organizations, and knowledge networks have long suspended the island in a cat's cradle of intersecting ties that extended far beyond its insular borders. Above all, its strategic location ensured that Rhodes was a complex site where people of various ethnicities and religions commingled, their networks, allegiances, and identities often blurring the borders of empire and nation. The ethnogynecology and ethno-obstetrics I describe in the next two chapters are a case in point. Part of a far-flung body of medical knowledge that washed over the island with each new wave of conquest and colonization, local Rhodian medicine was almost as global as the biomedicine that eventually replaced it. This chapter offers an overview of the island's history helpful for understanding the evolution of its medical systems, and traces the distinctive contours of its social and economic landscape today.

The Place

Rhodes is the largest and most populous island in the archipelago province known as the Dodecanese. The name, which means "twelve islands," refers to the dozen major islands first recognized as an administrative unit under the Byzantine Empire. Today, the province is composed of fourteen islands and many more uninhabited rocky islets, some lying in contested waters only miles from the Turkish coast (Kasperson 1966, 10). Annexed in 1947, the Dodecanese was the last region to join the Greek nation. Since the Ensomatosi, or incorporation, of the Dodecanese Islands into Greece, Rhodes Town has served as the provincial political and administrative center, just as it had for centuries before. With approximately half the island's total population of about a hundred thousand (Dhimos Rodhion 2002), Rhodes Town is also a hub of commerce, education, and medical care and, in recent decades, the destination of the vast bulk of the international tourism that is the economic mainstay of the region. Rhodes's pronounced dominance has endowed it with a diversity of opportunities unavailable on the other islands. Still, its economic and social life today is overwhelmingly defined by mass tourism. The dynamism of the tourist sector, together with the city's occupational diversity, has attracted migrants from throughout the archipelago, as well as from mainland Greece, and most recently from the Balkans, Eastern Europe, and South and East Asia. It has also drawn many native sons and daughters back to the island from North America, Australia, Argentina, Africa, and Western Europe. Thus, while most of the towns and villages of the Dodecanese have steadily shrunk over the last several decades, a few to the point of near abandonment, Rhodes Town continues to swell and sprawl.

Rhodes must surely rank among the most heavily touristed places in the world. Since the onset of mass tourism in the 1960s, the volume of visitors has been climbing unremittingly. In 1999, for instance, the island, with an area of just 1,400 square kilometers, hosted 1.2 million tourists, an astonishing one-tenth of Greece's total number for that year (Rollisson 2000, 3). The vast majority travel on package tours from Northern Europe aboard the parade of charter jets that roar overhead every fifteen minutes or so during the peak of the season. Charters enable tourists to fly to Rhodes directly from the smaller European cities, bypassing Athens and the mainland entirely. Because of this direct access, many tourists may know nothing of the rest of Greece, the island becoming, in effect, a metonym for the entire country. An Athenian travel writer barely conceals her irritation at this state of affairs when she describes her encounters with foreigners abroad who, discovering that she is Greek, smile broadly and sigh, "Oh, Rhodes!" (Boubouri 1999, 71). In fact, tourism, one of the most dynamic sectors of the Greek economy today, has been in decline in Athens for many years (Leontidou 1994, 91).

Drawing on their history for a handy metaphor, Rhodians sometimes jokingly refer to the tourists as the latest wave of occupiers in the island's long and nearly unbroken series of invasions and conquests. Throughout the early Middle Ages, their small size and crucial location along important trade routes of the Eastern Mediterranean rendered the Dodecanese vulnerable to perennial raids and devastating pillage by a succession of Persians, Arabs, Saracens, and Seljuks, among a host of others. Continuous attacks depopulated the coastal regions and forced the rural inhabitants to conceal their villages in the mountainous interior, tucked out of the sight of maritime marauders. The location and even the names of many of Rhode's twenty-two villages, such as Afantou, which means "invisible," still bear witness to this defensive strategy. In the sixth century, the archipelago began a long association with the Byzantine Empire, becoming a Byzantine province in exchange for protection from piracy (Kasperson 1966; Papachristodoulou 1994). In Rhodian popular memory, however, by far the culturally most prominent occupations are those of the Knights of St. John (1309–1522), the Ottoman Turks (1522–1912), and the Italians (1912–1943), a salience reinforced by the imposing and nearly ubiquitous material heritage left behind by all three.

The Knights of St. John imprinted their signature on the built environment of Rhodes in the form of the massively fortified medieval Old Town, today one of the city's major tourist attractions. After the Crusaders conquered Constantinople in 1204, Byzantine protection of Rhodes and the Dodecanese faltered and there ensued a fluid and unstable period of claims and counterclaims among a series of Latin-Western rivals. Rhodes and neighboring islands were prized for their potential as crusading outposts, as well as for their strategic military value in controlling the lucrative slave trade between Egypt and the Black Sea. The islands changed hands numerous times until the Knights of the Order of St. John finally captured them in 1309. Forced out of their famous hospital-fortress in Jerusalem, and later evicted from Cyprus as well, the Knights were finally able to establish a base on Rhodes from which they could continue to harass the "infidel" Turks over the next two centuries. The monastic order, also known as the Hospitallers, grew out of the hospice they founded in Jerusalem to provide medical care and charity to pilgrims and the poor. Eventually, the military functions of the order took precedence, but the tradition of caring for the poor and sick remained symbolically important for its impact on public opinion and economic support for the order in the Latin West (Luttrell 1999, 73). The hospital the order established on Rhodes, possibly inspired by Byzantine and Islamic prototypes, was an acknowledged showpiece of the time (ibid., 65; T. Miller 1997).

Under the Knights, Greek-speaking Rhodians were segregated in the *bourc*, an area within the medieval walled city of Rhodes but outside the heavily fortified castle and the inns, or residences, of the various tongues (*langues*) to which the brethren knights from different parts of the Latin West belonged. Other than that, Greek Rhodians do not appear to have been discriminated against in many other important ways. The order even gave some Greek men scholarships to study medicine in Italy and elsewhere in Europe (Tsirpanlis 1991). Rural Greek peasants, however, were obligated to provide the corvée labor and other services that helped build the impressive walls and defenses that made Rhodes Town one of the most heavily fortified sites in the world at that time (Riley-Smith 1999, 94). The Rhodian historian Christos Papachristodoulou (1994) credits the security the Knights provided against marauders with making their two-hundred-year rule a time of peace, religious tolerance, and economic prosperity for the island. In the fifteenth century, with the eclipse of the Byzantine Empire, Rhodes experienced a brief period of cultural florescence, and the city became a minor hub of Greek studies (Luttrell 1999, 219). By all accounts, Rhodes under the Knights was a cosmopolitan island, a busy commercial port of call. Within its walled town, a multitude of languages commingled, the regional tongues not only of the polyglot Order of St. John, but also of the resident Romaniot Jews, Maronite Syrians, Cypriots, and Turkish-speaking slaves (Luttrell 1999, 194, 220; Angel 1998, 9).

After a series of bloody sieges, Turkish forces under Suleiman the Magnificent finally succeeded in defeating the Knights in 1522. Understandably perhaps, Rhodian writers tend to portray this event in dark tones (e.g., Economopoulos 1990, 56). In fact, the sultan guaranteed the Dodecanese almost total autonomy, granting all but Rhodes and Kos the status of "privileged islands." He withheld this coveted status from Rhodes and Kos as punishment for their fierce resistance, which cost his forces some eighty thousand lives. But even there, islanders were permitted to keep their religion and their language, and most local institutions remained intact. Under Ottoman rule, a substantial number of Turks settled on Rhodes and Kos. Greeks were evicted from the secure walled portion of the city, in which now only Turks and Jews were permitted to live. A small number of Jews had long lived in Rhodes, but the community blossomed under the Ottoman policy of welcoming and resettling Sephardic Jews expelled from Spain and, later, Portugal. The Juderia, as the

Ladino-speaking community called itself, collected at the southernmost corner of the walled city around its central square, the Calle Ancha (Angel 1998; Varon 1999). Greeks, on the other hand, although allowed to conduct their business within the city, had to leave each day by sundown to return to the Greek quarters, the *marasia*, or suburbs, that huddled just outside the city's massive walls (Papachristodoulou 1994, 513).

Except for the collection of taxes, the local Turkish government interfered little with either the daily social life or even the local government of its constituent *millets*, as the mosaic of ethno-religious groups that made up the empire were called. This was true even on Rhodes, which served as the pasha's administrative headquarters (N. Doumanis 1997, 28). On the smaller privileged islands, which remained almost entirely ethnically Greek, there was only a yearly tax to be paid to the Turks, at least until the nineteenth century (D. Sutton 1998a, 17). The tax burden on Rhodes and Kos was more onerous and caused simmering resentment that grew over time. Taxes included a per capita annual assessment paid by all *rayades*—non-Muslim Ottoman subjects (sing. *rayah*, from the Turkish word for "herd" or "flock")—a customs tax, and a tithe on all agricultural produce. In the nineteenth century, additional taxes were exacted on land, animals, and even beehives (Papachristodoulou 1994, 410–11). These were especially burdensome for Rhodes and Kos, where agriculture and commerce were becoming increasingly important to the local economy. With some 85 percent of the arable land and the best water sources available in the Dodecanese, Rhodes and Kos were also fertile islands that specialized in the production of wheat, far and away the most important subsistence crop. By the end of the nineteenth century, these two islands were also exporting cash crops such as grapes, olives, currants, and citrus, particularly to Egypt, whose economy was booming at that time (N. Doumanis 1997, 20).

Rhodians also resented Ottoman rule for its neglect of areas of civic life other than tax collection. Public health suffered as epidemics took their toll on the local population. A small public hospital was built in the nineteenth century but ministered mainly to the very sick and the dying. Not surprisingly, it came to be known mostly as a place of death. Up until the middle of the nineteenth century, pirate raids continued to disrupt island life with little intervention on the part of the sultan's navy, which was only occasionally present in the Mediterranean during this period. Infrastructure, such as roads to link interior agricultural areas with the city and its port, was also neglected (N. Doumanis 1997, 22; Greene 2000, 6; Kasperson 1966, 19).

Many Rhodians, including local scholars, tendentiously read their local built environment as a kind of history text from which suitable morals and lessons can be gleaned. To support his portrayal of Ottoman indolence, for instance, the Rhodian historian Christos Papachristodoulou adduces as evidence the Hospitaller buildings of the medieval Old Town. Their Gothic magnificence, he asserts, was frozen by Turkish indifference to anything but tax collection. To these elegant buildings, the Turks added nothing more than the narrow wooden balconies (*kafosta*) from which their harems, sequestered behind latticed screens, could peer unseen at events in the street below. Appropriating the already existing Greek Orthodox churches, Papachristodoulou continues, the Turks did little more than append minarets (1994, 513–14). Through this catalogue of architectural detail, Papachristodoulou conjures familiar images of Ottoman rule as essentially static, derivative, and—as symbolized by their seclusion of women in the cagelike confines of the *kafosta*—oppressive and backward.

Popular and elite representations of the Ottoman period as one of stagnation and oppression notwithstanding, by the early twentieth century, Rhodes Town was the site of multiethnic and multilingual diversity where Greeks, Jews, and Turks undeniably inhabited a "shared world" (Greene 2000). In 1908, the number of Muslims experienced an important spurt with the resettlement on Rhodes of a contingent of refugees from Crete. Greek-speaking converts, these refugees were fleeing the bloodshed that had followed the Greek nationalist revolution on that island. The Ottoman administration built a new neighborhood of one-room houses for the Cretan refugees, a humble settlement by the sea known ever since as Ta Kritika (Papachristodoulou 1994, 478). Some locals feared that ethnic strife, such as had bloodied Crete, would ensue, but the resettlement of displaced Muslims occurred without incident. Rhodes Town's ethnic heterogeneity would later be drastically diluted by two epochal events: the roundup of Rhodian Jews in the Calle Ancha by the Germans in July 1944, and their subsequent deportation to Auschwitz; and in 1974, the hasty departure of approximately fifteen thousand Turks who feared the local eruption of violence as a consequence of the conflict on Cyprus (Saka 2003; Varon 1999).

But through most of the first half of the twentieth century, the ethnic mosaic laid down under the Ottoman regime remained in place. An Italian census of Rhodes Town undertaken in 1922, for instance, found that of the town's total population of 16,150, 40 percent were Muslim Turks, 33 percent were Greeks, and 25 percent were Jews (Armao cited in N. Doumanis 1997, 26). By this time, Rhodes also had a rapidly increasing population of Italians. With the Italian occupation, the old residential segregation of the *millets* began to blur and break down. Greeks moved into the Old Town, and Jews and Turks began to move out. For example, Kiria Lucia, the caretaker of the town's only remaining synagogue and one of the few Rhodian Jews to survive Auschwitz and return to the island, was born in a Greek neighborhood in 1926, her mother assisted in childbirth by a Greek midwife.[1] Kiria Dora and Kiria Vasilia, both in their seventies, exemplified the friendly and cooperative relations that often existed between Greek and Turkish women at the time. Unable to conceive after two years of marriage, Kiria Dora turned for help to her Turkish neighbor, a woman with considerable knowledge of herbal medicines. After she gave birth to a daughter, word spread of her successful treatment, and she was besieged by Greek women asking to be taken to her neighbor for treatment. On her part, Kiria Vasilia had taken an infertile Turkish friend to visit the miraculous Orthodox shrine of the Panaghia Tsambika, a popular local manifestation of the Madonna, instructing her first on how to make the vow that might result in a cure. Even intermarriage between Greeks and Turks appears not to have been rare during those years (Saka 2003, 32–33).

When the Italian army invaded the Dodecanese and wrested control from the Turks in 1912, they were at first enthusiastically welcomed as liberators. Local resistance was negligible because Greek Rhodians believed that the islands would be handed over immediately to Greece. The Italian government had originally promised as much. However, through skillful diplomacy, prevarication, and outright lies the Italians held onto the Dodecanese, which they regarded as a valuable bargaining chip in their negotiations with Turkey over other colonial territories, such as Libya (D. Sutton 1998a, 17; N. Doumanis 1997, 31–32). Ultimately, the Italians stayed until 1944. The policies pursued over the roughly thirty years of Italian colonial rule fundamentally transformed Rhodian society and economy.

In an apparent paradox, Italy was determined to develop this relatively insignificant string of islands despite the huge financial cost entailed by such an ambitious project. The social historian Nicholas Doumanis has lucidly explained why the Italians viewed this development as top priority:

> Those who ruled Italy believed that making her a Great Power was a moral imperative. Empire building was a quest to construct an identity which would locate Italy among the major nation-states. Her eligibility for such high status also depended on the way she ruled her empire. In this age of empires it was important for ruling nations to be seen as highly civilised, as cultures worthy of ruling other peoples. The colonies would therefore need to evoke the high standards of Italian civilization, as Italy's imperial record would substantiate her worthiness as a ruling culture. (1997, 35)

In pursuing this (self-) civilizing mission, the Italian occupation touched on nearly every aspect of life in Rhodes, and its effects still reverberate. In the next section, I follow one of the most significant threads of this colonial legacy, tourism, the stiff and increasingly inflexible backbone of the island's economic structure and social life today.

Tourism

The appeal of Rhodes as a mass tourist destination is related to a host of factors rooted in its geography and the vagaries of its history. The physical beauty of the island is undeniable, even after decades of untrammeled development that has blocked much of its coastline from view and cluttered the town with high-decibel bars and tourist shops whose outdoor displays of Greek souvenirs, commissioned from workshops in Thailand and China (Greek labor being much too expensive), have turned downtown sidewalks into obstacle courses. Of all the Dodecanese islands, Rhodes and neighboring Kos have the most fertile soils and reliable water sources, lending them a lushness entirely missing from the so-called *kseronisia*, the bare and heavily eroded "dry islands" such as neighboring Symi and Kalymnos. Despite the forest fires that erupt periodically in the hot dry summer months, the mountainous interior of the island can still boast scattered stands of fragrant pine forests, many of them remnants of Italian reforestation projects. But far more pertinent to the economically critical "sun, sand, and sea" component of the global tourist market, compared to the other Dodecanese islands, Rhodes has a (literal) wealth of beaches, long elliptical sweeps of sand or pebbles that interrupt its craggy limestone coastline with profitable regularity. Indeed, the entire northern tip of the city of Rhodes consists of a fine, broad beach, only a few minutes' walk from the city's densest concentration of hotels.

Rhodes's exceptional physical attributes led the Italian colonial regime to privilege it as the main site of tourist development. Although all the islands were part of the Italian dream of building a "new Roman Empire," they varied greatly in the impact and experience of Italian colonialism (N. Doumanis 1997, 17). Leros, for instance, with its many large and well-protected harbors, became the headquarters of regional Italian naval operations. Nearby Kalymnos, a *kseronisi* with little arable land whose economy, unlike that of Rhodes, relied on fishing and sponge trading, was largely ignored (D. Sutton 1998a, 18). In contrast, Rhodes, and to a lesser extent, Kos, were the sites of ambitious and wide-ranging modernization projects. As the administrative and political center of the Italian colonial administration, Rhodes benefited the most from the Italians' agenda to lay permanent claim to the region, first via the radical transformation of the built environment, and later through the systematic Italianization of its inhabitants (N. Doumanis 1997, 41). In this way, Rhodes became the site of the only hospital, a large, airy building staffed by Italian doctors and nuns that continued to serve as the regional medical center until 2000. The colonial government bankrolled a multitude of other costly public works as well, including schools, airports, ports, some three hundred miles of roads, agricultural colonies, aqueducts, theaters, and hundreds of buildings, including many dazzling architectural showpieces of the time, to house the Italian colonial administration and its functionaries (N. Doumanis 1997; Fuller 2007; Martinoli and Perotti 1999).

In particular, Rhodes was targeted for the development of a broad variety of attractions and amenities catering to the tastes of wealthy foreign travelers, as well as to the colonial ruling class, which counted many aristocrats among its ranks (Martinoli and Perotti 1999). After the war, the products of this phenomenal building boom were at hand to jumpstart Rhodians' timely entry into the nascent international tourist industry. Employing large numbers of Rhodian men, the Italians built and staffed luxury hotels, including the once famous Grande Albergo delle Rose. Often featured on postcards of the period with sailboats floating just beyond its waterfront, this hotel in its heyday was patronized by royalty from Europe and the Middle East. Today it is a casino in which waitresses in Playboy bunny costumes serve customers amid the continual dinging of its wall-to-wall slot machines. Just a few kilometers outside the city, on a spit of land known as Kallithea, the Italians built a health spa in the playfully Orientalized Art Deco style of Pietro Lombardi, celebrated at the time as the "architect of the Aegean" (Colonas 2002, 55). People with a variety of ailments flocked to Kallithea to take the *Trinkkur*, a form of nature therapy highly popular in Europe at the time. Ailing patrons headed first to the spa's central fountain, jauntily festooned with stars, to imbibe a few cups of its cathartic mineral waters. After waiting a half-hour or so for the waters to take their violent effect, they hastily repaired to the endless rows of toilet stalls built over the spectacular cliffs of the Kallithea cove. Despite lying in ruins for years, the spa has remained a major tourist attraction, as much for the continuing appeal of its graceful architecture as for the beauty of the cove.

Even the island's archeological tourist attractions owe much of their existence to colonial Italian aspirations. The Archeological School established on Rhodes by the Italians in 1914 was responsible for the extensive if partial, and by some expert accounts, fanciful, reconstruction of the Acropolis of Rhodes town. They also excavated ancient Kamiros, one of the island's three city-states that reached their apogee during the classical period, and an important tourist draw to the eastern side of the island. Paradoxically, these ambitious archeological excavations were part of the colonial project to permanently annex the Dodecanese to the Italian state. As Doumanis (1997, 36–37) explains: "Italian enthusiasm for local antiquities usually had a political subtext, as new findings were meant to confirm historical connections with Italy, supposedly legitimating her presence in the area." Be this as it may, in contemporary popular memory, the archeological projects executed by the Italians are still appreciated as important sources of tourist revenue, while the Greek Archeological Service, which severely restricts building and remodeling of sites deemed to be worthy of historic preservation, is regarded with considerable hostility and resentment.[2]

The walled Old Town of Rhodes, which has been declared a UNESCO World Heritage Site, is another major attraction that owes much of its continuing touristic appeal to Italian reconstruction. For most of the twentieth century, the Old Town was a distinctively lower-class, multiethnic neighborhood of the city. In the Old Town's cramped maze of low-lying single-family residences lived Greeks (after 1912), Turks, and Sephardic Jews who made their livings as artisans, petty merchants, and, on the once notorious St. Fanourios street, the town's prostitutes (St. Fanourios's mother, it is said, was herself a prostitute). Today, the Old Town is solidly packed with tourist establishments, although very recently, its intensely picturesque ambience—the dim cobbled alleyways, slender Ottoman-era minarets, and partially excavated classical ruins overgrown with acacias and morning glories—has attracted intellectuals and artists to the neighborhood as well.

The Italian ruling elite, who preferred to build their residences and villas in the wide open spaces of the New Town, Niokhori ("new village"), at the northernmost tip of the island, was interested in the Old Town mainly for the ruins of the Hospitaller Order. These Gothic structures were symbolically important as local links with the Catholic, Latin West (N. Doumanis 1997, 51). Their centerpiece was the Palace of the Grand Master, the Castello (the Italian word by which it is still popularly known), once the seat of government of the order. Demolished by a gunpowder explosion in 1856, this lugubrious castle was imaginatively rebuilt, complete with imposing crenulations and turrets (Disneyfied, *avant la lettre*), according to Italian architect Vittorio Mesturino's controversial notions of what a medieval castle *should* have looked like (Kasperson 1966, 15; Martinoli and Perotti 1999, 88, 444). Inhabitants of the Old Town like to joke that today the Greek Archeological Service uses these turrets to police their building activities for infractions of the strict and roundly resented preservation code. The Castello lies at the highest point of the Old Town, at the end of Street of the Knights. Along this steep, highly photogenic cobbled lane are found the inns, or residences, of the various tongues that once composed the polyglot order. This site, reconstructed by the Italians along with the Castello, also bears little kinship to the buildings erected during the Knights' long rule. It is, however, a must-see attraction for tourists visiting Rhodes. In the summer, it becomes particularly difficult to navigate the heavily congested street, as dozens of tour groups, assorted by their modern tongues, clot around their guides to hear their various versions of the street's history.

The colonial administration's mission to Italianize the local population in preparation for permanent absorption into the metropole also inadvertently helped prepare Rhodians for the tourism boom that took off in the 1960s. Of special relevance was the policy of compulsory language instruction that enabled many to become fluent in Italian. Colonial social policies were generally resisted for the threat they were perceived to pose to the islanders' Greek Orthodox identity. But acquisition of Italian was often regarded in a positive light, at least in hindsight. Beginning in 1926, the first governor of the Dodecanese, Mario Lago, began the Italianization process by introducing compulsory Italian language instruction in the schools. The policies of the second governor, the widely resented Cesare De Vecchi, were far more drastic: he replaced the Greek schools altogether, and declared an offense the speaking of Greek in public (N. Doumanis 1997, 56). Punishment could be harsh. Kirios Antonis, a Rhodian musician in his seventies, for instance, remembered how one day in the third grade he had been castigated for speaking "three words of Greek." Spying a classmate eating fresh figs, he blurted impulsively, *"Ela re, dhos mou ena!* Come on, you, give me one!"* Overhearing him, his Italian teacher sent him to sweep up the ubiquitous olive pits that littered the schoolyard and made him kneel on the pile with bare knees for over an hour in the noonday sun. Although Kirios Antonis still resented his teacher for this punishment, he was also obviously proud of his bilingualism. Like many of the oldest Rhodians I interviewed about this period, he peppered our conversations with Italian phrases, immediately translating them into Greek for my benefit.

With the onset of mass tourism, such bilingualism represented social capital that could be converted into economic advantage as well. An example was Kirios Kostas, a lawyer also in his seventies who still practiced law with his son. Over the years, he had maintained a substantial Italian clientele interested in Dodecanese vacation real estate. Our interview, in fact, was interrupted by a phone call from one such client, with whom Kirios Kostas conversed in effortless Italian. Business had picked up considerably, he told me, after the release of the Academy Award–winning Italian movie *Mediterraneo* in 1991. Set on the Dodecanese island of Kastellorizo, the film piqued Italian demand for local properties and helped revitalize that woefully depopulated island. Another example was my neighbor Kiria Kirania, who found that being fluent in Italian helped her run her highly profitable pension. Like other Rhodians who entered primary school after De Vecchi's language policy was instituted in 1936, Kiria Kirania could not read or write Greek at all. She relied on her husband, who was a few years older than she and had attended school under Lago's regime (and so could read Greek as well as Italian), to read her official correspondence for her. But her knowledge of Italian proved a bankable skill as she attempted to communicate with her multinational clientele. In fact, Kiria Kirania spoke to *all* her guests—Scandinavian, British, Japanese—in Italian. Using it as a sort of all-purpose Romance language, she assumed, often correctly, that any foreigner was bound to figure out the meaning of at least some of the words.

In short, by the end of the Second World War and the Ensomatosi, the Italians had left in place a substantial infrastructure of roads, harbors, tourist facilities, and attractions, as well as a cadre of bilingual Rhodians trained in service work. As importantly, they had created the idea and image of Rhodes as a desirable and prestigious tourist destination. When international tourism gained momentum in the 1960s, the island was in an excellent position to become a major player in the burgeoning European mass tourist market. This advantage was recognized by the Greek state as early as the 1950s, when it earmarked Rhodes for a major share of credit and other financial incentives for tourist development (Galani Moutafi 1993, 250). A decade later, the military junta that ruled Greece from 1967 to 1974 offered another significant installment of incentives. After Greece's accession to the European Common Market in 1981, EC (and later, EU) grants and loans with generous terms once again poured into Rhodes. This staggered series of incentive packages offered Rhodians multiple entry points into the tourist boom that took off spectacularly after the 1960s.

Sprouting in the shadow of the large hotels and other tourist enterprises generously nourished by subsidies from the government and the European Union was also a tangle of small-scale, sometimes unofficial, family-owned and -operated businesses. In Rhodes, these pensions, rooms to let, and tavernas tended to be largely in the hands of women. Beginning in the 1960s, women in tourist areas throughout Greece took advantage of new opportunities by opening businesses based in their homes (Galani Moutafi 1993, 1994; Kasimati, Thanopoulou, and Tsartas 1999; Koussis 1989; Leontidou 1994). At that time, gender ideologies and norms, at least among the middle class and aspiring middle class, ideally restricted women's activities to unpaid labor in and around the house. As Galani Moutafi (1993, 1994) explains in her study of tourism on the island of Samos, several factors conspired to enable women to seize the new economic opportunities without overtly challenging prevailing notions of feminine respectability. For one thing, managing a small pension or restaurant from her house was seen as a logical extension of a woman's domestic responsibilities, notably cooking and cleaning. Women in Rhodes, like women elsewhere in the Aegean islands, are closely associated with the house, which, moreover, is often their inalienable dowry property. Managing an enterprise from her home, then, could be seen as an extension of the deep historical connection between woman, house, and domestic labor and, unlike waged work, posed no overt challenge to the gendered division of labor. For another thing, women themselves did not regard their businesses "as a means either to achieve personal enrichment or to enhance their identity" (Galani Moutafi 1994, 118). Rather, they viewed their entrepreneurial activities primarily as a way to contribute to the long-term parental project of helping finance the ever-increasing cost of their children's education and dowries and thus of successfully establishing them in society (Galani Moutafi 1993; 1994, 121). In the end, women's involvement in the tourist industry was valued and endorsed because, far from challenging established norms, it in fact "enabled [women] to conform to the ideal model of a housewife" that prevailed at the time (Galani Moutafi 1994, 118).

Even so, and despite their humble beginnings, over the years many of these businesses have flourished and proved quite profitable. Litsa, for instance, started up a food stand by carving a window out of the side of her house from which she sold *souvlakia*, kebabs, prepared by her widowed mother to passersby on the street. Nearly two decades later, Litsa's initially modest enterprise was practically unrecognizable: it now comprised a spacious indoor air-conditioned dining room as well as an outdoor patio and had become a popular tourist taverna that employed her entire family. Kiria Kirania, whom I introduced earlier, launched her pension with a couple of rooms to let added on to her house. Over the years, she steadily acquired all the adjacent properties as they came up for sale, eventually more than quadrupling the number of her rooms. Profits from the pension enabled her to underwrite the university education of both her daughters (one of them abroad) and purchase substantial additional properties for their dowries.

According to older Rhodians who had worked in tourism for decades, the first wave of postwar tourists was distinguished by its "good quality" (*kalis piotitas*). These were well-heeled travelers who spent money freely and tipped well. They included many Italians as well as mainland Greeks curious to see for themselves the vaunted material legacy of the Italian occupation. Beginning in the 1970s, it was commonly lamented, "quality" tourists declined in number, and a different kind of second-class (*dhefteris kateghorias*) tourism came to predominate. Although the numbers of tourists are in continual ascent, Rhodians characteristically complain at the end of each season that they didn't make much money, after all, because the tourists that came were "poor, they don't spend money, *ine ftokhi, dhen ksodhevoun.*"

Not all tourists are regarded in the same light, however. Rhodians have developed a taxonomy that roughly differentiates and ranks nationalities according to their putative characters and habitual touristic behaviors. By most accounts, the British lie at the bottom of this list: they are said to be the poorest and the rowdiest. As one Englishwoman living in Rhodes for over a decade complained to me: "They [Rhodians] always say, 'The English haven't got the money.' They don't say anything about the Germans—well, they do, but the first people they say something about is the English. I think it's because of the yobbos." The latter, as she explained this unfamiliar British term, are the young men who come in groups, get drunk, and sometimes destroy property, such as the car that was set on fire one summer in my neighborhood. Scandinavians, far more numerous but less obtrusive, come primarily to drink duty-free liquor and bask in the sun. German and French tourists, also classified as poor spenders, are known for preferring to get off the beaten path, in terms of both where they stay and when they come. For instance, Germans tend to be more plentiful during the spring and fall shoulder seasons. Thus despite their alleged frugality, they are appreciated as the economic mainstay of otherwise slow periods in the tourist cycle and of the more neglected villages of the island. The Japanese and, in recent years, the Russians are praised for their avid shopping, lavish spending, and indifference to bargaining. And everyone seems to like the Italians.[3]

Despite their complaints, Rhodians are nearly unanimous about the economic benefits of tourism. Indeed, by the early 1990s, Rhodes was one of the wealthiest regions of Greece, with official income a hefty 40 percent above the national per capita average (Karasoulli 1994, 1).[4] Nearly banished from the island was what the Anglo-Irish writer Lawrence Durrell, who lived in Rhodes between 1945 and 1947, had romantically if carelessly extolled as "the tenth muse," that is, poverty. Whereas, in the immediate postwar years, as he reported, "everywhere . . . conversation revolves around food" (1960, 61), today it is likely to revolve around the tourist season: how well or poorly it was going, how much money was being made this year as compared to last, and so on. One reason that Rhodians' average income is so high is that so many of the hotels and other tourist businesses are locally owned (in fact, only one major hotel was entirely foreign owned). In most Greek resort areas, the smaller, lower-category hotels, pensions, and rooms to let tend to belong to locals, often to local women, as mentioned earlier, while the larger, higher-quality hotels are owned by nonlocals or by the state. Rhodes is distinctive in that the majority of its higher-quality hotels are also in local hands (Loukissas 1983, 533). As is well documented for other areas, local ownership and control of tourist facilities helps stanch the leakage of economic benefits to the outside so often bemoaned in socioeconomic analyses of tourism, and fosters the local redistribution of these benefits. Many other tourist-related services offer very good income opportunities as well. For example, taxi driving is so lucrative that permits in Rhodes cost nearly double those in Athens. Drivers may earn the equivalent of hundreds of dollars a week or more and, not surprisingly, some opt not to work at all during the off-season.

Yet Rhodians' grievances and dissatisfactions with the economic returns of tourism accurately speak to their relatively unfavorable position in the global political economy of contemporary mass tourism. For, although nearly all the tourist infrastructure lies in local or at least Greek hands, the terms for a large portion of the critically important package tourist trade are set by tour operators based in Northern Europe. Tour operators retain up to half the price of a vacation package (Leontidou 1994, 98). Rhodian hoteliers and their organizations may attempt to bargain for better rates, but the fungibility of tourist destinations predicated on "sun, sea, and sand" leaves them vulnerable, and means that tour operators can without too much difficulty divert large numbers of tourists to more compliant resort areas. Turkey, its Anatolian coastline visible from Rhodes Town even on a hazy day, has been one such especially irksome competitor.

Of course, not all tourists stick to the bottom line in deciding where to spend their vacations and other sentiments may also apply. A Norwegian man told me (in the mid-1990s) with evident pride that he continued to come to Rhodes, even though Turkey was cheaper, because of the latter's poor human rights record. A good many tourists I met had developed emotional and social ties to Rhodes, fostered by repeated visits to the same pensions, tavernas, and shops. Returning year after year, sometimes twice a year, they kept a meticulous account of their trips that reminded me of the way many Greeks kept track of the number of swims they'd taken over the course of a summer. Twenty-two visits, thirty-seven trips, forty-four times, tourists would tell me to my initial astonishment. As the number of my own visits mounted, I began to see the same people on the street or in a cafe, and we would greet each other as old acquaintances. Comparatively high salaries, the enviable vacation benefits European workers have managed to wrest from their welfare states, and a highly organized tourist industry (favoring the North) have all helped make these multiple repeated visits possible.

On Tourist Time: The Saison and the Rhythms of Rhodian Social Life

As a result of the massive influence of tourism, both space and time have been profoundly reconfigured on Rhodes. As is generally true of the Mediterranean, the annual calendar is popularly divided into two contrasting halves: winter, rainy and overcast, stretching from late fall to the spring; and summer, predictably cloudless and bone-dry. However, in Rhodes, as in all Greek tourist areas, there exists a notable reversal of meanings usually attached to these seasons elsewhere:

> Tourism here re-establishes the dominance of nature and the seasons, but in an inverse manner from the one familiar to Western societies: work and overpopulation during the summer, pause and depopulation during the winter. (Leontidou 1994, 82)

Summer in Rhodes, also known as the *saison*, the French loan word used throughout Greece to refer to the period of intense tourism, is a time of hectic work pace and punishingly long hours. Winter, in contrast, is a time of initial quietude and repose born of exhaustion, and later, gradual recuperation and social reconnection.

On Rhodes, the saison begins in May and ends in late October, with increasing numbers of businesses staying open into November as long-standing efforts to diversify tourism and extend the season have met with some degree of success. This is a very long season. It is long in absolute terms, as people's tolerance for the exhausting pace of work is stretched to its limits. Tourist businesses typically open early in the morning and stay open until late at night, seven days a week; restaurants and bars stay open until two AM and hotels and pensions remain open all night. Until mid-June when school lets out, parents must also juggle their hectic schedules to accommodate their children's continual need for tutoring and chauffeuring to afternoon tutorials, language classes, and extracurricular activities. During *mesimeri*, the quiet midafternoon siesta hours, mothers, and often fathers too, can be seen in the tourist shops helping their children plow through their mounds of homework.

As it happens, the Rhodian season is also long in comparison to the rest of the region's islands. For instance, the island of Leros, despite the zealous efforts of its local business people, has a saison that lasts a single month, August, during which most of its tourists visit (a total of 2,900 in 1998). As Lerians complain, a saison that short, no matter how profitable, is simply not sufficient to live the year round. Tourism there must of necessity be combined with other generally poorly paid and precarious activities, such as fishing the seriously depleted Aegean waters. The somewhat larger island of Patmos, with its attractions for religious tourism—it is the site of a famous monastery, as well as the cave in which St. John is alleged to have written the Apocalypse (Kasperson 1966, 14)—received a heftier fifteen thousand visitors in 1998. Yet when I traveled there in early October one year, I was unable to find an ice cream cone for my daughter anywhere. "But, madame," the owners of the shops that were still open offered by way of explanation, "the saison is over." Spoiled by the extended Rhodian season, which most often coincided with my own fieldwork saison, I hadn't realized the myriad ways in which even the most trifling aspects of everyday life are affected by the rhythms of the tourist calendar, especially on the less popular islands.

In the winter, the frenetic pace of the saison comes to an abrupt halt, as hotels and shops shut down from one day to the next. As soon as the saison ends, many Rhodians promptly leave the island. Some reoccupy apartments in Athens that lie empty most of the year. For Rhodians, as for other provincial Greeks, owning an apartment in Athens is desirable on many counts: as a home base when seeking the superior medical attention which brings many to the capital on a regular basis (some Rhodian women have Athenian gynecologists whom they visit even for their routine checkups, for example); as an excellent investment, given that the price of apartments there continues to soar; as a temporary home for children attending university. Many of those employed as waiters, dishwashers, and chambermaids have come to Rhodes from other parts of Greece, or from local villages on the island, to which they return to spend a quiet winter with their families. If they have worked "on the books," they have collected stamps from their employers, called *ensima*, which entitle them to unemployment payments at the end of the season. Others, especially the owners of tourist businesses, board up for the winter and themselves become international tourists, their turn now to invert the conventional meanings of winter and summer. Some may visit Northern Europeans they have come to know well from their annual vacations on the island. Some older Rhodians go to Italy to reunite and stay with childhood friends made during the Italian occupation. Others, embracing international tourism as a sign of modernity and distinction, travel to such far-flung tourist destinations as the Seychelles or Maldives Islands, Bali, and Thailand. I was sometimes taken aback by how well-traveled even many older Rhodians were: I remember in particular one man in his sixties wearily describing to me his round-the-world tour, taken in just twelve days, and a woman about the same age, observing how much she liked mangoes, which she'd first eaten on a trip to Cuba.

Although winter is a time of repose for most Rhodians, for some the end of the saison is a time when work picks up. Construction projects on hold during the summer begin or are resumed, as hotel owners make repairs they had postponed, proprietors of pensions expand their rooms, and parents plow their tourist earnings into houses and apartments for their children. Some Rhodians still use the word "dowry" (*prika*) to describe the housing that most parents try to provide for their daughters, and today occasionally for their sons as well, upon marriage. But others, like Kiria Kirania, who generously dowered her daughters with property when they married, eschew the word for its traditional connotations. The dowry institution was formally abolished under the highly gender-egalitarian Family Law that was passed in 1983. Today, Rhodians may simply refer to this nonetheless resolutely persistent practice, described in more detail in Chapters 3 and 7, as "a help" (*mia voithia*) that every parent "naturally" wants to offer their offspring, and this desire fuels a good portion of the demand for new construction (see also D. Sutton 1998a, 100–102). The winter is therefore the busy season for architects, carpenters, plumbers, electricians, and, in recent years, interior decorators, and a profitable time for stores selling furniture and appliances. Time-consuming (and costly) ritual events, such as baptisms and weddings, in the past typically took place in the summer. Now, they are postponed until winter when people have the time and money to plan and attend them. In April, shopkeepers and owners of tavernas and bars engage in a burst of spring cleaning, freshly repainting the facades of their businesses and making minor repairs and improvements. After the quiet and slow-paced winter months, there is a jaunty sense of expectation in the air, of a performance about to begin. As Lila Leontidou, in an optimistic endnote to her otherwise critical study of tourism in Greece, observes of the annual onset of the saison: "The sound of foreign languages in public urban spaces is welcome and pleasant; it feels like welcoming the summer again" (1994, 99).

The Fourth Occupation:
Intimate Invasions, New Configurations

Despite the acknowledged economic benefits of tourism, and the social ties that many Rhodians have forged with tourists, their sheer numbers were often perceived as overwhelming, especially as the long season dragged to its exhausting conclusion. To a certain extent, this sense of being overrun could be mitigated on a large island like Rhodes by the high degree of spatial segregation that exists between natives and tourists (as Loukissas [1982] also found to be the case on Corfu). Rhodians rarely patronized tourist restaurants, bars, and shops and vice versa. Still, as I noted at the beginning of this chapter, Rhodians occasionally referred to tourists as the island's "fourth occupation." Beyond and behind the humorous tone, the metaphorical use of "occupation" (*katokhi*) hints at a threatening sense of continuity between contemporary tourists and those outsiders who in the past used the island for their own benefit. The occupation metaphor is found elsewhere in Greece as well. Stewart (1991, 48), for instance, reports its use on the Cycladic island of Naxos. It is also in evidence in the following unusual prayer invented by the Greek Orthodox Church in the 1970s:

> Lord Jesus Christ, Son of God, have mercy on the cities, the islands and the villages of this Orthodox Fatherland, as well as the holy monasteries which are scourged by the worldly touristic wave. Grace us with a solution to this dramatic problem and protect our brethren who are sorely tried by the modernistic spirit of these contemporary Western invaders (Smith and Turner 1973, 55, quoted in Crick 1989, 334).

While this prayer reflects the official xenophobia and social conservatism of the junta years, when Greece was under the control of the right-wing colonels with the support and cooperation of the Church hierarchy, vestiges of these sentiments and tropes linger on today. A recent example can be found in a travel article on Rhodes that appeared in the popular Athens weekly *Athenorama*, a publication akin to the *Time Out* series. The article's title, "I dhiki mas Rodos," literally means "Our Rhodes" (Boubouri 1999). A literal translation, however, does not do justice to the intricate web of culturally specific meanings upon which the title draws. As many ethnographers of Greece have observed, "dhiki mas" is a common rhetorical strategy used to both index and construct insider status. In affirming Rhodes to be "dhiki mas," the title draws on this homely strategy of inclusion to redraw social boundaries so that what was formerly "outside" and foreign (*kseno*) now finds its way to a socially intimate "inside." At the same time, in her bid to reclaim Rhodes from the tourists and make it "ours" again, the author appears to evoke (with considerable bathos, no doubt) the famous irredentist slogan that Constantinople would be freed from its Turkish occupation and become "Ours Once More" ("*dhiki mas pali*"; see Herzfeld 1982a, chapter 6).

Although in her title the author of the *Athenorama* article rhetorically reannexes Rhodes to the rest of Greece, the occupation metaphor continues to lurk just below the surface:

> I, as I imagine many other Greeks did, "left" the two islands [Rhodes and Corfu, the second most popular destination for package tours] to foreign hands . . . I turned up my nose (*snobara*) at the image from thousands of post cards, the hordes of blond Scandinavians, and of course, the *kamakia*. (Boubouri 1999, 71, my translation)

In this excerpt, Boubouri also reveals some common class and gender assumptions about international tourism and its impact on Rhodes, and on Greece more generally. In her use of the loan word "*snobara*," a verb adapted from "snob," she distinguishes herself and "many other Greeks" (of a class background similar to hers? The *Athenorama* has a largely middle-class readership) from the "hordes" of implicitly working-class European foreigners who have invaded, and consequently "declassed" Rhodes (a sentiment that echoes in Rhodians' own laments over the decline into "second-class" tourism). Rhodes has become too expensive for many working-class Greeks. But even the middle-class Athenians I knew who could afford to do so had rarely vacationed on Rhodes (or they had visited only once during adolescence on the annual spring-break group tours, *penthimeres*, that Greek high school students are indulged in before graduation) and tended to prefer the smaller, less crowded, and less accessible islands.

Class and gender assumptions about mass tourism also underpin Boubouri's reference to the "kamakia" she disdains in the last line of the quote. It is a popular belief among Rhodians that many foreign women come to Greece specifically looking for sex, along with sun, sand, and sea—the fourth of "the four s's" that are commonly credited with driving global tourism today (Crick 1989; Eisner 1991). Kamakia (sing., *kamaki*) refers to a subculture of generally marginal Greek men who, sharing this assumption, devote themselves to the serial seduction of tourist women. Derived from the word for harpoon, kamaki connotes a hunt, the intention of which "is to metaphorically spear the 'victim'" by means of a fairly conventional bag of romantic tricks (Zinovieff 1991, 208). According to Sofka Zinovieff, who studied this subculture in the mid 1980s, the poor and working-class men who engage in kamaki derive a sense of domination from these sexual encounters, a reversal, however fleeting, of Northern European hegemony over Greece (see also Buck-Morss 1987). Thus, tourist women, often richer and better educated than the kamakia with whom they have sex, "can be seen as crossing many symbolic boundaries." In the popular imagination, such boundary crossings lend a dangerous aura of confusion and even pollution to these encounters (Zinovieff 1991, 213), and by extension, to the sites, such as tourist areas, in which they occur. *Kamaki* subculture had its heyday in the early decades of mass tourism. Today it is essentially defunct—undone by a combination of fear of HIV/AIDS, Greece's increasing affluence, and the dramatic changes in sexual expectations and behavior among young Greek women and men—though sex and romance between individual Rhodian men and tourist women certainly still occur. Nevertheless, as the *Athenorama* excerpt suggests, at least for some audiences, the intimate and transgressive traffic across the borders of foreign and native has left Rhodes with the vestiges of a "spoiled identity" (Goffman 1986).

What is intriguing about Rhodes and other heavily touristed areas of Greece is that it is strictly the native men who have been eroticized and exoticized. For many foreign women traveling to Rhodes, the expectation of encountering a "Greek god" remains in fact an integral part of the vacation package (Smith 2002). In marked contrast, there is no counterpart "Greek goddess" figure among male tourists. This asymmetry is especially puzzling because historically, tourism has been associated almost exclusively with masculine notions of pleasure, adventure, and a *feminine* exotic Other (Enloe 1989, 20). Greece is too far above the level of economic despoliation and desperation that drives sex tourism in other parts of the world, although in recent years there has been a steep increase in the number of women from the Balkans and the former soviet republics fleeing war and economic disarray who may end up as sex workers in Greece. In any event, the absence of female sex tourism cannot explain why it is exclusively Greek men who have been eroticized.

Underpinning this asymmetry is what Jill Dubisch identifies as an "intra-European hierarchy of difference" in which exotic masculinity is often stereotypically embodied in the Mediterranean male (1995b, 35). Within this hierarchy, the Mediterranean male is figured as "more sensual, more passionate, more emotional, more 'primitive' than his Northern European counterpart, a stereotype which he himself may play into and use as a means of self contrast." The sources feeding this stereotype, however, remain cloudy. In part, it builds upon the linkage Western European thought has long made between climate and sexuality. This association found expression in the literary work of generations of male European writers who documented their sensual awakening under the influence of the Mediterranean sun (as evidenced in the multiple meanings of the word "sultry" [Littlewood 2001]), and whose writings have played a major role in fostering and disseminating cultural stereotypes within Europe (Borneman and Fowler 1997, 502).

The *specific* linkage between the Mediterranean male and a purer, less inhibited form of sexual expression, however, ultimately may owe much to the figure and writings of Byron. Among the reasons Byron went South was to find an "escape from Anglo-Saxon attitudes [toward homosexuality] and a vantage point from which to challenge them" (Littlewood 2001, 118). Byron was followed by generations of writers, "for the most part homosexual, who have quite consciously used the pursuit of forbidden fruit [in the South] as a form of guerilla warfare against the conventions of their own society" (129). Toward the end of the nineteenth century, the trial and conviction of Oscar Wilde spurred a new wave of terrified homosexual men to follow Byron's path to Italy and Greece (131). In Byronic fashion, the writings of these sexual rebels often extolled the superior sensuality of the southern male. In the twentieth century, a new generation of philhellenic writers, most famously Lawrence Durrell and Henry Miller, traveled to Greece and produced works that continued to portray Greek men in stereotypically rapturous terms—oddly enough, it would seem, given Durrell's and Miller's rather ostentatious heterosexuality. In an unmistakable echo of imagery made popular in the nineteenth century by Byron and the "Byronish" writers who followed him, the men that populated the "new geography of Greece" created by Miller, Durrell, and other writers in the interwar period were portrayed as proud and lusty Dionysian or Pan-like figures. Greek women, in contrast, were peripheral or completely absent (Roessel 2002, 257). When large numbers of single women began to travel abroad after the Second World War, these enduring literary images of the sultry Mediterranean male were at hand in the popular imagination to fold into their own heterosexual scripts of holiday romance. Today, echoes of this Greek male stereotype also circulate among both Rhodian men and women. Many of the women I spoke with, for instance, readily understood why a foreign woman would prefer a Greek man: Northern Europeans, like their climates, tend to be *krii* (cold), less affectionate and demonstrative than Greek men.

If Greece, as a part of the sunny Mediterranean South, connotes otherness in the Northern European imagination, this sense of the exotic appears to be amplified and even more irresistible when located on an island. Islands occupy a special place in Western imaginings of otherness: as "backwaters to large economic centers, as sites of romantic idealism and of untamed nature" (Parman cited in Casteneda 1993, 206). This association is not only the stuff of travel brochures and advertising, but has a surprisingly long pedigree in literature and science writing as well (Beer 1989). Furthermore, in popular Western thought, notions of "islandness" and "Paradise" are often closely linked (see, e.g., Buck 1993). This chain of signifiers is immediately evident in Lawrence Durrell's loving memoir of his two years' sojourn on Rhodes, *Reflections on a Marine Venus*. On the very first page of the book's first chapter, tellingly entitled "Of Paradise Terrestre," he describes himself as an "islomane" or person "who find[s] islands somehow irresistible" (1960, 15). By quirky coincidence, the Rhodes airport, gateway to the island holiday fantasy, is located in the town of Paradisi, obviously derived from the Greek word for paradise. By deplaning in Paradise, as it were, the Western traveler is poised to partake of the timeless authenticity of the Greek island experience.[5]

On the ground, these stereotypes and romantic narratives have coalesced into a phenomenon also found in other heavily touristed areas of Greece: the relatively large number of marriages between local men and Northern European women who arrived as tourists, fell in love with a local man, stayed, and settled on the island. On Rhodes, by one estimate there were some four thousand such cross-cultural marriages (Smith 2002).[6] Even among the men studied by Zinovieff (and belying her bleak portrayal of predatory kamaki subculture), half eventually married foreign women (Placas 2001). In contrast, there are only a handful of cases in which foreign men have married Rhodian women. A Danish man who was married to a Rhodian woman told me he knew of only four such marriages. Like himself, they had all met their wives abroad, in his case when they were both university students in Germany. Clearly, cross-cultural marriage is sharply bifurcated along the trenches of class and gender.

The common view is that unions between Greek men and foreign women, skewed by disparities of culture and class, are inherently fragile and inevitably slated for divorce. This was indeed the fate of many cross-cultural marriages, but there were also many others that succeeded. Foreign wives put down roots on Rhodes: they learned Greek, often quite well, many converted to Greek Orthodoxy, and some stayed on even after their divorce. Some have become successful local entrepreneurs, running Swedish bakeries, English pubs, and Danish restaurants. The salesclerks and waitresses employed in these businesses were often the bilingual offspring of such North-South marriages. Over the years, foreign wives have also established a variety of social clubs and associations organized by their nationality. These associations meet regularly to celebrate the national or cultural holidays of their countries of origin, sponsor civic improvements in Rhodes (the first ultrasound machine in the Maternity Department of Rhodes's public hospital was donated by the English-speaking association), and organize language classes for their children. Most of the Swedish, Finnish, British, Belgian, and Dutch women I met went to great lengths to raise their children bilingually and biculturally. They spoke to them exclusively in their native tongues, packed them off to their home countries for summer vacations, and sent them from a young age to the language classes sponsored by their organizations. In 1999, the mayor's office of Rhodes, recognizing the asset that these bilingual and bicultural Rhodians represented for the island, began to subsidize foreign language classes for the children of the eight major nationalities of women living in Rhodes. For many of these women, seeing that their children learned their native tongue was a way of keeping their citizenship options flexible (Smith 2002). Above all, foreign mothers wanted to ensure that their children were sufficiently proficient to be able to attend university in their home countries, as a backup to failing to pass the highly competitive and gruelingly difficult Greek university entrance exams, or to spare them that ordeal altogether.[7]

Memory, Countermemory, and Rhodian Identities

On a warm June night in 1999, I strolled with Kiria Olga Stamos alongside the massive facade of Italian-era buildings that line Rhodes's central Mandraki harbor. Kiria Olga, a widow in her seventies, is a former dressmaker whose knack for reproducing the latest French couture had guaranteed her a wealthy clientele, first in Rhodes and later in Athens. That evening, dressed in a black linen suit, her auburn hair meticulously coifed and her make-up impeccable, she was easily the more chic of the two of us. As we walked, she began to reminisce about her childhood during the years of the Italian occupation. When we reached the building that today houses the National Theater, she paused to inform me that it was once known as Il Teatro Puccini, and that, twice a year, it hosted performances of La Scala's opera company. During the intermezzo, she continued, using the Italian word, couples in elegant evening dress would cross the street to the nightclub called La Ronda, dance a single dance, and then return to the performance (Fig. 1). Listening to her narration, I was both entranced and amused; I had known that whimsically round building only as the Elli, a tourist nightclub specializing in the limited repertoire of Greek songs ("Never on Sunday," the Zorba theme) that are perpetually recycled in such establishments. Then, with a sweep of her arm that took in the imposing harbor front, Kiria Olga told me something I had heard from other Rhodians as well: "*Tote, i Rodhos itan ena komati Evropis.* Back then, Rhodes was a piece of Europe."

The symbolic significance of Kiria Olga's claim that Rhodes was once a part of Europe and thus, by implication, at some remove from the Orient is one that any Greek can recognize, if not necessarily agree with. Rhodians often strategically use the same binaries as other Greeks (Europe/Orient, East/West, etc.) to negotiate that shifting and unstable terrain called identity formation. But, as one might expect, their use of these terms is also inflected by

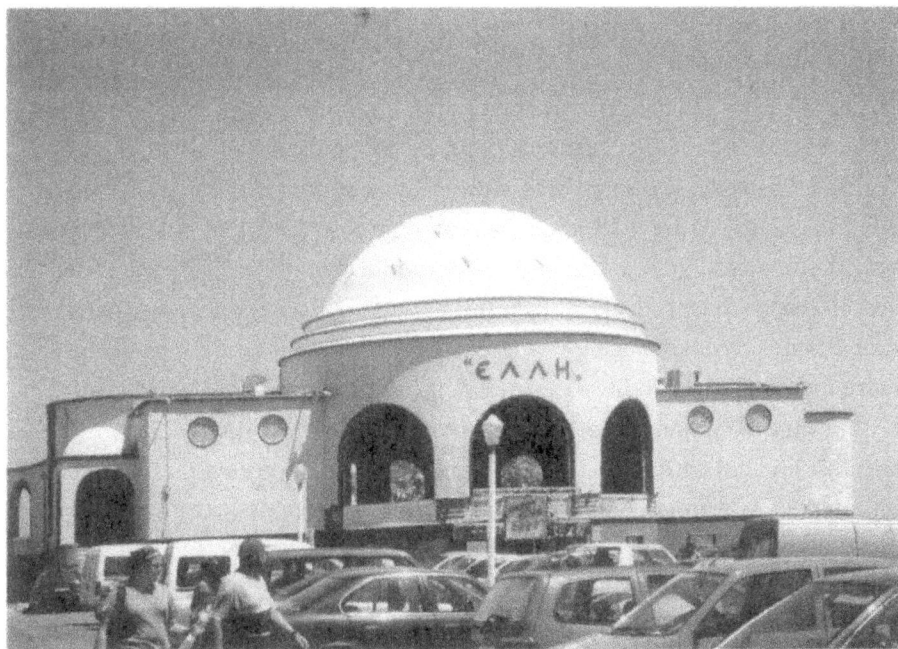

1. The Elli, formerly La Ronda Sea Baths. Designed by A. Bernabiti, 1935, in the Mediterranean Modernist style.

the particulars of their location and history—of the experiences, stories, and local environments they share as Rhodians. Place, in other words, is integral to the ways in which Rhodians, like all people, shape, articulate, and experience their identities (Kelly 2003). On Rhodes, the Italian occupation and its lasting imprint on the local environment are among the most salient ingredients in local constructions of identity.

For Rhodians, as Kiria Olga indicates, the Italian occupation is most often deployed as a sign of Rhodes's European valence. With the exception of some of the island's intellectual and political elite, it represents the cornerstone of Rhodians' claims to a degree of cultural superiority and sophistication associated with being more Europeanized (*eksevropaismeni*), in comparison not only with the rest of the Dodecanese, but with other Greeks as well. Like the Greek Cypriots described by Vassos Argyrou (1996, 2) who attempt "to capitalize on the 'civilizing experience' of British colonialism," Rhodians draw on the Italian colonial presence as a strategy to distinguish themselves from mainland Greeks. Like Kiria Olga, they point to the imposing material legacy of the Italian occupation as literally concrete support for these claims. Multiple ironies are at play here. For their part, the Italians, another Mediterranean people at the "margins of Europe" at the time, saw Rhodes as a privileged stage upon which to enact their aspirations to move from a "belated" to a fully modern status on a footing equal to the Great Powers. Against the galling skepticism of the rest of Europe, the fascist state staked its reputation on not simply ruling over, but "civilizing," "modernizing," and "developing" its backward colonies at least as well as, or better than, the Great Powers had theirs. Ultimately, the grandiose scale these imperial aspirations acquired in Rhodes proved to be a formidable economic loss for Italy, but an enduring source of material gain and symbolic capital for Rhodians. Ironically, then, Italy's decision to definitively Europeanize itself via its enlightened imperial rule over Rhodes dovetailed snugly with the Europeanizing aspirations of this even more marginalized Mediterranean region (N. Doumanis 1997, 47ff.).

For elite Rhodian historians and politicians with a vested interest in nationalist and patriotic principles, however, the Italian occupation is invariably represented as a time of injustice, oppression of Greek culture and language, and heroic resistance on the part of the local population (N. Doumanis 1997). This perspective is very much in evidence, for instance, in a speech given by the late Ioannis Zighdis, a Rhodian politician and former minister of industry well known throughout Greece, to inaugurate a new cultural center. In his speech, Zighdis remembered the Italian occupation as a time in which "Dodecanesians were the 'guinea pigs' of the Fascists for the imposition of new means of tyranny and terror, to which they resorted continually." Putting a finer point on his argument, he went on to recount the example of his father, "a true apostle of Faith and the Fatherland [*patridha*]" who was forced to drink "a kilo of castor oil" for his subversive activities against Italian imperialism (1993, 18, my translation).

For many others, in marked contrast, the occupation is remembered in positive terms for leaving in place a legacy that continues to benefit Rhodes. Nicholas Doumanis (1997) has documented this idealization of the colonial past through what he calls the "countermemories" of the ordinary Dodecanesians who lived through this period. In their narrated recollections, his interviewees compose a portrait of the occupation that is radically at odds with official representations of elites and public figures such as Zighdis. The stories I heard from older Rhodians who had experienced the occupation reverberate with many of the same idioms used by Doumanis's interlocutors: the Italians were a civilized people (*politismenos laos*), who brought "order" to Rhodes, and an unprecedented burst of "development" that generated abundant and well-paid opportunities for employment. As Doumanis persuasively argues, these countermemories gain much of their rhetorical force from the explicit comparison of the Italian occupation with the period of Ottoman rule that preceded it, popularly remembered as a time of official apathy and disinterest in anything but the extraction of taxes, and the long anticipated but ultimately disappointing incorporation into Greece once Italy's imperial schemes crumbled. The years following the incorporation were exceedingly hard ones not only in Rhodes, but throughout Greece, when some three hundred thousand people died of famine and the mainland was devastated by a protracted civil war (Mazower 1993). Wracked by scarcity, hunger, and unemployment, Dodecanesians remember this time as a return to the black life (*i mavri zoi*) that had blighted the Ottoman period (N. Doumanis 1997, 199). In the decade of extreme hardship that followed the war, massive numbers of young Rhodians streamed off the island in search of livelihoods. Entire villages were decanted of their most productive members. For many Rhodians, a good deal of the blame for their woeful social and economic plight was attributable to what they perceived as the Greek government's neglect and disarray.

Doumanis (1997, 198) suggests that during the civil war years and their divisive aftermath, when explicit criticism of the government was politically dangerous, nostalgia for the Italian period represented an indirect way of venting disappointment with Greek rule. Thus, Rhodians' generally positive memories of the Italians are based in part on their lived experiences of the colonial largesse of the past, but they also reflect and give voice to dissatisfaction with the present. The narratives of older Rhodians like Kiria Olga who came of age under the Italians are rife with fondly remembered details about the past that simultaneously point a finger at the contemporary shortcomings of the state and Greek civil society. As Kiria Olga reminisced:

> When you ate *pasatempo* [a popular snack consisting of a variety of unhulled seeds], you had to put the shells in your pockets, not throw them on the ground like now. You couldn't hang out your laundry after nine AM. If you forgot to bring your laundry in, the *vigilo urbano* would pass by and remind you: "*Proibito, signora.*" If you continued to do it, they'd fine you.

In a similar but more extreme example, Doumanis (1997, 132) quotes a woman from Kos Town who recalled approvingly how her future husband was arrested by the carabinieri and *beaten* for serenading her:

> "Why are you singing at this hour . . . , it is illegal." They took him to the gaol house, and the maresciallo asked them what he had done. «Che cosa fate», he said, what did he do. The soldiers said that he made loud noises at an illegal time.

As Doumanis (134) insightfully observes of these stories, respondents remember such petty infractions and disproportionately harsh discipline in a positive light at least in part because of their implicit comparisons with the present, when littering is common and bars catering to tourists blare loud music late into the night.

In Rhodes today, as it happens, it is not only the old-timers who lived through the Italian occupation who indulge in this strategic nostalgia. Rhodians of all ages, including young people born well after the incorporation, would point out this or that building, this or that grove of trees and, using a stock phrase I heard repeated many times, lament: "Look what the Italians built [or planted]; the Greeks don't build [or plant] anything!" The built environment left behind by the Italians, impossible to avoid in Rhodes Town, was always, it seemed, at hand to underscore a moral lesson. Often, this entailed a critique of the perceived deficiencies of the contemporary Greek state. One of the most popular targets of such critiques was the old health spa at Kallithea, perhaps because unlike so many of the other Italian buildings, it had not been recycled for contemporary use. Lying in ruins on the outskirts of Rhodes Town, it had become a local symbol of what is perceived as the irresponsibility and indifference of an otiose Greek state. This reading of Kallithea even finds its way into the travel article on Rhodes discussed earlier, when the author, advising Athenians on what to see in Rhodes, lists it in first place: "Where to Go: Kallithea, so you can see the frightful condition of the spa (a work of the Italians, naturally) and curse the Greek public sector" (Boubouri 1999, 75, my translation). In such locutions, the Greek state is reified and critiqued as implicitly Oriental, in unflattering comparison with how a truly modern European state would behave (Herzfeld 1992, 1995).

Attesting to their multivocality and versatility, but also to their widespread internalization, these pervasive binarisms are used in everyday speech in a variety of thrust and parry maneuvers by "the humblest of local social actors," as well as by the "agents of powerful state entities" (Herzfeld 1997, 31). Elites deploy them in an attempt to shift the onus of disorder and backwardness away from the state, where it is so often placed in everyday discourse, and onto the fundamental character flaws of ordinary citizens. This rhetorical strategy, which Michael Herzfeld (1997, 96) has aptly termed "practical orientalism," is apparent in the continuation of former Minister Zighdis's speech. Note especially how he faithfully reproduces these idioms even as he instills them with specifically Dodecanese inflections. According to Zighdis, one of the principal objectives of the new cultural center he was helping inaugurate was to provide a venue in which

Greek scientists, but also the inhabitants of the islands, will come into closer contact with foreign scientists and tourists of high status so that they will understand that the lower returns and lack of competitiveness of our economy are owed to a large degree to the retention of the mentality (*nootropia*) and behavior of a preindustrial society, and not always to the lack of modern technology. . . . Thus, they will be obliged to abandon this mentality and to adopt that of modern postindustrial societies. In other words, we will stop acting like "*rayadhe*s" or "levantines," and become true, modern Europeans (1993, 23, my translation).

Nootropia (mentality) has become something of a keyword that, as Herzfeld (1997, 79) has also observed, "enjoys enormous currency . . . as a term of popular speech" to encapsulate stereotypical attributes of national character (see also Paxson 2004, 99). In 2000, even then–prime minister Simitis used it to make his case that reform of Greek public institutions demanded "a change of mentality and culture" on the part of the Greek people (quoted in Close 2002, 287). In Zighdis's speech, the Turkish word *rayah*, meaning bondsman or subject of the Ottoman Empire, iconically indexes the Oriental ("levantine") attributes allegedly internalized during the infamous "four hundred years" of occupation. Once again, it is the taint of Greeks' "Oriental" past that is blamed for braking their movement toward modernity. In this case, however, the onus is deflected from the state and, as in Simitis's usage, strategically placed on Greeks as individuals. Consistent with the idealism that underpins this perspective, Zighdis implies that it is only through the diffusion of European culture and contact with higher-status Europeans (as opposed to the "poorer category" of the mass tourist?) that Greeks can obtain the "cargo" of a progressive, modern mentality (see Papagaroufali and Georges 1993).

As should now be clear, these rhetorical usages are ubiquitous. However, if their use often reveals "the best evidence of the reproductive menace of hegemony," it may also "provide the weak with a protective wall of practical discourse" (Herzfeld 1997, 158). That is to say, while the meanings attributed to "Europe" and "European" are on the whole associated with positively valued and desired qualities and ends, they are always multivocal, deployed strategically and shifting shape and content according to context and audience. On occasion, their positive associations can be inverted and even reversed. I have already mentioned that a certain characteristic coldness is believed to limit the Northern European capacity for spontaneity, intimacy, and *jouissance*, and is widely adduced to make sense of the attraction that Greek men have for foreign women. David Sutton (1998a, 43), in his ethnography of neighboring Kalymnos, reports that islanders there evince a distinct ambivalence toward the idea of Europe. While they might agree with Rhodians that their island was more European than was Kalymnos (due to the Italian legacy and to tourism), they also criticized Rhodians as suffering from what they regarded as the undesirable sequelae of such Europeanization: materialism, loss of the old ways, and the promiscuity of the women (37ff). More generally, the vaunted European attributes of progress, order, rationality and so on, were seen as yoked to a "dull, robotic way of life" with little time or desire for socializing (41). Rhodian identity discourse generally ignored Kalymnos—Karpathos was the preferred primitive Other, as we have seen. But, at times Rhodians expressed a very similar critique of the Western way of life. Occasionally, they too referred to Northern Europeans (in the abstract) as living like "robots." Elaborating on this mechanical metaphor, Rhodians, like Kalymnians, might stereotypically distinguish their approach to life by pointing out that, for them, work was a means to living life more fully, not an end in itself. Indeed, a Rhodian might remind me, if the Greek lifestyle were not superior, why would so many tourists and retirees flock to the island?

By highlighting the negative and undesirable entailments of a machine metaphor like "robot," Rhodians and Kalymnians can be seen as engaging in a variety of "reverse discourse" (Foucault 1978 [1990], 101), a rhetorical strategy whereby the same vocabulary of power, and the same categories by which a practice is disqualified, are used to challenge hegemonic ideas and practices. By this logic, the technical, positivist rationality usually deployed as a sign of cultural superiority is represented as ensnaring people within its iron cage and converting them into joyless machines—robots. Thus, if Western Europeans and Greek elites have stereotyped ordinary Greeks as unruly, incapable of rational organization or planning, and so forth, then these same qualities can be appropriated, their meanings inverted, and their bearers celebrated.

Such reversals are by no means confined to Greeks, of course; they draw on the broader legacy of romanticism, which alongside positivism provided many of the key dualities that informed nation building in the eighteenth and nineteenth centuries (McDonald 1993, 229). Today they can also be found among other Southern Europeans—Spaniards, for example, also assert that Northerners "do not know how to live" and claim the Spanish lifestyle as superior (Douglass 1992, 75; Ruiz Jimenez 2004)—as well as among Northern Europeans themselves. Without necessarily relinquishing their views of Southerners as undependable, unruly, etc., Northerners may simultaneously stereotype themselves, as in the Swedish view, as "gray and boring, obsessed with order, punctuality, and the control of emotions, characterized by a total lack of spontaneity and esprit-de-vie" (Lofgren, cited in Moutsatsos 2001, 126).[8] In sum, the flexible deployment of national stereotypes founded on the putative dominance of reason versus emotion, control versus spontaneity, and so on is a widespread phenomenon; ultimately, it reflects the enduring influence of both positivist and romantic currents of thought on European identity discourse (McDonald 1993).

The Rhodian Diaspora

Rhodians, like Greeks generally, have long been "a diaspora people" (Clogg 1999, 1). For more than a century, successive waves have streamed off the island in search of opportunities not locally available. Over the last few decades, smaller, but still significant, numbers of Rhodian migrants and their foreign-born children have returned to the island to live. In an unprecedented turn of events, more recently still, Rhodes has become the destination of considerable numbers of immigrants from Albania and other Balkan countries, Eastern Europe, and Asia. Together with tourism and the large number of cross-cultural marriages between local men and foreign women, this variety of new immigrants, return migrants, and their multicultural offspring have nourished the island's intensely transnational ambience. On Sundays at the popular Swedish bakery in my neighborhood, for instance, Tagalog and Sinhalese could be heard alongside Greek and the usual mix of European languages, as young Filipina and Sri Lankan domestic workers mingled with the tourists to enjoy their sole day off in the company of their compatriots.

The first large-scale exodus of Rhodians began at the end of the nineteenth century. This early wave was predominantly composed of young men whose preferred destination was the United States. Many headed directly to the Greek enclaves of New York City, but others founded Rhodian neighborhoods in such cities and towns as Baltimore, Maryland, and Aliquippa, Pennsylvania, that endure today. Smaller numbers also migrated to Argentina and Africa. It has been estimated that between 1880 and 1912, one in four men aged fifteen to forty-five left the Greek kingdom (Clogg 1999, 6). The numbers for Rhodes are unknown, but they are surely no less substantial. In fact, Rhodians and other ethnic Greeks under Ottoman rule had an additional impetus to leave their communities. When Kemal Ataturk and his party seized power, the Ottoman ancien régime and its long tradition of differential treatment of the non-Muslim *millets* was abruptly overturned. With the goal of modernizing the faltering empire, the young Turks declared equal rights for all citizens of the nation of Turkey. This newly bestowed equality meant that Greeks were no longer exempt from military service as had traditionally been the case. Almost immediately, this reform motivated a substantial pulse of emigration, as alarmed young men fled to the United States and elsewhere to avoid conscription into the Turkish army and the possibility of fighting and killing fellow Greeks in the looming Balkan Wars of 1912–1913 (Papachristodoulou 1994, 479; Papataxiarchis 1995, 231–32). This was in fact the story of my own grandfather's migration. Born a Turkish subject in the town of Kirk Kilisse (Saranta Ekklisies) in Eastern Thrace, he was "temporarily" shipped by his family to New York City when he turned eighteen to sit out the war. He eventually met my Kalamata-born grandmother in Wichita, Kansas, married her two weeks later, and never returned.[9]

Although Greek migrants are often stereotypically represented as illiterate and bewildered peasants abruptly transplanted to New York City at the turn of the century, in fact they came from a variety of backgrounds, in terms of class as well as rural and urban origins (Clogg 1999). Even before the massive outpouring of young men to the United States, Rhodians had been migrating to Egypt to pursue the opportunities created by the cotton boom that took off in the 1860s. The Greek diaspora in Egypt, which was concentrated in Alexandria, was a diverse and stratified community comprised of industrialists, merchants, and professionals as well as workers and petty bourgeoisie (ibid., 12). Wealthy Alexandrine Greeks were among the most prominent benefactors of the Greek kingdom in the nineteenth century. Alexandrine Rhodians closely followed this pattern of conspicuous philanthropy to their communities of origin. They underwrote a variety of major civic projects on the island, the most important of which was the rapid expansion of secondary education that occurred in the 1870s and 1880s. Each year, wealthy Alexandrine families returned to Rhodes to summer in the elegant seaside villas they built in the village of Trianda. Located just a few kilometers outside Rhodes Town, Trianda eventually came to be known as the "Kifissia of Rhodes," after the Attican village that was a favorite spot for the country houses of the Athenian bourgeoisie at that time.

After the United States placed highly restrictive quotas on immigration from Southern and Eastern Europe in 1924, the Rhodian exodus trickled to a halt. In their search for alternative destinations, a number of Rhodians turned to the then-Belgian Congo, where by the 1960s the total number of Greeks had mounted to about twenty thousand (Clogg 1999, 14). Some of these migrants managed to amass considerable wealth by acting as go-betweens for the colonial government and the native populations, a lucrative niche in which Greeks typically specialized elsewhere in sub-Saharan Africa as well (Gerasimos Makris, personal communication). When, in the mid-1960s, Mobutu Sese Seko seized control of the newly independent state of Zaire and began to expropriate the property held by foreigners, Rhodians were abruptly forced to flee and many returned to the island. It was always easy to spot the houses of these return migrants: their living-room curio shelves inevitably displayed the delicate ivory carvings, egg-shaped chunks of polished malachite, and bas-relief copper sculptures carried back with them from Africa. Those fortunate enough to be able to hold on to their Zairian-generated capital (some lost almost everything) found themselves in a good position to take advantage of the generous incentives being offered by the junta to enter the tourist industry as more than minor players.

After World War II, transnational migration took off spectacularly once again. Large numbers of Rhodians, now for the first time as likely to include women as men, streamed off the island to find work in Western Europe, Australia, and Canada. After Australia changed its restrictive immigration policies and began to accept Greeks in 1949, but especially in the 1960s, Rhodians, along with other Dodecanesians, migrated to the urban centers of Australia (Doumanis 1999). This postwar migration, unlike earlier ones to Egypt and Zaire, was largely working class in nature (Clogg 1999). In a revealing example of how class and the notion of Europe may be conflated, many Rhodians who migrated to Africa considered themselves more Europeanized than both nonmigrants and those who had actually lived for decades in Europe. This distinction was largely based on the fact that guest workers to Western Europe tended to work in semi- and unskilled jobs and cluster in rundown immigrant neighborhoods, whereas African Greeks were merchants and go-betweens who lived in the segregated expatriate European enclaves of the colonies, spoke French, and often managed to accumulate considerable wealth.

By the 1970s, Western European countries that had once recruited Greek labor began to restrict emigration as their economies experienced recession. In Rhodes, the return of a sizable number of migrants during these years coincided happily not only with the expansion of the tourist industry, but also with an unprecedented economic growth and impressive improvement in the standard of living that was occurring throughout Greece. Some returnees established small businesses in town; others simply retired to their villages to live off their pensions or the remittances sent by their children still living abroad. Expansion of education and of the public sector also attracted back to the island a number of well-educated migrants' children who had been living abroad.

Migration, return migration, and tourism combined to transform communities throughout Rhodes into transnational spaces with startlingly novel configurations. The village of Ermia, in which I lived for a total of about four months, is an especially lively example of these transformations. Until the end of the Second World War, most Ermiot families relied for their survival on subsistence agriculture, above all on the cultivation of wheat. Today, only a couple of households use their tractors to grow wheat on just a handful of the village's most fertile plots of land. The sandy fields bordering the seashore, once scorned for their poor yields, are now the preferred sites for the lucrative hotels, tavernas, and bars that have sprung up in ever-increasing numbers in recent years to become the mainstay of the local economy.

By the 1970s, substantial numbers of Ermiots, like other Rhodians, began returning from their sojourns abroad. Because nearly all economically active return migrants have settled in Rhodes Town, the village's permanent inhabitants today are by and large quite old, mainly grandmothers who spend their evenings gathered on the steps of a friend's house, and who were among my principal sources of information about reproductive knowledge and practices before the introduction of biomedicine, and grandfathers who pass most of their day in the coffee shop watching television and playing cards and backgammon. The majority of the village's approximately five hundred whitewashed houses appear empty (Fig. 2). This tranquil scene is routinely overturned every Friday night and Saturday morning and on all holidays, as Ermia's native sons, daughters, and grandchildren make the forty-five-minute drive from Rhodes Town to spend the weekend in the village. And so, for a few days each week, the village becomes a vibrantly multigenerational internal resort in which the distinctive cadences of Australian, Canadian, and American English are as likely to be heard in the village's narrow alleyways as is the equally distinctive village dialect.

This transformation has been facilitated by a new village tradition that since its invention has become a significant component of Ermiot identity and social life (although it is found in other villages throughout Rhodes as well). Sometime in the late 1960s, an Ermiot woman who had lived in Australia for many years decided to give her daughter as dowry not only an apartment in Rhodes Town, but also a second house in the village. Buying an apartment in town was itself a "new tradition." It replaced the older practice in which parents gave up their house to their eldest daughter when she married and moved into a small annex, in some instances an abandoned shed or stable (see du Boulay 1983; M. Clark 1995). Today, Ermiot women typically receive two residences when they marry, an apartment or house in town and a house in the traditional style in the village next to or near their parents.[10] Despite their generally modest exteriors, which help maintain the compact, whitewashed Greek village ambiance that attracts growing numbers of foreign tourists to Ermia each year, these dowry houses are often far from rustic. The traditional hearth, encased in the *panga*, a raised platform where birth always took place

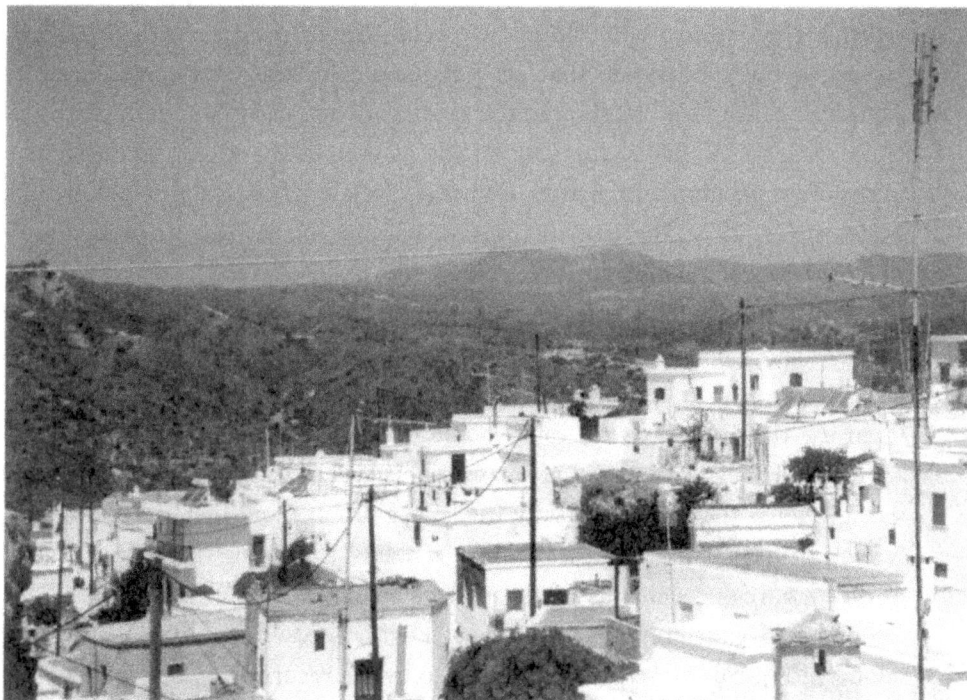

2. Ermia.

in the past, remains the centerpiece of the kitchen. In the newer houses, however, it is apt to be surrounded by a microwave, late-model electric range, and ice-making refrigerator. Rhodian-made ceramic plates invariably decorate the kitchen walls, but the floors are usually of Italian tiles.

It would be easy to read the second dowry house in the village as a sign of distinction, mimetic of the villas that wealthy Greeks, like the Alexandrine Rhodians of Trianda, have long kept in the countryside. I believe they also point to the diffusion of a new cluster of meanings that the rural village has recently acquired in Greece (see also Dubisch 1993; Hart 1992). Now that the hardscrabble agrarian and pastoral way of life is almost extinct, the countryside has come to signify in the popular imagination a refuge from, even at times a critical negation of, the disenchantments of urban, modern life. Up through World War II, village life was widely associated with hardship, hunger, and what Marx famously derided as the "idiocy of rural life." Today, these negative associations persist: *khoriati* (villager) is still a derogatory epithet that connotes ignorance, superstition, and backwardness (Stewart 1991; Argyrou 1996). But, as the identity of villager has been widely "renounced, transcended, or muted for the sake of a place in the urban social landscape" (Bakalaki 1997, 512), older meanings are accompanied, and sometimes even superseded, by other highly positive ones. These new connotations resonate with the idealization of the countryside that, as Raymond Williams discovered, came to characterize English literature in the nineteenth and early twentieth centuries. According to Williams, the countryside at that time was reconfigured as a place of cooperation with nature, unmediated experience, and the "old, human ways" (1973, 297). The city, in contrast, became increasingly associated with the negative values of competition, alienation, and isolation.[11]

When my daughter entered second grade in our neighborhood school on Rhodes and I helped her with her homework, I found many of these images and ideas at play in her language textbook. Throughout Greece, all schoolchildren use the same texts for each course, rendering them obviously powerful vehicles for socialization and normalization (Avdela 2000). *I Ghlossa Mou* (My Language) is the text universally used for grammar and literature lessons in Greek primary schools. Greek feminist scholars, subjecting this text to critical scrutiny, have uncovered its subtle gender stereotypes and implicit assumptions of procreative heterosexual destiny (Delighiani-Kwimsi 1993a).[12] Reading along with my daughter, I was struck also by the recurring ideological opposition between country and city. Throughout the text, city life was uniformly represented in dark tones, while the countryside was consistently idealized. Thus, for instance, lesson 6, "The Sky," begins: "In the apartment we live in, I don't see the sky." Kosma, the little boy narrator, only comes to understand the meaning of "sky" when he goes to visit his grandmother in the village for a month (Velalidhis et al. 1996, 29). In the very next lesson, a poem entitled "How Can We Be Happy?" another child stuck in an apartment in the city empathizes with the caged bird confined to his balcony (32).

As Raymond Williams (1973, 294) also observed, for the new bourgeoisie, the contradictions between country and city were spatially resolved by the country house, and temporally by the division of time into the week and the weekend. Middle-class, as well as many working-class, Greeks have increasingly emulated this bourgeois division of space and time—of work, weekday, and city on the one hand, and leisure, weekend, and country on the other. Ironically, the mass postwar migration to Athens and other cities that so effectively evacuated the countryside also helped create the conditions for the redefinition of the latter. As Roger Just (2000, 28) has pointed out, in Greece, as opposed to other parts of Europe, the second house in the country is most often a legacy. The patrimonial house (*to patriko*) emptied by migration or abandoned for other reasons could be repaired, remodeled, and renovated, or patrimonial land built upon, to accommodate the redefinition of the village as weekend and holiday resort. Today, those without patrimonial land might even buy plots in villages to which they have no kin ties and construct there what

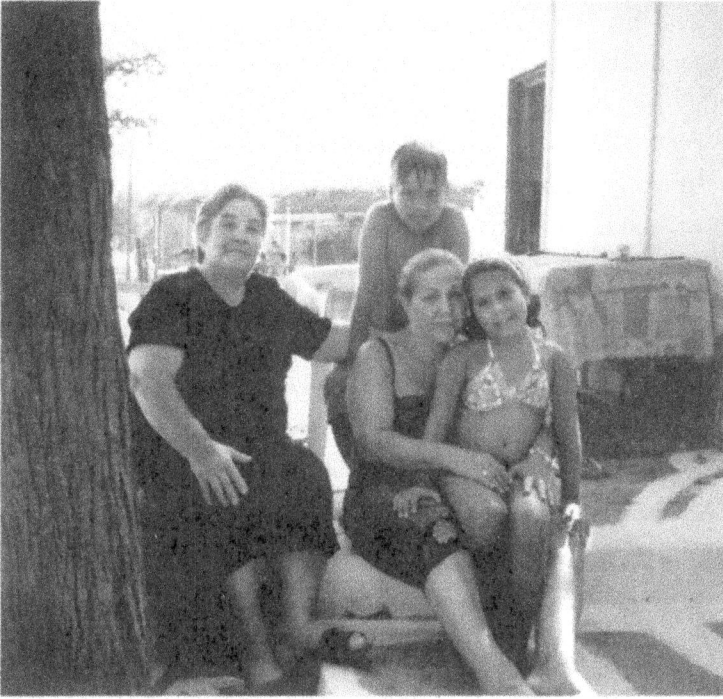

3. Family weekends in Ermia with Grandmother.

one Athenian friend, a professor of architecture, called, with tongue firmly in cheek, their "neo-patriko."

This recent reconfiguration of time and space divided into the workweek in Rhodes Town and the weekend in the village has special implications and meanings for women with children. Going to the village marks a welcome rupture in women's everyday work routines, a holiday from the heavy demands of the intensive model of mothering that I describe in Chapter 7, and a break from the stress and anxiety that so many described feeling as a result of juggling their numerous responsibilities. Almost as soon as the family arrives in the village, children hive off from their parents and disappear to join up with their *parea*, their groups of age-mates, which, given the strong tendency toward village endogamy, usually includes a large number of their cousins. Children spend the weekend freely roaming the village in the company of their *parea*, finding rides with co-villagers to the beach to fish or swim and, when hungry or tired, dropping by their grandmother's house for a meal or a nap (Fig. 3). In the event that parents really want to find them, children can easily be tracked down with a few cell-phone calls. Mothers thus may see little of their children until it's time to return to Rhodes Town on Sunday night. Heavily subsidizing this maternal holiday are women's *own* mothers and mothers-in-law who live permanently in the village. Grandmothers usually prepare the weekend meals for the extended family and mind the babies and toddlers while their mothers go for a swim or out with their own *parea* in the evening to one of many clubs, bars, and restaurants that have sprung up locally in recent years.[13] Finally, on Sunday night, elderly parents load up their children's cars with enough fresh vegetables and seasonal fruits from their gardens to last them until they return the following week.

With their children finally packed off to Rhodes on Sunday night, grandmothers were once again free to return to their placid weekday routines, tending their gardens and visiting with their own *parea* of elderly women in the evenings. It was usually only on these quiet weekdays that they had time to talk to me about their lives in the past and about the very different place that Ermia was just a generation ago.

Chapter 3

Menstruation, Procreation, and Abortion in Prewar Rhodes

Dedicated to the Dormition of Mary and dating from the eleventh century, Ermia's church nestles snugly in the spatial and social heart of the village. The tiny limestone basilica is composed of three sections, each crowned by a low dome and each entered through its own door. The door to the central nave was for the exclusive use of men. The one on the right was used by most women. The entrance to the left, known as the *atsalos tholos*, "the disorderly dome," was reserved for women who were menstruating or had given birth within the previous forty days (Fig. 4). As in all the religions derived from the Abrahamic tradition—Christianity, Judaism, and Islam—menstrual blood and the lochia of the postpartum period were regarded as ritually unclean substances. This quality of uncleanliness, moreover, was not contained by the boundaries of a woman's body, but radiated like a hazardous aura into her immediate environment as well. Because of this, contact with the disorderly body of an unclean woman could cause all manner of havoc. It could make feta cheese turn yellow, bread fall flat, wine go sour, oil turn rancid. Within the church itself, her touch could defile the sacred objects of Orthodoxy. For this reason, menstruating and postpartum women should not venerate the icons (which involved kissing them), light a candle, or take Holy Communion.[1]

Kiria Sofia, a wiry Ermiot grandmother of four in her seventies, has been explaining to me why women in general are healthier and have more endurance than men. Their advantage, she tells me, is due to their ability to menstruate. Like most women of her generation, she uses the term *taksi*, which means "order," to refer to menstruation.[2] Within the local model of health and illness that she is describing, the orderly flow of menstrual blood is appreciated because it regularly eliminates unhealthy impurities, the internal "filth" and "dirt" that naturally accumulate in the human body over the course of each

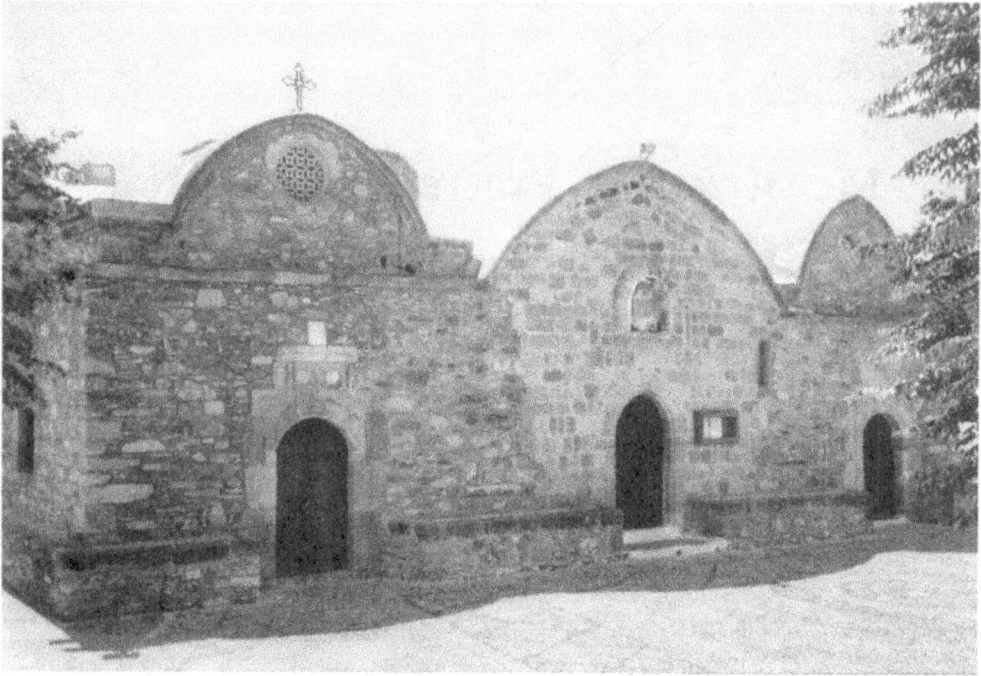

4. Ermia's church, dedicated to the Dormition of the Mother of God (Kimisis tis Theotokou).

month. By expelling this dirty blood, women's bodies are regularly cleansed, refreshed, and renewed. Men, along with women who do not menstruate whether because of age or sickness, lacked this advantage and their health consequently suffered. Thus, in notable contrast to the perspective of Orthodoxy, in which menstruation indexed the essentially disorderly and disruptive nature of women's bodies, from the humoral perspective, menstruation signified order, health, and well-being.

Well into the middle of the twentieth century, these two distinct discourses, one thoroughly secular and mechanical, the other religious and spiritually charged, provided the most influential conceptual frameworks with which women in rural Rhodes made sense of their bodies and negotiated their corporeal practices. Of the two, the tenets and teachings of the Greek Orthodox Church represented the dominant discourse. The Greek Orthodox Church has been intimately identified with, and supported by, the nation-state since its inception in the nineteenth century. It represents a long and valued literate scriptural tradition. Its all-male hierarchy buttresses in multiple ways the androcentric bias that threads through much of Greek culture and society. Without the rituals of Orthodoxy, neither the collective life of the village nor the life course of each individual within it could acquire its proper shape and meaning. Indeed, it was only through these rituals that a person's full humanity and social identity were gradually achieved over time.

When juxtaposed to the palpable presence and authority of the Church, the ethnomedical discourse concerned with women's bodies and health was, in de Certeau's sense, "quasi-invisible" (de Certeau 1984). It is perhaps partly for this reason that it has been almost entirely ignored by ethnographers and why Orthodoxy, in contrast, has been privileged as "the ultimate reference point for 'local' gender meanings" (Cowan 1996, 65), as well as for local illness beliefs and practices (cf. Machin 1983). Unlike Orthodoxy, Rhodian ethnogynecology lacked a "proper locus" in either space or canonical text. Rather, it was dispersed and embedded in women's bodily practices and prescriptions (de Certeau 1984). Although associated in intricate ways with the long and respected literate tradition of Galeno-Hippocratic gynecology, as I show in this chapter, by the twentieth century this body of knowledge circulated almost exclusively within the oral lifeworlds of women. Because it was diffusely dispersed, pragmatically deployed, and controlled by women themselves, this knowledge was available for occasionally subversive and secretive ends, such as abortion. It would not be entirely accurate, however, to portray women's body of ethnogynecological knowledge as a muted or subjugated alternative to the dominant discourse of the Church, at least not from the perspective of villagers. Humoral knowledge was neither secret nor stigmatized, and its practices were grounded in a logic that was distinct from the Church's. Rather, women (and men) valued *both* humoral medicine and religious healing, using them hand in hand to address their concerns with procreation, illness, and health.

From a feminist theoretical perspective, the coexistence of these two discourses, conceptually at odds with each other in many ways, offers an intriguing opportunity to grasp how women who came of age in the prewar period moved between complex and often starkly contradictory symbolic orders as they met the practical challenges of maintaining health and enhancing or limiting fertility. One of my central concerns in this chapter, then, is to explore how women navigated these discourses, negotiating their key idioms and reinterpreting their moral imperatives as they confronted the corporeal exigencies of their everyday lives. Because everywhere ideas and practices concerned with procreation reflect and are embedded in mutually constitutive ideologies of gender and kinship (Yanagisako and Delaney 1995), I begin with a description of the local understandings of appropriate behavior for the women and men who came of age before the war.[3]

The Prewar Demographic Regime: The Marriage Imperative and Procreative Destiny

Despite their fundamental differences, Greek Orthodoxy and the humoral model of health shared a profoundly pronatalist orientation. The Church regards as sinful all attempts to limit fertility, with the exception of the rhythm method, which in any case was unknown to the oldest generation of rural Rhodians. Abortion is categorized by the Church as a major sin and equated with murder. For its part, the humoral model represented pregnancy and birth as desirable events that triggered permanently salutary changes in a woman's body. Together these discourses informed and shaped community values in ways that strongly upheld a moral mandate to marry, procreate, and produce large families.

In Rhodes, as elsewhere in Greece, marriage was seen as the destiny of each person (Hirschon 1989). Well-wishers conventionally greeted the birth of either a girl or a boy with the phrase "*ke stis khares tou*," which roughly translates as "may we be present again at his/her wedding." (For boys only, another conventional Rhodian wish at birth was that they grow up to become "a priest, a bishop, a doctor," *ke papas, ke dhespotis, ke ghiatros*.) In the past, and to a limited extent still today, it was only through marriage that one could establish an independent household, engage in legitimate sexuality and procreation, and ultimately, gain full social personhood in the eyes of the community. By this logic, men and women who remained unmarried past a certain age were in some sense anomalous, incomplete beings who had failed in the project of becoming fully mature adults (Argyrou 1996, 61; M. Doumanis 1983; du Boulay 1974).

However important a threshold in itself, marriage was above all the means to fulfilling one's procreative destiny as a human being and an Orthodox Christian. For both men and women, marriage constituted a sacred as well as a social bond, whose ultimate purpose was producing children. "That's why you marry, to have children. *Ghi'afto pantrevese, na kanis pedhia*," I was often told by Rhodian men and women of all ages. This sacred procreative mandate is reflected in the Greek Orthodox wedding ceremony, in which God himself is called upon to bless the marriage and endow it with "the gain of well favored children" (Harakas 1996, 129). The children that result consequently represent sacred "gifts from God."

Implicit in the procreative imperative is a processual and relational understanding of personhood. Having children transforms the status and identity of both women and men in ways that permit them to live up to moral understandings of what it means to be fully human. The links between procreation and the attainment of full social personhood are forged over the course of the life cycle and assume many dimensions. Through their children, men and women are able to achieve the valued social identities of "mother" and "father." As mothers and fathers, they are able to carry out the moral mandate to perpetuate "the house," *to spiti*, that is, the family, and by extension, life on earth (M. Doumanis 1983; du Boulay 1974, 62). Children also represent an important spiritual and physical link between the generations. In the naming system that prevails on Rhodes and throughout Greece, Christian names are usually passed between alternate generations (Herzfeld 1982b). When a child receives a grandparent's name, it is said that the name continues "to be heard" for another generation. This continued voicing and hearing of the grandparent's name is a highly valued form of commemoration (Hirschon 1989; D. Sutton 1998a). As Walter Ong (1982) observed, where literacy was uncommon and orality the norm, as in much of rural Greece before the war, the spoken word of necessity represented the primary means of remembering.[4] Under conditions of orality, as Ong (67) also insightfully pointed out, the spoken word acquires "a high somatic component," that is, it implicates and engages the body in a variety of ways. This somatic dimension of orality, and of the arts of memory under conditions of orality, is dramatically enacted in Greek naming customs. When a child receives a grandparent's name, it is believed that something of the grandparent's unique character and personality are also physically passed along to the grandchild. Thus, both through the spoken name that continues to be voiced and heard in the community and through the body and person of their namesakes, the grandparents leave traces materially present in the world of the living long after they die (Stewart 1991, 58). Additionally, but not least, children infuse each person's life with ultimate meaning and joy because, quite simply and categorically, as I was often told, "children are happiness" (*ta pedhia ine eftikhia*).

Although procreation is an essential ingredient in the life project of both men and women, this was most emphatically true for women. It is through the bearing of children that women are fully "completed" as female persons (*oloklironese san ghineka*). This commonly heard phrase points to the cultural salience of motherhood in transforming women from persons of relatively little social worth into persons of respect, a process often remarked in the ethnography of Greece (M. Doumanis 1983, 35–36; Dubisch 1986; Paxson 2004). But there is also another, corporeal dimension to a woman's completion through marriage. From the local ethnogynecological perspective that I describe in this chapter, sexual intercourse, pregnancy, and birth were necessary for effecting desirable transformations to her body. Together, they functioned to "open" a woman's body in ways that completed her development as a physically mature (and more attractive) adult female. For men, in contrast, sexual intercourse, while essential to mental and physical health, as also discussed here, was irrelevant to the completion of their physical development and maturation.

As Renée Hirschon (1978) first observed, "openness" is an auspicious idiom found across diverse domains of Greek culture. A highly productive trope, "open" works against the mirror of its undesirable opposite, "closed," to reinforce implicit hierarchies of value. In Greek, one's heart "opens" in a joyful state but "closes" in sorrow. A person's luck may "open" and her desires be fulfilled, or it may "close" and leave her mired in misfortune. One's prayers are heard when "the heavens are opened." Conversely, *stenokhoria*, a negative emotional state signifying worry, anxiety, and depression, literally paints a word picture of a narrow, confined space, *stenos khoros* (ibid., 77; Danforth 1989, 122ff). An important subset of usages involving the contrast between "open" and "closed" is highly gendered. For Rhodian women of the oldest generations, the auspicious state of social "openness" was attainable only through marriage. To leave the confinement of maidenhood and the close supervision and scrutiny it entailed, to emerge into society, to "open her house," that is, to establish her own household and family, to bear the children that "completed" her and marked her entry into full adult womanhood—all of these highly desired ends were, through the first half of the twentieth century, contingent upon her marriage (Hirschon 1978; Dubisch 1986).

The idioms of "open" and "closed" were not only "good to think" about the social order. As anthropologists since Mauss have observed, cultural idioms used to express the proper functioning of society are often mirrored in notions about the healthy body (Lock and Scheper-Hughes 1996, 57). Given the gendered associations of the open/closed binary, it is also not surprising that these social values were primarily inscribed on the bodies of women. In rural Rhodes, as throughout much of Europe until recently, women and houses were symbolically closely linked. The house was a common metaphor for the woman's body and, more specifically, for her womb (Benthien 2002). As it was only through marriage that a woman was able to "open her house," so it was through marriage that her body also began "to open" (*anighi to soma tis*).[5] As a consequence, first, of sexual intercourse, and later, of pregnancy and childbirth, a woman's womb became wider, her hips assumed their broader and rounder adult shape, and she became plumper (Hirschon 1978, 78), formerly a most pleasing feminine attribute.

Sexual intercourse, pregnancy, and birth had positive entailments for a woman's physical well-being on at least three counts. First, in causing the womb and hips to expand and become permanently wider, they made the bearing of subsequent children easier. Second, the womb's new roominess eased the congestion and pressure exerted by pooled-up menstrual blood, and thus helped mitigate or even eliminate painful menstrual cramps. Finally, giving birth left women physically refreshed and "renewed" (*tis ananeoni*) and enabled them to reach their peak of physical attractiveness. Explaining these benefits, Kiria Sofia adduced an adage I heard from other women as well: "The woman who gives birth is reborn, *i ghineka pou ghena, ksanagheniete*." "Because of her happiness?" I asked. "That is part of it," Kiria Sofia replied. "But in her body, too, a woman is refreshed when she gives birth. That's why you see that many women become prettier afterward." Thus, a husband was doubly essential to the process of becoming a mature woman. A husband was the key that made it possible for a woman to "open her house" and emerge into society as a social adult. Equally important, he was the instrument by which her body achieved the auspicious quality of openness that was the hallmark of a physically mature woman at her peak.

Blessed by God and Church, and firmly upheld by community cultural norms, this procreative imperative dictated that pregnancy should follow as soon as possible after a couple married. Typically, if a woman hadn't become pregnant within a couple of months of her wedding, she began to worry. As discussed later in this chapter, she embarked on a quest for therapy that often started with a visit to the local midwife for a thorough "shaking," a procedure designed to shift her womb to a position more favorable to conception.

Nevertheless, despite the multiple discourses that so powerfully promoted procreation, there were other considerations at play that also influenced the ultimate size and composition of families and the spacing of births. Although medical means of contraception were not known, and families were indeed larger than they are today, it would be a mistake to label the prewar demographic regime in Rhodes "natural" or "traditional," as demographers are wont to do. As Susan Greenhalgh (1995, 17) has cautioned: "Like the dualisms of modernization theory, the traditional/modern and natural/uncontrolled labels in demography may serve to mystify more than to clarify a complex reality." As a growing body of ethnographic literature has documented for women in many parts of the world, Rhodian women engaged in a variety of practices aimed at tinkering with procreative outcomes over the course of their reproductive years (e.g., Bledsoe 1995, 2002). In prewar Rhodes, these practices included menstrual regulation, abortion, selective neglect of newborn infants, and fosterage. Guiding these practices were both tacit and explicit understandings about the particular kinds of persons and social identities that were morally worth reproducing (Moore 1994, 93). These understandings, in turn, were intimately bound up with the agrarian political economy of rural Rhodes in the first part of the twentieth century, and with the historically specific cultural ideologies of motherhood, fatherhood, and childhood characteristic of that time.

Mothers, Fathers, and Children in Agrarian Rhodes

Among the oldest generation of women, pregnancies were numerous and families tended to be fairly large, although their size was continually susceptible to reduction by the high infant and child mortality common to all of rural Greece in the prewar period (Emke-Poulopoulou 1994, 62; Hionidou 1995). Many village women explicitly attributed their desire to have numerous children at least partly to the fairly commonplace experience of infant and child death. Diarrhea and respiratory disease were childhood scourges, but tuberculosis, malaria, and other unspecified "fevers" also took a heavy toll. Besides the burden of infectious diseases, Greeks in general, and Rhodians in particular, are characterized by extraordinarily high rates of lethal genetic diseases. Between 7 and 10 percent of the Greek population carries the genes for the blood disorders thalassemia, G6PD deficiency, and sickle-cell anemia, all of which have been linked to the region's long history of endemic malaria. Amplified by a strong preference for village endogamy, the frequency of these traits in rural areas of Rhodes is higher still. In some villages, over one-third of the population may be carriers for the G6PD trait alone (Trakas 1981). In the prewar period, children who inherited the thalassemia trait from both parents inevitably died painful deaths at a very young age (ibid.). Kiria Eleftheria lost her second child, a son, to thalassemia in 1952, although she didn't know the cause at the time:

> What did we know back then? Now couples have tests and they don't get married if they both have the *stigma* [i.e., carry the thalassemia trait]. But we didn't know that then. Later I went to a doctor and he told me that both my husband and I have the *stigma*. We didn't know. My boy died when he was three years old. He was so beautiful that everyone said that someone must have given him the evil eye, and that's why he died. But later the doctor told me what it was.

Whether from genetic or infectious causes, most women in their seventies and eighties had lost at least one or two children at an early age. Some were particularly unfortunate. Kiria Maro, who worked alongside her husband in the family's wheat fields and olive groves, gave birth to nine children, four of

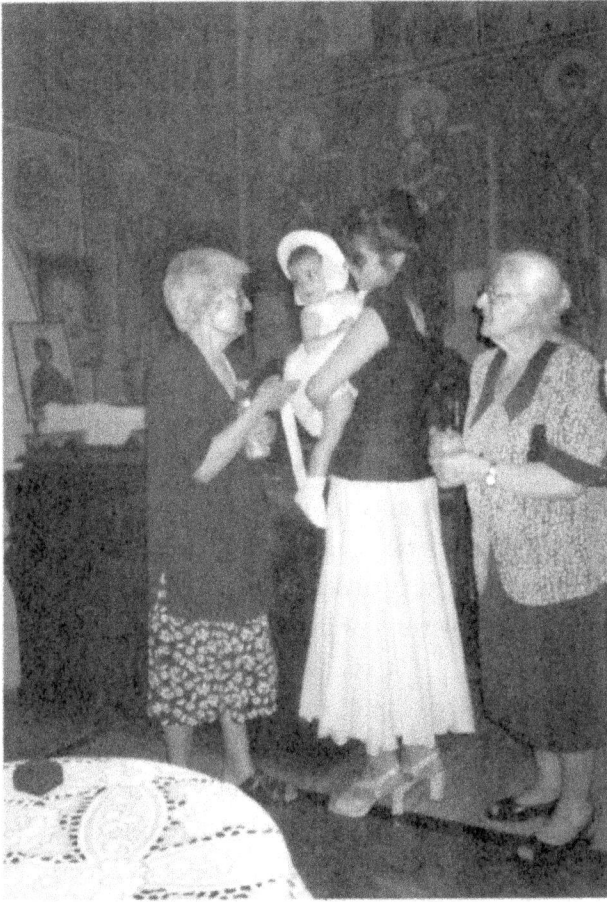

5. Newly baptized baby with her mother and grandmothers.

whom died at a young age. Of Kiria Popi's eight children, five died before reaching adulthood. Kiria Maro's and Kiria Popi's reproductive histories capture with grim accuracy a common saying of the time: one [child] is no better than none, *ena dhen ine kanena*; two is equal to one, four is equal to two. (This saying is found in other areas of Greece as well. See Beyene 1989 for Evia; Schneider and Schneider 1991 report a similar saying for Sicily.) In prescribing abundant childbearing as insurance against childlessness or unacceptably small families, common sayings and proverbs can be seen as encoding a kind of practical epidemiology. Distilling the experiential knowledge of countless women about child survival, and setting the parameters of worst-case scenarios, they offered a rough rule of thumb for thinking about childbearing across a woman's reproductive years.

Perhaps because of their tentative hold on life, newborns were ambiguous creatures whose humanity, initially only partial, gradually unfolded over time. The not-yet-human quality of the unbaptized infant was reflected in the terms with which it was addressed. Even when a name was already selected, an infant might be simply called by the generic terms *moro*, baby/infant, or *beba* if a girl or *bebis* if a boy (Stewart 1991, 55; Hirschon 1989, 204; Kenna 1976, 33). Baptism, the Orthodox ritual through which the infant formally acquired its Christian name, was the first major step toward its incorporation into the human community (Fig. 5). As Stewart (1991, 55) eloquently explains: "Baptism is the portal through which humanity is entered. At this rite the child is forcibly separated from the realm of the demonic by means of a series of exorcisms." Or, as Kiria Eleftheria put it in homelier terms, "Until it is baptized, the baby is a Turk." Her pithy pronouncement also points to the historical centrality of religion to Greek identity during the Ottoman period (which in Rhodes lasted until 1911), when "Greek Orthodox Christianity versus Islam . . . constituted the cornerstone of the distinction between 'Greek' and 'Turk'" (Just 1989, 82). Even though infants and children only gradually emerged as Greek Orthodox Christian persons, their deaths were nonetheless often recalled as grievous events. This was particularly true if the child had managed to survive beyond the first few years of life to "become a person," *na anthropefsi*, in village parlance.

Under the harsh conditions of village life in the past, often remembered as a time of deprivation and exhausting workloads, having a large number of children was an important strategy for ensuring a favorable mix of surviving boys and girls. As has been documented elsewhere in rural Greece, sons were highly valued as the economically important "hands" of the household (e.g., Galani Moutafi 1993). In Ermia, sons helped their parents with the heavy physical labor required to eke a living from the rocky, worn-out village land. Fathers and sons worked together to plow and plant food crops in the family's many small fields, often scattered over dozens of hilly kilometers. This typically Rhodian agrarian pattern was due largely to local norms of partible inheritance. Under this system, all children were entitled to roughly equal shares of their parents' property, either upon marriage in the form of dowry, for girls, or after the parents' death, in the form of fields and animals, for boys (Herzfeld 1980). It was due also to the absence of the large, seigneurial landholdings known as *tsiflikia* that dominated many other parts of Greece (Dimitriou-Kotsoni 1993). Most of a family's land was devoted to the cultivation of wheat, far and away the most important subsistence crop. Olive trees and grapevines also required careful attention, but wheat was the staple on which the family's survival vitally depended throughout the year. Prepared in different ways, wheat was eaten three times a day, every day, supplemented with meat perhaps once a month and on feast days.

Beyond their economic contributions, sons were also highly valued because it was through them that the family surname continued to be heard for another generation. Lack or loss of sons "closed the house" because it "erased" the paternal surname (*zvini to onoma*) and ruptured the continuity of the family line (Hirschon 1989, 147; D. Sutton 1998a, 183ff). Girls and boys were both desired because they perpetuated the Christian names of one's mother and father, respectively. But it was only through a son that *both* the Christian name and the surname of the paternal grandfather would be exactly reproduced. Kiria Eleni explained why she had wanted her first and second children to be boys: "I wanted to give my husband's father's name to our [first] son, *na vghalo to onoma tou patera tou*, to please him. I wanted to name my second after my father. He had just had a serious operation and I was afraid he might die soon, and I wanted to please him, too." Finally, she wanted a daughter to name after her mother, so that her mother's name "would continue to be heard" after her death.

Not least, sons were appreciated because, unlike daughters, they did not entail the obligation of a dowry house. When a son married, he moved into the house provided by his bride's parents. In contrast, the birth of a daughter, as Kiria Eleftheria explained,

> was heavy, *itan vari, poli vari*, very heavy, because her father had to build a house for her. Always, when a girl was born, the father's face would fall a little. "I'll have to make another house," he thinks. . . . My husband wanted a boy, to give him his father's name, and he was a little upset when our first child was a girl.

Typically, the village midwife was given an especially lavish gift if the first baby born to a couple turned out to be a boy.

But daughters were valued too, especially by women, despite the heavy parental obligation to provide them with a dowry house when they married. The following Rhodian proverbs would seem to contradict the stated preference for boys:

> The fortunate woman's first child is a daughter.
> *Tis Kalomoiras to pedhi, to proto ine koritsi.*

> The good mother's first child is female.
> *Tis kalomanas to pedhi, to proto ine thiliko.*[6]

Kalomoira, referred to in the first proverb, is one of three quarrelsome sisters known as the Fates who visit the newborn infant seven days after birth to bestow its lifetime share of luck, both good and bad. Kalomoira, which literally means "good fate," is the beautiful sister who metes out all that is desirable in a person's life. Because the value placed on male children was palpably strong, I sometimes suspected that women regaled me with such proverbs as consolation when they learned that my only child was a girl.[7] Be this as it may, they had no difficulty giving reasons for preferring their firstborn to be female. After describing the general preference for boys, especially as the firstborn child, Kiria Eleftheria continued:

> But the mother is happy when a girl is born. Because she helps her mother. She is more tied to her mother, closer to the family, *ine tou spitiou,* she is of the house. Boys are a different thing entirely.

Although, as just noted, the midwife was handsomely rewarded when the firstborn was a boy, she also received an especially nice gift when the couple already had a couple of boys and the birth resulted in a girl.

From an early age, daughters acted as important adjuncts to their mothers' labor. Women in particular appreciated having a girl as their firstborn because it eased the burden of mothering the children that would follow. That is why, in the second version of the proverb, having a girl as a firstborn is said to enable a woman to perform as a "good mother," *kalomana.* Daughters helped their mothers not only with child rearing, but with the cooking, cleaning, weaving and myriad other onerous and time-consuming chores essential to life in the prewar rural context. The following excerpt from the life history of Kiria Rena, a mother of four in her sixties, gives some idea of the style of mothering that formerly prevailed in the villages and of the vital assistance daughters provided in the running of the household:

> Our parents woke up at five every morning and went to the fields. My brothers and I would wake up after they left and make our breakfast— goat's milk or mountain tea [made from wild herbs such as sage and marjoram] and a piece of bread spread with pork fat and a little sugar. We'd go out and feed the chickens and pigs, and I, since I was the girl, *san koritsi,* would wash the dishes and pack our snack of bread, almonds, or figs. After morning classes, I'd come home, make the fire and heat up the lunch my mother had left for us from the night before. We fed the animals again, and I'd clean up—sweep, wash the dishes—and then I would study for the afternoon classes. In the afternoon, we had history and religion, and we'd go back to school til six PM. On my way home, I'd stop by the coffee shop my father ran, and I'd sweep up and light the fire to have it ready for the coffees he would make his customers when

he returned from the fields. Then, I'd go home to make dinner, feed the animals again, study, and wash the dishes. On Saturdays, I got up early to go clean my father's coffee shop: I whitewashed the walls, lined the cupboards with fresh newspaper, and rinsed the glasses with vinegar so they would sparkle. Then I went home to help my mother bake the loaves of bread that would last us the week.

One night, I remember, I was so tired and sleepy, I said, "I'm not going to wash dishes now," and went to bed. And my mother, God forgive her, returns from the fields, and she comes and wakes me. . . . "Rena, my daughter, why didn't you wash the dishes? Tomorrow the sink will be too full. Get up, light the fire, and heat the water." My father protested, "*Kale, Maria mou*, Goodness, Maria dear, leave her be." "No," my mother answered, "she must learn that she shouldn't leave the dishes in the sink at night." And from that day forward, I never again left the dishes.[8]

This story, which Kiria Rena recounted without apparent resentment, was intended to instruct me as a mother on the importance of assigning chores and responsibilities to my daughter. Although I had explained the objectives of my research to her in some detail before our first interview, Kiria Rena herself redefined our several encounters as opportunities to offer me advice on how to properly raise my child. Along the way, Kiria Rena's narrative also reveals much about the nature of mothering and of the relationship of mothers, fathers, and daughters in the village life of the prewar period.

For rural Rhodians of Kiria Rena's generation and older, to father was to work long and hard to provide materially for one's family. However, rainfall agriculture was often too precarious or insufficiently productive to allow a man to fulfill this obligation. To eke out their families' living, many men, like Kiria Rena's father, had to combine agriculture with a variety of other part-time or seasonal work. Some engaged in interisland trade; others seasonally migrated to the nearby coast of Turkey to find work; some worked on the various large-scale construction projects underwritten by the Italian colonial government. Other men left the village altogether. Beginning in the early decades of the twentieth century, they migrated abroad, where they stayed for years at a time. Fathers with multiple occupations, or fathers absent temporarily or for long periods, often increased the workloads of the wives and daughters left behind in the villages.

For the generation of women who came of age in the prewar period, to mother essentially meant providing the physical care required to ensure their children's sheer survival—which, as previously noted, was by no means assured—as well as the labor to run the household and contribute to the family's subsistence. In practice, as Kiria Rena's narrative reveals, mothers too spent long hours away from their children, working alongside their husbands in the fields or tending goats and sheep alone in remote pastures.[9] The extent of a mother's absence varied with the agricultural calendar and the demands of the olive trees, grapevines, and wheat fields, as well as with the father's occupation. It was especially prolonged during the all-important wheat harvest. If the past was sometimes remembered as a time of endless, backbreaking work and scarcity, *all* of the old women I spoke with singled out the wheat harvest as the time of greatest hardship. Because their survival literally depended on completing the harvest before the winter rains began, to save valuable time families left their homes in the village and camped out in their fields for weeks at a time. Day after day, wives and husbands toiled side by side under the late summer sun to bring in the crop on time. The intense heat and discomfort of harvesting were made worse still, I was told, by the high leather boots men and women wore to protect themselves from the ubiquitous scorpions and poisonous snakes, and the cotton scarves that swathed their faces to keep them from choking on the dust they kicked up as they worked their way through the desiccated fields.[10]

To accommodate this heavy lien on women's time and labor, child-care practices in the prewar periods were of necessity "mother centered" (Ross 1993). That is, they were designed to help women cope with the often-competing demands of subsistence work and child rearing. For example, even up until the 1960s, infants were tightly swaddled from neck to toe, primarily, I was told without apology, because this immobilized them and made them easier to mind. "Wherever you put your baby, that's where you'd find it later!" Kiria Sterghoula exclaimed, with an air of satisfaction at having solved a vexing problem. As long as an infant was still nursing, it was taken along to the fields with its mother. Mothers carried their infants in a special device called a *naka*, a sling made of a piece of cloth suspended between two wooden reeds. While she worked, the *naka* was hung from the bough of a nearby tree to rock in the breeze, safe from the poisonous snakes said to be irresistibly attracted to the infant by the scent of milk.[11] Mothers dislodged their babies from this perch only to nurse them and change their soiled clothes. Older children were left behind in the village under the light supervision of a sister or other female relative and neighbors. Most infants were nursed for a year or two, but one man in his seventies told me that his mother continued until he was five. Well after he was old enough to be left alone in the village, his mother dragged him along to the wheat harvest so that she could give him the breast. "Leave the child with me," his grandmother urged her, arguing that it would be a hardship, a *taleporia*, for the boy to be camping in the fields for several weeks under the hot sun amid the snakes and the scorpions. No, no, his mother responded, he recalled with a chuckle, she needed him at her side to keep nursing so she wouldn't get pregnant again.

As the excerpt from Kiria Rena's narrative reveals, even though mothers might have been physically absent much of the day, they were nevertheless figures of considerable respect and not a little fear. Kiria Rena remembered her mother fondly, like many of the oldest women I spoke with. But, like a number of women, she expressed a special affection for her father. Women often remembered their mothers as being strict, "*afsteri.*" Mothers had a strong claim on their daughters' lives, and it was often they who made the key decisions that determined their course. On occasion, a woman's need for her daughter's labor was factored into these decisions, overriding her daughter's own desires and preferences. In the case of Kiria Tsambika, a seventy-eight-year-old woman from a village in eastern Rhodes, this need affected the amount of education she was able to receive. Kiria Tsambika recalled that despite her strong desire to learn how to read and write, she did not go school. She did manage to attend the first grade for a few days, but after that her mother pulled her out and kept her home for good. "What, you're going to go to school *every* day?" she remembered her mother rebuking her, implying that she was shirking her household responsibilities. Another woman told me the story of her first cousin, who at eighteen was engaged to a young man with whom she was in love. Her mother later broke off the engagement to keep her daughter home a few more years because she needed her help raising her five younger children.

Even with their daughters' help, women's responsibility for the household's subsistence often demanded that they curtail their own consumption and sacrifice their own needs in order to meet those of others in the family. As many ethnographers of rural Greece have noted, maternal identity drew heavily on the cultural ideology of sacrificial maternalism. Up to the recent past, and still to some extent today, the gendered idioms of "pain," "suffering," and "sacrifice" were salient features of the poetics and performance of motherhood (Dubisch 1995a; Papataxiarchis 1995; Seremetakis 1991). This poetics, as Jill Dubisch (1995a, 217) has argued, can be interpreted as a vehicle through which women "demonstrate to and remind others of the difficulties inherent in the performance of their roles." The moral claims underlying the poetics of maternal suffering drew authority from their intimate association with the sacred imagery of the Panaghia, the Mother of God, as Mary is known in the Greek Orthodox tradition. Ethnographers have typically represented the trope of sacred motherhood as an important resource and strategy in the self-presentation of rural Greek women; its pragmatic dimension, however, has received less attention. If, on the one hand, it was a cultural resource that gave meaning and dignity to women's lives otherwise seen as marginal or disempowered, on the other, it served to morally obligate children to lifelong recognition of a mother's efforts on their behalf. This recognition, and the reciprocity it entailed, was expected from all of one's children. But daughters in Rhodes were expected to provide emotional and material support that endured all their mothers' lives. "Always, the girl is more tied to her mother than the boy," Kiria Eleni told me (see also Dubisch 1995a).

Related to this ideal is the cultural expectation that daughters will shoulder the primary responsibility for taking care of aging parents (*na tous ghirokomisi*) worn out by the hard labor demanded for survival in the agrarian prewar economy. On mainland Greece and Crete, this duty fell to the son and his wife (e.g., du Boulay 1974). On Rhodes, local dowry customs and inheritance rules facilitated and made almost inevitable the cultural mandate that daughters maintain emotional bonds with parents and care for them in their old age. Because daughters were given dowry in the form of houses, into which grooms were expected to move, the resulting residence pattern was strongly matrilocal and matrivicinal. That is, closely related female kin tended to cluster near each other (Loizos and Papataxiarchis 1991a, 9; Dimitriou-Kotsoni 1993). Ideally, each daughter should receive a dowry house, but meeting this costly and onerous obligation was not always possible. Birth order was not officially taken into consideration in dowering daughters on Rhodes, as it was on some of the other Dodecanese islands. On the small mountainous island of Karpathos, for instance, only the eldest daughter, called the *kanakarisa*, was entitled to dowry and thus able to marry. Other daughters were effectively disinherited (Vernier 1984).[12] On Rhodes, despite the egalitarian ideal, eldest daughters were also at something of an advantage. This was because parents often met the dowry obligation by simply giving up their house to their firstborn daughter when she married. Parents moved into an addition or small adjacent structure, sometimes a converted stable or shed, known as the *gherontomiri*. Such an arrangement kept them in close proximity until their deaths to at least their eldest daughters. Parents provided their other daughters with such houses as they could afford, sometimes with the contributions of their sons, sometimes with the help of family members who had migrated abroad.[13]

Taken together, the various reasons for desiring both male and female offspring were compelling enough that if a woman had only sons, she attempted to acquire at least one daughter, and vice versa. Kiria Paraskevi, for example, had given birth to five daughters and was desperate for a son. "What did you expect," her mother-in-law told her husband, "you married a *thiliko-ghena*, a woman who only bears girls, what else is she going to give you?" Kiria Paraskevi, one of five sisters herself, conceded that the women in her family did indeed have a tendency to give birth only to female children. Her first cousin, who had four boys in a row, was equally desperate for a girl. They agreed to exchange their youngest children and raise them as their own. Fosterage, almost unheard of today, was not uncommon among close relatives in the recent past and sometimes served to tinker with and balance out the gender composition of a family (or provide a child to couples with no children). Other women with only boys or only girls might deliberately keep having children until they finally got the gender they wanted. Gender composition of the family also influenced some women's decisions as to whether to keep a pregnancy. When Kiria Koula was overwhelmed by the birth of her third son within five years of her marriage, she decided to stop for a while, aborting several subsequent pregnancies. After several years, she became unexpectedly pregnant with her fourth child. This time, she felt ambivalent about having another abortion—what if it was a girl? She decided to keep the pregnancy, she explained, in part because of her own desire for a daughter and in part because both her husband and her mother were strongly urging her to have another try at a girl: "'Leave it,' my mother said, 'maybe it will be a girl. A house without a girl isn't a "house" [a family]. It's not complete.' And so, not to disappoint them, *na min tous khalaso khatiri*, I kept it. And I made my Popi!" Kiria Koula told me with evident satisfaction.

Hippocrates, Galen, and Byzantine Medicine: Tracking the Humoral Sources of Rhodian Ethnogynecology

To meet the procreative imperative of marriage, to shape the size of their families, and to maintain or restore their health in general, women routinely turned to a body of local medical knowledge known as the iatrosophia. The iatrosophia ("medical wisdom") provided the conceptual framework and practical interventions for addressing the health concerns of both men and women. In the following sections, I focus on that portion of the iatrosophia that was directly related to women's procreative health. I employ the terms "ethnogynecology" and "ethno-obstetrics" (the focus of the next chapter) to distinguish this largely oral medical tradition from other, canonical medical traditions, whether Byzantine or biomedical (Inhorn 1994; Sobo 1993).

As it happens, learned medicine in the Byzantine Empire was also referred to as "iatrosophia" (Temkin 1962). Beyond their shared name, the similarities between Rhodian and Byzantine medicine are numerous and surprisingly exact. Both medical traditions are clearly related to the corpus of Hippocratic writings that began issuing from the neighboring Dodecanese island of Kos and coastal Ionia in the fifth and fourth centuries BCE (Jouanna 1999). Given the limited scholarship on the history of popular Greek medicine, the precise nature of this relationship is presently obscure. It is possible that Rhodian ethnogynecology is derived in a direct line of descent from ancient medical traditions that anteceded the Hippocratic writers. Midwives, after all, served as important sources of gynecological information for the ancient Hippocratic doctors. As the medical historian Leslie Dean-Jones (1994, 40) has sensibly argued: "In developing their theories of female physiology, [ancient] male authors who espoused scientific principles would have had to turn frequently to women for their data, and their images would have had to be ratified to some extent by women." Their similarities may therefore be due to a common foundation in pre-Hippocratic midwifery and ethnogynecology.

Be this as it may, in its details, Rhodian ethnogynecology hews with remarkable precision to the particular version of Hippocratic medicine resurrected by Galen in the second century AD. It was this distinctively Galenic version of the Hippocratic corpus that eventually came to dominate the canonical gynecological texts of Byzantine medicine (Temkin 1962). Later on, Galenic medicine became the official medicine of the Ottoman Empire as well. Supplemented by advances made by renowned Islamicate physicians, Ottoman medicine continued to remain "attached to its Galenic roots" until well into the nineteenth century (Ze'evi 2006, 20).

Galen's theories of the body, health and illness pervaded Byzantine gynecology. A tireless systematizer and prolific popularizer of the Hippocratic authors, Galen (130–200 AD) was a pivotal force in the restoration, preservation, and elaboration of their medical theories. After the fall of the Western Roman Empire and the disappearance of city life and centers of formal learning, Galeno-Hippocratic medicine dissolved into the folk or popular sector of the Latin West. However, it remained vitally central to the teaching and practice of learned medicine in the Byzantine Empire over the next millennium (Green 1985; Temkin 1962). Byzantine medical teachers, called iatrosophists, distilled Galen's texts into handbooks and encyclopedias that served as canonical summaries of the medical wisdom of the time (Temkin 1962). By far the most influential of these encyclopedias was the seven-volume *Pragmateia* written by Paul of Aegina (flourished ca. 640). The immense popularity of the *Pragmateia* is attested by its existence "in more pre-thirteenth century Greek codices than any other text, with the exception of the Bible and some patristic writings" (Green 1985, 79). Paul's encyclopedia, which contained numerous chapters devoted exclusively to gynecological and obstetrical topics, played a major role in the transmission of Galenic approaches to women's health.[14] Alongside earlier medical encyclopedias written by Aetius, Oribasius, and others, the

Pragmateia was an essential reference work for the Byzantine iatrosophists. It was also a standard text for physicians and teachers in the renowned medical school at Alexandria, where Paul taught and practiced, as well an influential model for subsequent Arabic encyclopedias devoted to women's illnesses (Green 1985, 80ff; Jouanna 1999, 360–61; Temkin 1962).

For ease of use in teaching and to provide a handy reference guide for medical practitioners, the voluminous Byzantine encyclopedias and other medical texts were further distilled into brief handbooks. These too were called iatrosophia. Often roughly composed and anonymously written, this lowly genre has been described as "the literature of everyday practice . . . [with an] emphasis on quick orientation and application, rather than on theory" (Temkin 1962, 113). Iatrosophia handbooks appear to have played an important role in the diffusion of medical knowledge throughout the Byzantine Empire (Sonderkamp 1984; Temkin 1962).

Information about Byzantine medical practice and the transmission of medical knowledge outside Constantinople is lamentably thin (T. Miller 1997; Nutton 1984; Scarborough 1984). For provincial regions like Rhodes, it is completely lacking. There is, however, a telling piece of evidence that the island maintained some significance as a regional center of Byzantine learning. After the Latin conquest and pillage of Constantinople in 1204, the emperor John Vatatzes (1222–1254) hired the most brilliant scholar of the time, the monk and former doctor Nikephoros Blemides, to scour the provinces for ancient manuscripts in order to restore Byzantine learning. Stopping over in Rhodes, Blemides wrote a letter to his imperial patron describing "the rich library with important books" housed in the Artamite Monastery there (Papachristodoulou 1994, 258, my translation; see also T. Miller 1997, 191). In the Byzantine Empire, as in the Latin West in the early Middle Ages, monasteries and ecclesiastical schools were sites "where medicine as a science and art found a modest refuge" (Temkin 1962, 111). If Rhodes was the site of a monastic library rich enough to impress the learned Blemides, it is perhaps not unreasonable to assume that the lowlier genre of the iatrosophia handbooks also circulated locally at that time.

When the Knights of St. John captured Rhodes in 1309, they brought with them their own version of Galenic medicine. In the hospital they built to provide the medical care for which their order was famous, Hospitaller doctors practiced in the Salernitan tradition that dominated learned medicine at that time (Riley-Smith 1999, 26). Beginning in the eleventh and twelfth centuries, the celebrated medical school at Salerno in southern Italy became the major point of entry and diffusion into the Latin West of Arabic translations of Byzantine Galeno-Hippocratic medicine (Porter 1997, 106–7). Some prominent

Arab interpreters of Galen, such as Humain ibn Ishaq, were even given Hel-
lenized names (Iohannitius) to make their work more palatable to the abbots
and monks of Salerno. Under cover of such Greek disguises, Arabic texts introduced into the Latin West a flood of Galenic knowledge that eventually
swamped and replaced the largely pragmatic and atheoretical approaches that
had prevailed through the early Middle Ages (Jacquart 1991, 188). In the late
tenth century, leading Arab physicians such as al-Majusi, drawing many of
their gynecological principles directly from Galen, as well as indirectly from
Paul of Aegina and other Byzantine writers, made numerous advances in
women's medicine (Green 1985, 110–11). This thoroughly "Galenized" gynecology also eventually entered the West via Salerno. From there, the growing
body of Galeno-Arabic medical knowledge was transmitted to the universities and medical faculties being founded in the thirteenth century at Bologna,
Montpellier, and Paris (ibid., 116; Jouanna 1999, 362). Hospitaller doctors
were trained in this elite Galenic Salernitan tradition, which dominated European medical teaching and practice after the eleventh century. Among the
doctors practicing in the hospital were ethnic Greek Rhodian men who had
been sent to study medicine in Italy on scholarships provided by the order
(Tsirpanlis 1991).

When the Ottomans, led by Suleiman the Magnificent, finally drove the
Knights out of Rhodes in 1522, they in turn brought with them their own version of Galenic or Galenized Arabic medicine. Although little is known about
the teaching and practice of medicine in Ottoman-era Rhodes, the numerous parallels with the learned iatrosophic tradition described here later suggest a fluid and complex interplay of oral and literate routes of transmission.
It is known, for example, that Greek iatrosophic texts and popular reference
manuals circulated widely during the Ottoman period. They appear to have
been especially abundant in the Aegean region, where itinerant practical doctors often traveled from island to island plying their skills. Comprising what
one scholar has called "an ignored category of manuscripts," the approximately
150 Ottoman-era iatrosophic manuals that have been catalogued so far were
typically written in plain language, often peppered with regional, Italian, and
Turkish words (Tselikas 1995, 63). As the medical historian Armin Hohlweg
asserts, it was "from these iatrosophic texts that [local] doctors who did not
have a theoretical medical training drew their knowledge" (1995, 38, my translation). Surviving iatrosophic texts range from humble handwritten notebooks
to the prominent and enduring *Geoponicon*, a manual written by the Cretan
monk-doctor Agapios Landos and issued in twenty-six editions between 1623
and 1919. In addition to the practical agricultural advice it offered, the *Geo-*

ponicon contained a wealth of thoroughly Galenic knowledge on health and illness, including a section specifically devoted to gynecological problems and therapies (Hohlweg 1995, 39). At the other end of the spectrum, there is the handwritten notebook completed in 1930 by the rural Cretan practical doctor Nikolaos Theodorakis based on the medical knowledge he had learned from his father. Patricia Clark, who has analyzed the many striking stylistic and substantive parallels between Theodorakis's manual and classical Greek medical texts, describes it as "an incarnation once removed from [the] older, more formally scripted iatrosophia handbooks" (2002, 341). Without dismissing the role of oral routes of transmission, it seems reasonable to assume that popular texts such as these also had an important role to play in the preservation and transmission of Byzantine medical knowledge during the Ottoman period among those who spoke Greek. Finally, although even less is known about the relationships among ethnic Greek populations, their popular practitioners, and both official and popular Ottoman medicine, the privileged and authoritative status of Galenic medicine in the Ottoman Empire may have also helped disseminate and reinforce this medical tradition among its Greek-speaking subjects.

Ultimately, although much remains to be learned about the routes of transmission of humoral medicine to Rhodes, this much is clear: through long historical exposure to Byzantine, Latin Western, and Islamic influences, and possibly also from local knowledge and midwifery traditions that may have preceded and nurtured all these "Great Traditions," Rhodians had a long history of exposure to an essentially Galeno-Hippocratic understanding of the body. In the following section, I describe some of the components central to the maintenance and restoration of women's procreative health shared by Galenic medicine and Rhodian ethnogynecology: the flow of humoral substances, the most important of which was blood; the therapeutic manipulation of opposites to restore balance; and a practical corpus of therapeutic interventions and pharmacopoeia with which to confront the critical concerns of fertility regulation and the general maintenance of health.

Enduring Principles of the Humoral Medical Tradition

Humoral medicine derives its name from one of the fundamental physiological principles of Hippocratic medicine, to wit, that the body was composed of essential fluids known as humors. Of the four humors described in the Hippocratic Corpus—black bile, yellow bile, phlegm, and blood—blood played the most significant role. To prevent disease and restore health, blood needed to flow without obstruction. Such unimpeded flow of blood promoted its periodical replenishment and renewal. In Galen's (re)formulation of Hippocratic medicine, this principle acquired an even more emphatically critical function. For Galen, *plethora*, an imbalance in which excess blood pooled and putrefied in the body, posed the greatest threat of all to health. If untreated, it led to inflammation (*phlegmone*), a state of bodily derangement and disorder that encompassed a broad range of serious diseases (Kuriyama 1999, 213). In Galen's view, prevention of inflammation and other deleterious consequences of plethora was far preferable to cure. Bloodletting thereby became the Galenic "cornerstone of therapy," the prophylactic procedure of choice against plethora as well as a host of other conditions and ailments (200).

Expelling excess that "overfilled" the body and renewing the blood were processes crucial in maintaining and restoring the health of both genders. At the same time, Galen recognized that because women menstruated, they possessed a natural bloodletting mechanism. As Kuriyama explains: "Close ties between blood and sickness explain . . . why in Galen's view, women menstruating normally don't suffer severe illnesses, whereas all kinds of disorders arise from suppressed menses (1999, 200)." By this logic, menstruation was central to woman's health, a position espoused by Kiria Sofia at the beginning of this chapter. Each month, for some four or five days before and after menstruation, the healthy woman's womb opened to permit the discharge of potentially pathogenic excess blood. It followed, then, that if menstruation was the central means of maintaining and protecting health, the *absence* of menses was a potential harbinger of disease. Amenorrhea, the lack of menstruation, indicated that the flow of excess blood was somehow being obstructed. Blood forcibly retained in the body could putrefy and precipitate serious pathology. For this reason, amenorrhea demanded immediate therapeutic intervention (Green 1985, 29).

Because the developing fetus absorbed a woman's excess blood, pregnancy was another means of relieving menstrual "overfilling" and promoting health. For the Hippocratic authors, pregnancy also brought long-term benefits to a woman's body. In their view, pregnancy and birth caused a woman's pelvic region to expand, creating more open space to accommodate the volume of her blood. As the author of a Hippocratic gynecological text put it:

> I say that a woman who has never given birth suffers more intensely and readily from menstruation than a woman who has given birth to a child. For whenever a woman does give birth, her small vessels become more easy-flowing for menstruation. (Quoted in Green 1985, 18)

As noted earlier, in the prewar period, rural Rhodians also believed that pregnancy and birth had salubrious consequences because they "opened" a woman's body. Although the oldest generation of Rhodian women spoke of pelvic "openness" in more general terms and made no reference to "easy-flowing small vessels," the anatomic logic is the same: bodily expansion mechanically eased the pressure and alleviated the pain caused by blood accumulating in a too-constricted area.

Another fundamental principle of Galeno-Hippocratic medicine held that health depended crucially on the balance between a linked set of oppositions, in particular, those of hot/cold, wet/dry, and left/right. Balance was modulated and restored by following the Hippocratic maxim of *contraria contrariis curantur*, the principle of opposites. By this therapeutic logic, "hot" illnesses were treated with "cold" remedies, and vice versa (Foster 1994; Green 1985; Temkin 1962). Each of these binaries was further linked to a hierarchical understanding of gender. Wet and dry held special significance for understanding the healthy functioning of women's bodies, which were always theorized as more problematic than those of men's. Because the flesh of a woman was softer and more porous than that of a man, it was more absorbent of fluids and thus naturally more "wet." This spongelike quality made women especially susceptible to the accumulation of humidity, which, if not eliminated, resulted in pain and illness (Green 1985, 13–16).

On the other hand, the womb should not become too dry either. Excessive dryness was largely due to a lack of sexual intercourse and the revitalizing moisture provided thereby. The Hippocratic writers argued that if the womb became too dry, it would be compelled to wander the body in search of moisture. If it wandered too high, it bumped into and exerted pressure on the lungs, causing the malady known as "hysterical suffocation." The therapy of choice for a wandering womb was frequent and regular irrigation through sexual intercourse with a man (Green 1985, 19–20).

Sexual intercourse was not the only therapy prescribed for a wandering womb, however. The Hippocratic writers also believed that the womb had a sense of smell. To coax a wandering womb back to its proper place, sweet-smelling herbs and spices that appealed to this olfactory sense were administered in the form of pessaries (vaginal suppositories) and fragrant fumigations of the vulva. Attracted by these pleasant fragrances, a womb wandering too high in the body migrated back down to its proper place. Alternatively, fetid or acrid odors might be applied near a woman's nose. Offended by their foulness, the womb recoiled with displeasure and likewise retreated downward. The Hippocratic Corpus offers no formal rationalization for this extraordinary sensory attribute, which appears as a kind of orphan idea within its anatomy and physiology (Green 1985, 21). Attribution of sentience to the womb appears to be very ancient and may have predated the Hippocratic authors by at least a millennium. Egyptian medical treatises devoted to issues of women's health (and veterinary medicine), such as the Kahun and the Smith papyri (ca. 2100–1900 BCE and 1700 BCE, respectively), also prescribed aromatic fumigations and pessaries as treatments for a wandering womb (Thompson 1999, 21). The association between womb, olfaction, and olfactory organs was also an exceedingly long-lived one in Western medicine. In 1671, Jane Sharp, the first Englishwoman to write a midwifery guide, made note of the womb's sensitivity to smells (Hobby 1999). The belief continued to circulate in Stuart England (Eccles 1982), and traces appear to have persisted even into the twentieth century (Laqueur 1990, 36–37). Wilhelm Fliess, a colleague and friend of Freud, for instance, derived a treatment for female masturbation—removal of the turbinate bone of a woman's nose—from his theory of nasal-genital spots (Bordo 1993, 162).

Hippocratic theorists and practitioners were often locked in acrimonious debate and competition with a variety of alternative schools of medical thought. Soranus of Ephesus, who practiced around 100 AD, was after Hippocrates the most influential writer on gynecology and obstetrics in antiquity. Distinguishing himself from the Hippocratics, Soranus considered absurd both the theory of the wandering womb and the notion that the womb had a sense of smell. Soranus and the Methodist medical sect with which he was associated completely rejected these ideas, along with many other Hippocratic beliefs about women's health. However, their fate over the next nearly two millennia was ultimately determined by Galen in the second century AD (Green 1985).

Galen is often credited with the renaissance of the Hippocratic corpus, but his "Hippocratism," while enthusiastic and thoroughgoing, was nonetheless selective. On the one hand, Galen redeemed and reinstated the idea that the womb possessed a sense of smell. However, like Soranus, he jettisoned the theory of the wandering womb. As it happened, Byzantine medicine concerned with women's health bifurcated into a gynecological arm that drew heavily on this Galenic understanding of women's anatomy and physiology, and an obstetrical arm that also relied on Soranus (Green 1985). Soranus, like others of the Methodist school, distinguished himself by rejecting or inverting nearly all the organizing principles of Hippocratic gynecology. Not only did Soranus scoff at the concept of uterine olfaction; in an obvious reversal of core Galenic principles, he regarded menstrual *retention* as health promoting. In general, Soranus and those who followed him prescribed gentler external therapies such as massage over the harsher internal medicines and aggressive phlebotomy advocated by Galeno-Hippocratic doctors (Green 1985, 29ff). As discussed in the following chapter, the ethno-obstetrical practices of midwives in rural Rhodes featured many commonalities with Soranus's teachings. Ethnogynecology, on the other hand, closely concurred with the precepts of Galenic medicine.

Blood, Sexuality, and the Humoral Body in Prewar Rhodes

In Rhodian regimes of the body in the prewar period, menstruation occupied the same central place and carried much the same meaning as it had in Galeno-Hippocratic medicine. Menstrual blood was regarded as a "dirty" or "filthy" (*vromiko, akatharto*) substance laden with noxious impurities. Because of its pathological potential, the regular elimination of this "dirty" blood through menstruation was considered essential to the maintenance of a woman's health and fertility. Consistent with this logic, copious menstruation was a good thing: the greater the flow, the more impurities were excreted, the greater the benefits to a woman's health (as Beyene 1989 also reports for the island of Evia). Thus, when her period ended each month, a woman said of herself, "I was cleansed," or "I became clean" (*katharisa*) and referred to this time as *ta katharismata*, the "cleansing."

Yet blood was nonetheless fraught with ambivalence and multiple, often contradictory, meanings. If from a humoral perspective menstrual blood signified health, bodily order, and fertility, from an Orthodox perspective it was closely associated with sexual knowledge, sexual activity, and carnal sin. Like open/closed, the clean/dirty binary so prominent in discussions of menstruation is richly polysemic (Dubisch 1986; Hirschon 1989). This polysemy reflects the symbolic salience of blood common to the otherwise distinct discourses of Orthodoxy and humoral medicine. Thus, the cyclical appearance and disappearance of blood indexes, on the one hand, the state of a woman's ritual purity, which is regularly suspended by the unclean effects of menstruation. On the other hand, it indicates the regular accumulation and purging of potentially pathogenic dirt and the renewal of bodily health and fertility.

Because only women who shed blood were able to conceive, menstruation was also highly valued as a sign of fertility. By the same token, however, the onset of menstruation marked an unmarried girl's new vulnerability to shame and disgrace. And menstruation periodically cycled married and unmarried women alike through the embodied experience of ritual uncleanliness and its associated proscriptions. These negatively charged associations were mostly tacit; by and large, they went unspoken. As du Boulay explains, the sense of ritual danger and uncleanliness attached to menstrual blood was realized "not by specific vocabulary, but by a series of prohibitions and the ideas of causation which lie behind them" (1991, 64). On du Boulay's view, these prohibitions were embedded in a network of Greek Orthodox Christian beliefs and practices that aimed to safeguard the boundaries between sacred and profane categories. Women's blood is spilled as a consequence of Eve's sin and is thus associated with the Fall. Because of its origins in this primal sin, "menstrual blood should not be juxtaposed with the sacrificial spilling of Christ's blood" (ibid.). Thus, menstruating women should not enter a church, take communion, worship the icons, or light candles. The dangerous uncleanliness of menstrual blood also threatens those substances intimately associated with Orthodox ritual—wine, bread, and olive oil—even when these are found in a secular context. In short, a web of embodied and largely implicit meanings and valences linked menstrual blood to Eve's sin and ultimately to sexual knowledge and sexual shame.

The fundamentally opposed meanings associated with menstrual blood may help explain the otherwise puzzling fact that among the oldest generation of women, menarche was generally blanketed in secrecy and silence. Such secrecy is found elsewhere in Greece and was probably the norm up to the first half of the twentieth century. In her unique study of menarche in Evia conducted in the 1970s, for instance, Yewoubdar Beyene found that half the women in the village she studied knew nothing about menstruation at the time of their first menses. Because their mothers considered the passing on of such information to be a sin, "they did not know what it was and were frightened at the time of their first menses" (Beyene 1986, 107). The discourse of sexual shame, minimally glossed as "*dropi*," also kept many Rhodian mothers and daughters from speaking about menarche.

Like the women in Evia, many Rhodian women of the oldest generation experienced their first menstruation with no idea of what was happening to them. Terrified by the blood, some spontaneously ran to tell their mothers. Kiria Rita's mother responded joyfully, telling her, "Now you are a woman!" Then, to her daughter's further amazement, she gave her a smart slap on the face, as mothers sometimes did, to cause her cheeks to become permanently rosy. Other girls, out of shame or fear, tried to hide their periods. Kiria Sotiria hid hers for nearly a year, waiting until others weren't around to wash her undergarments in secret. All the while, she later discovered, her mother worried in silence because she believed that her daughter's periods hadn't yet begun. Kiria Voula's mother noticed some stains in her daughter's underclothes as they hung out to dry, and summoned her eldest daughter to speak to her because, as Kiria Voula explained to me, it was *dropi* for her to speak to her daughter directly about menstruation. Kiria Despina's story was the most extreme and the most poignant:

> EG: Did you know about periods before you got them?
> Kiria Despina: No, I didn't know about those things, I didn't understand anything. In those years, we didn't have television, people were closed, *itan klistos o kosmos*, we didn't have contacts [with the outside] . . . we didn't know anything about it.
> EG: Did your mother tell you anything?
> Kiria Despina: *A pa pa*! No way! I had a mother who was very strict, *i afstiri tou kosmou*. I got my period and I didn't know what it was. I was going to catechism class and when I returned home, I felt like I was wet. I look and I said, "Blood! God have mercy, *Kirie eleison*!"

At this, Kiria Despina broke off her story and glanced at the tape recorder on the table between us. "Maybe I shouldn't be saying this now?" I reassured her and she continued:

> I look, *eh Panaghia mou*, what is this? I take off my underpants and hide them. [Why did you hide them? I asked.] I hid them because we respected our mother, and feared our mother. . . . By the time I put on another pair of underpants, more of the same! Then we didn't have washing machines, bleach—however much you washed it, the stain wouldn't come out. So I took the scissors and cut out the part below. My mother saw the clothes when she washed them. But it didn't occur to her to say, "Come here, my child, thus and so"—nothing. She only asked, "Why are your underpants cut with a scissor?" "I don't know, maybe a rat ate them." What could I say now? And she had this inside her. She never said, "Go wear a cloth," or whatever.
> EG: How long did this go on?
> Kiria Despina: Until they married me. Until I was seventeen, my mother never saw my period. The only thing she saw—she saw my virginity, *ti parthenia mou* [the bloody towels and garments shown first to a girl's mother after her wedding night and later to her mother-in-law and other close kin and ritual godparents]. Nothing else.

The implicit association between menarche and a girl's sexuality hinted at in the last line of Kiria Despina's narrative is more explicitly made in the following story Kiria Nota, an energetic and astonishingly spry sixty-nine-year-old grandmother, told me:

> I was ten years old when I got my period for the first time. I woke up one morning and saw the blood. I was very frightened, and I woke up my siblings—it was winter and all five of us were sleeping together in the *ghonia* [the raised platform that surrounds the hearth and is therefore the warmest spot in the house]. When my oldest brother woke up and saw the blood, he said to me, "*Katse mori!* Hey you, wait a minute! Who did you go with? [Who did you have sex with?]" My aunt came by the house a little while later and my brother told her what happened. She took me and locked me up in the *patara* [the large storage cupboard in the back of the house] for several hours as "punishment" for having sex. She was joking—she knew of course that I hadn't had relations with a boy. Later she let me out and told me what it was.

No woman could offer an explanation for the prohibition on telling girls about menarche that articulated much beyond Kiria Despina's embodied sense of fear, shame, and respect for her mother. It would appear that although the humoral discourse of health maintenance offered women a positive set of meanings with which to make sense of menstruation, these meanings were generally unavailable to them before marriage. For girls and maidens, a deeply embodied sense of sexual shame dominated the topic and often dictated silence. In other words, at least until they married and could engage in legitimate sexuality, the dominant discourse of the Church seems often to have trumped and suppressed the positive value attributed to menstruation by the humoral model. These menarche narratives further expand the range of meanings that attached to menstrual blood and indicate how profoundly these meanings might vary according to the specific circumstances of a woman's life (Gottlieb 2002, 386).

Although some mothers did talk with their daughters about menstruation, apparently very few had discussed sexual intercourse with them before their marriage. Sexual ignorance and virginity were the cultural expectation for unmarried girls in prewar Rhodes. Kiria Ariadni, in her early sixties, told me that the only thing her mother told her before she married was that she should be careful not to sleep with her husband for several days immediately before and after March 25, the holy day known as Tou Evangelismou, so that she wouldn't give birth around Christmas. If a child were born right before

Christ's birthday, her mother warned her, it would become a *kallikantzaros*, a sleepwalking demon (see Stewart 1991). All Kiria Eleftheria's mother told her was to expect a visit the day after her wedding from her mother-in-law, who would come to see the bloody towels that ratified her virginity and bring her sweets to eat, "*na ghlikani ti nifi*, to sweeten the bride."

Most of the oldest women I spoke with told me they were unprepared for their wedding nights. Without implying the exercise of bad faith, such statements of course can be construed as narrative performances of the sexual modesty and innocence morally appropriate to women until they married. But although young women in the prewar period may have had some knowledge, it did not seem to be very extensive. Kiria Despina, who warned me at the beginning of our interview that if her life were made into a movie, everyone would leave the theater crying, once again provided the most poignant story of her wedding night:

> EG: Did you know what would happen?
> Kiria Despina: No, *no*!
> EG: But you lived in a village—hadn't you seen any animals mating?
> Kiria Despina: I had seen a little dog, but I didn't understand. Eh, OK, I
>   might have suspected something, but I didn't want. . . . As a girl, my
>   mind didn't dwell on such things. A pure ox, *sketo vodhi*, I'm speaking
>   to you seriously.

I asked Kiria Despina to tell me about her wedding night:

> So, they take us to our room, accompanied by the violin, the clarinet,
> the musicians playing. And then my mother locked us in the room, and
> I pulled and tugged at the door. On the other side, I could hear my aunt,
> God forgive her, who was crying. She loved me a lot, and she was drunk
> [women in rural Rhodes routinely drank a good deal at weddings]. And
> my uncle was crying too, because I was leaving the house [the groom lived
> in Rhodes Town]. And I, I was supposed to make love, when on the other
> side of the wall you hear them all crying and singing.
>
> A little while before, they had taken my husband aside and had told
> him to be careful, to go slowly, gently. And near the bed they had put
> ouzo, cologne, and rosewater. They said to him, "She's young, she may
> faint, throw something in her face!"

Later, when Kiria Despina saw the large amount of blood, she thought it was her period:

Once again, that thing had come to me. My husband wiped some up with the little towels my mother had put out, and I thought, "How can my mother see these now?" Around eight AM the next morning, I heard an accordion at the door and songs outside. I hid under the covers—how could I get up? I was ashamed. I had done dirty work, *skatodhoulia* [literally, "shit work"], it wasn't right, I was afraid. I was ashamed. Then, they all entered the room—aunts, uncles, brothers, sisters—and they threw roses and rosewater. My husband gave them the bloodied towels and they put them on a silver tray, and everyone piled money, dried roses, and cologne onto the tray. I felt such shame that I thought the heavens had fallen on top of me.

Kiria Despina's narrative reveals with almost heartbreaking poignancy how difficult it was to suddenly reconcile the embodied sense of sexual shame culturally appropriate to girls and young women with the joyous associations of legitimate married sexuality.

Ideally, like Kiria Despina, brides were virgins. I was told that nevertheless, even in the past, a number of brides were pregnant when they married. As Dimitriou-Kotsoni (1993, 70) points out in her review of the distinctive features of the "Aegean cultural tradition" of which Rhodes is a part, honor killings and physical violence over infractions of the sexual code were absent in the Aegean islands, in marked contrast to Mani and some other parts of Greece (see, e.g., Seremetakis 1991). Nevertheless, a girl's virginity was expected (and inspected) and the consequences of sex before marriage could still be serious, if not life threatening. To illustrate these consequences, Kiria Dimitra told me the story of her aunt, whose daughter was in love with a young man of whom her parents didn't approve. Visiting her secretly in the remote mountain pasture where she tended the family's goats, he managed over time to "fool her, *ti ghelase*," that is, to convince her to have sex with him. Eventually, her mother noticed the girl's regular vomiting and correctly guessed that she was pregnant. After a thorough tongue-lashing from her mother, her parents went to speak to the boy's family about arranging a wedding as quickly as possible. Exploiting their advantage, the boy's family demanded a much larger dowry than would otherwise have been given. By the time negotiations were concluded, much of the other children's shares of the family wealth had been promised to the groom.

Conception: Two Seeds or One?

Kinship ideology in Rhodes, as throughout Greece, is bilateral. Both mother's and father's sides are recognized in the reckoning of kin relations. Bilateral kinship is supported by duogenetic procreation theories in which both the mother and the father are recognized as contributing essential substance to their offspring. Children, who are said to be of "two bloods," thus inherit qualities and characteristics from each parent (Loizos and Papataxiarchis 1991a, 8). This duogenetic principle is also consistent with Galeno-Hippocratic procreation theory, which posited that both men and women contribute the "seed" or generative substance required for conception. Alongside the duogenetic two-seed or two-blood view, however, there coexists another, monogenetic theory of procreation, the fundamentals of which Carol Delaney thoroughly describes in her 1991 ethnography of rural Turkey, *The Seed and the Soil*. As Delaney observes, the association of men with the creative seed and women with the nurturant soil is common to all three of the monotheistic and patriarchal religions of the Abrahamic tradition. In the monogenetic view, the role of the father in procreation is to actively create life, the role of the mother to passively nurture its growth and development. In antiquity, this view was most famously championed by Aristotle, who regarded semen as the purveyor of the essence, or soul, of humanity (Laqueur 1990). Throughout the Middle Ages, as the eminent historian of Byzantine medicine Oswei Temkin (1962, 108) has noted, "there remained a latent tension between Aristotle and Galen" on this point. The monogenetic procreative theory has not previously been reported in the ethnography of rural Greece. Among Rhodians of the oldest generation, it could be found alongside the more symmetrical duogenetic theory.

The ancient debate between Galenic and Aristotelian perspectives is unwittingly reproduced in the following discussion that took place between Kiria Eleftheria and her husband, Kirios Manolis, both in their early seventies. Using imagery identical to that reported by Delaney for Turkey, Kiria Eleftheria explained to me the fundamentals of an essentially monogenetic theory of procreation:

> *I ghineka ine to khorafi*, the woman is the field. The man is the farmer, he sows the seed, *o andras ine o gheorghos, aftos sperni*. You had a girl? Well, we say to the man, whatever you sowed, that's what you'll reap, *oti esperes tha therisis*. The woman isn't to blame, *dhen ftei*, if you have a girl or a boy; the one who sows is responsible. As my mother used to say, if you sow

barley, you won't get wheat. Only if you sow wheat, will you get wheat. That's why they say, to be true siblings, you have to have the same father.[15]

Defending the Galenic position, Kirios Manolis adamantly disagreed with his wife's monogenetic exegesis. Kirios Manolis, a slight, courteous man, had been listening quietly throughout most of the interview. Occasionally, he attempted to interject his own thoughts, but each time, Kiria Eleftheria, easily the more formidable of the two, interrupted and reclaimed the floor. Now, though, Kirios Manolis felt strongly enough about the subject to ignore his wife's interruptions and assert his opinion. In his view:

> The child takes equally from the mother and the father. That one little seed the father gives? That little thing? The mother has that little seed in her stomach for nine months. She feeds it, she waters it with her blood, she does lots for it. So I think both its mother *and* its father give equally to the child.

In this exchange, local versions of the Aristotelian one-seed and the Galenic two-seed theories of procreation not only compete but also, and perhaps more to the point, are differentially mobilized in the discourse of blame over who is responsible for the gender of the child.

The duogenetic theory of procreation reflects an implicitly Galenic understanding of sexual difference. Galen's one-sex model, which dominated both Ottoman and Western thinking about the body until the modern period, held the two genders to be versions of a common anatomical design (Laqueur 1990; Ze'evi 2006). More precisely, women's bodies represented inversions of the basic male pattern. According to Galen and the countless medical theorists who followed in his footsteps, the female's generative organs were identical to the male's, only turned inside out. The vagina or cervix, for example, was an inverted, interior penis, the uterus an internal scrotum. Although a woman's organs were by reason of this inversion seen to be less perfect than a man's, they were nevertheless essentially alike in structure and function. Following the logical thread of this fundamental identity, conception required the emission of generative fluids by both sexes. Therefore, in the one-sex model, conception was possible only when men and women each experienced orgasm (Laqueur 1990, 38ff).

It was rare for a woman of the oldest generation to openly and directly speak of her intimate sexual experience, at least to me. The women who did, however, implied that for conception to occur, both the man and the woman had to experience climax. References to women's sexual pleasure were usually oblique and euphemistic, but in the context of their narratives, I think, unmistakable. Kiria Panaghiota, a pale woman in her late seventies with piercing blue eyes, insisted that conception required that both women and men feel *khara* (joy) during sex; only when they did would both emit *ta igra* (the moisture) essential to conception. Kiria Eleftheria insisted that if a woman didn't feel *oreksi* (desire; literally, appetite), for sex, she couldn't conceive a child. Quoting a common saying to support her view, she explained: "They say that 'a woman can go with ten men, but if she doesn't have *oreksi*, she won't get pregnant.'" [Why?] "Because then her womb opens, and it pulls in the seed, *to travai.*" On her part, Kiria Marianthi used the word *kefi*, a Greek idiom notoriously difficult to translate that among its many usages may be deployed to index "a heightened form of experience" (Caraveli 1985, 263). As Kiria Marianthi explained:

> If you didn't want your husband, didn't want him to approach you, . . . if a husband and wife don't both feel *kefi*, then you can't make a baby. . . . A close friend came to me one day and said to me, "Marianthi, I don't know how I made these children. I don't feel anything with my husband." "Don't you embrace your husband? Don't you kiss him on the mouth?' I asked her. "*Thou!* [spitting sound]" she said to me, "never, never!" "Don't you 'play' with him?" I asked her. "Never, not at all," she told me. I told her that if I don't "play" with my husband for a while, I don't reach my *kefi*, in other words . . . [trails off]. I can't understand myself how she made those babies.

Not far beneath the surface of Kiria Marianthi's implication that both men and women must experience sexual climax (*kefi*) for conception to occur is the Galenic one-sex understanding of the procreative body.[16]

Just as the anatomy of men and women in the Galenic model was basically one, so was their physiology. Following this logic, blood, semen, and milk, the fluids essential to procreation, were simply different versions of the same fundamental substance. In Laqueur's memorable phrase, they represented "fungible fluids" in the corporeal economy of health and fertility (1990, 35). This Galenic logic was also evident in the rough equivalence that the oldest generation of Rhodians attributed to blood and semen (milk was generally ignored).[17] Just as the elimination of menstrual blood cleansed women, the regular expulsion of semen was necessary to rid men's bodies of their accumulated impurities, "male dirt," as it were. More specifically, Galen warned that a lack of regular sexual intercourse caused men to "feel heavy in the head, become nauseated and feverish, have a poor appetite and bad digestion" (quoted in

Kuriyama 1999, 228). In a particularly lively interview, one couple in their late sixties, Kiria Paraskevi and her husband, Kirios Sterghos, clarified for me the relationship between health and the regular discharge of men's and women's bodily fluids:

> EG: You have explained to me how women get rid of dirt through menstruation, but how do men do this?
>
> Kiria Paraskevi: That's why they have to go with a woman, to get rid of that. Why does a man have to be with a woman? To cleanse himself! *Na katharisi!*[18]
>
> Kirios Sterghos: A man who's thirty years old, is it possible for him never to have gone with a woman? Is it, I ask you? *No*, it's not. He can't do it, something will happen to him, he will get sick, *tha pathi kati*. He will lose his mind, *tha tou stripsi to mialo*. [Kiria Paraskevi interjects: "That dirt, all that dirt!"] There is the need, he *must* get rid of this. That's why boys, from the age of fifteen or sixteen, must go with a girl.
>
> EG: Is it dirty?
>
> Kirios Sterghos: It's natural, but he must get rid of it. That's why so many men resort to self-service [using the English term, laughing].
>
> EG: Is a man's body renewed by this?
>
> Kirios Sterghos: Yes, of course.
>
> EG: Does a woman need this [regular sex] too?
>
> Both: *No!*
>
> Kiria Paraskevi: A woman has her period every month. We have our own self-service. [Everyone laughs.]

The rough conceptual equivalence and fungibility of semen and menstrual blood is evident in this exchange in the humorous use of the English loan word "self-service," usually restricted to the cafeteria-style restaurants that cater to tourists, to describe both masturbation for men and menstruation for women. This exchange is also notable for the perspective it offers on the old maxim that "a woman can last a thousand years" but a man can't rein in his sexual urges for very long. Underpinned by the cultural belief that "[a] man's sexual drive was held to be physiologically imperative, uncontrollable, and diverted only with dire consequences" (Hirschon 1989, 149), this adage has sometimes been taken as evidence of the fundamentally *different* and separate natures of men and women in Greek gender ideology. When examined through the humoral lens, however, the sexes are seen to be essentially similar in their experience of desire. As Hirschon observed among the Asia Minor refugees she studied in Piraeus, youthful blood was recognized as being "hot" (*vrazi to ema*), regardless of gender; it "boils" equally for girls and boys, "provoking parents of adolescent girls into thoughts of early marriage" (ibid.). The humoral perspective adds another dimension to our understanding of older Greek beliefs about gender difference. From this perspective, the anatomy and physiology of women and men are basically the same, although their outlets for eliminating the noxious build-up of heat and the resulting bodily impurities differ. For women, this was accomplished through regular menstruation, and for men, who lack this mechanism, through ejaculation.[19]

The Humoral Body and Women's Fertility in Prewar Rhodes

Because "you get married to have children," pregnancy was expected to follow soon, if not immediately, after a woman's wedding. Typically, if a woman did not become pregnant after a couple months of marriage, she paid a visit to the *mammi*, the local midwife. Practical midwives were first and foremost obstetrical specialists whose services were normally restricted to the time of birth and the postpartum period, as I describe in the next chapter. But they were also often consulted as the first resort when women were having difficulty becoming pregnant. In small villages such as Ermia, where the mammi was one's neighbor, aunt, or sister-in-law, such consultations might simply take the form of an informal chat or chance meeting.

The therapies at the mammi's disposal were exclusively external and manipulative. Internally administered herbal therapies for infertility, discussed shortly, were common knowledge among women and did not require a specialist's assistance. When asked to help, the mammi first examined the woman by palpating her abdomen to determine the position of her womb. She then selected between one of two kinds of therapies. In the treatment known as *sintinaghma*, or *tinazma*, roughly translatable as "shaking," the midwife took the woman by the waist, lifted her slightly in the air, and gave her a several firm shakes. "*Me tinakse*, she shook me," women would say. Or the midwife, assisted by two or three other women and possibly by the woman's husband, might drape the woman over the edge of one of the tall platform beds typical of village houses of the period. Holding her upside down by her legs, they shook her repeatedly. Alternatively, the midwife might decide to give her an abdominal massage. In this case, a woman would lie down, with her legs high up against a wall, while the mammi massaged her belly with warm olive oil. The exclusive focus of both *tinazma* and massage, as for all ethnogynecological interventions, was the womb. Both approaches had the same objective: "to bring the womb back to its proper place"; "to bring the womb back to the center"; "so that the womb is straight"; "to raise up the womb" (*na pai i mitra sti thesi tis; va feri ti mitra sto kentro; na ine i mitra isa-isa; na anipsosi i mitra*). After administering these therapies, a mammi might also advise the woman to bind her abdomen with a kerchief into which two bars of soap were placed, one on either side. Worn for two or three weeks, the bars helped sustain the uterine "lifting" effected by the mammi's treatments. Some women were unsure of how this helped a woman conceive, but others said that these therapies worked by correcting a womb that was situated too low (never too high) or tipped to one side and that had to be restored to its proper place for conception to occur.

At first blush, the idea that conception was impeded by a uterus that was somehow out of place calls to mind the Hippocratic notion of the wandering womb. However, women did not believe that the womb could roam the interior of the body. It could only fall too low or lean to one side, problems a few women compared to a prolapsed or tipped uterus. Nor, as I discuss in this section, did the manipulative therapies midwives used to correct the condition follow the therapeutic logic dictated by Hippocratic approaches to the treatment of a wandering womb.

If the mammi's treatments failed, then a woman's inability to conceive was most commonly attributed to a womb that was suffering from a cold. A womb cold (*na kriosi i mitra; krioma tis mitras*) could be diagnosed by the presence of abdominal pain, especially painful menstruation, or by the absence of menstruation. Most insidiously, a womb cold could occasionally be asymptomatic, working its damage without a woman's awareness. A woman became afflicted by a womb cold, as one woman explained, "just like a person gets any cold—from cold water or cold air, let's say, or from lingering in a wet bathing suit after a swim—that's how your womb gets a cold." In Greek usage, one does not "catch" a cold, as in English. Today, one can "catch" other illnesses, such as the flu (*kolisa ghripi*) or, even before germ theory circulated widely, a dreaded disease such as tuberculosis. To suffer from a cold, however, one "becomes cold" (*kriosa*, or *ekho krioma* or *kriologhima*, "I have a cold," but rarely *kolisa kriologhima*). In the first instance, there is a sense of penetration by an active external agent or foreign element that directly causes a state of disease. In the second usage, colds result from the internal chilling of the body caused by exposure to cold assaults. Implicit in this usage is the humoral notion that disruption of the body's thermal balance is pathogenic, or at least potentially so.

Colds usually attack specific parts of the body, according to the form taken by the cold insult and the nature of a person's vulnerability at the time. Such insults could be literally cold, as in a cold current of air or of water in the ocean, or metaphorically so, as in the symbolic valence of particular substances regardless of their physical temperature. Foods such as lemons, for example, were classified as "cold" (as also reported by Beyene 1989 for Evia). Illness causation usually followed a two-step process. In the first, necessary but insufficient, step, the body's optimal thermal balance somehow became disturbed, rendering a person susceptible to illness. Vulnerability to cold, for instance, increased when the body became overheated through sweating or being out in the sun. The second step required exposure to an additional assault of excessive cold that tipped the thermal balance sufficiently to precipitate an illness episode. Draughts or currents of air or water, both referred to as *revmata* (sing., *revma*), could cause the dangerously chilled bodily state known as *puntiasma* (from *punta*, a current). A current of air hitting a person in the head, for example, could cause a painful condition known as *psiksi*, in which the face sometimes becomes temporarily frozen in a distorted grimace (akin to Bell's palsy). A womb cold could result from a draught of cold air or water directly hitting the abdomen or entering "from below" (*apo kato*), that is, through the genitals. A cold insult could also affect the womb by entering the body through the feet or buttocks, as a result of walking barefoot or, most unwisely, sitting or lying on a cold floor.

A woman was particularly susceptible to a womb cold when her uterus was in an "open" state. Such openness increased her vulnerability and placed her at risk because it allowed cold insults to penetrate her body with ease. As discussed earlier, the events of marriage and childbirth caused a woman's womb to open. This auspicious opening was not, however, a permanent or irreversible state. Over the course of her life, a woman's womb regularly opened and closed in response to many different stimuli. During sexual intercourse, for instance, her womb opened and remained open for a brief while. For this reason, after sex, a woman should take care to dress warmly "down below," *apo kato*, and avoid going out into the cool night air. Similarly, after each birth, the womb opened, and stayed vulnerably open, throughout the forty-day postpartum period that followed. For her own protection, the *lekhona*, as the postpartum woman was called, should ideally remain secluded in her house with her newborn, dressing warmly and drinking plenty of infusions made of metaphorically "hot" substances such as cinnamon, sage, cloves, and honey. Every month, a healthy woman's womb opened to allow for the discharge of menstrual blood. That is why, as Kiria Artemis explained to me, "they say that a woman who has her period is like a woman who has just given birth." Consistent with Galeno-Hippocratic theory, women believed the womb opened a few days before menstruation began and remained so during menstruation and for some three to five days afterward. During this period of openness, women should strictly avoid bathing, washing their hair, and eating metaphorically "cold" foods. Some women would not sprinkle lemon juice, a key condiment in Greek cuisine, on their food when they menstruated. Others, to be on the safe side, avoided eating lemons altogether until menopause. In accord with Hippocratic beliefs, it was during this week or so of unobstructed openness that Rhodian women believed they were most likely to become pregnant. Finally, illness such as a cold could cause a woman's womb to close.

When a woman suffered from a womb cold, the consequences for her health and well-being in general, and for her fertility in particular, were always adverse, usually serious, and potentially devastating. Womb colds were cited by women of the oldest generation as the single most important cause of female infertility. They could also lead to lifelong painful menstrual cramps and, eventually, to a difficult menopause and assorted health problems in old age. For these reasons, women should be tirelessly alert to cold insults, not only to their own bodies, but also to those of their daughters and other young women in their circle of intimates. Because of the procreative imperative and the role of motherhood in "completing" a woman and enabling her to achieve full personhood, protecting oneself from the cold is not merely a matter of preventive health care; it is a moral obligation as well. Although from an early age children of both sexes are bundled to a degree that most Americans would consider excessive (D. Sutton 1998b), in my experience, young girls were kept under an especially watchful eye. Still today, girls may be reprimanded with alarm if they sit on a cold tile floor or walk with bare feet in cold water, especially if they were already vulnerably warm and sweating from the sun or from their physical activities. Kiria Voula recalled her mother's tireless remonstrations when she was growing up:

> Women protected themselves then. Would my mother let us bathe when we had our period? *A pa pa*! She was always watching out for us not to get cold. "Dress well!" "Watch out for the cold! "Don't get wet [when washing clothes]!" "Don't sit on the ground!" "Something will happen to your womb, you'll get a cold and you won't have any children." Today, I see girls go bathing every day with their periods. It seems so strange to me. Then, they used to watch out for us, *tote, mas prosekhane*.

Such vigilance was, in effect, part of women's moral responsibility for the physical care, health, and well-being of their children. Although, as Kiria Voula indicates, the range of preventive practices is attenuated today, mothers still take very seriously their duty to protect their children from the cold. Both popular stereotypes and scholarly representations of Greek mothers have often focused on their dedicated, even zealous, feeding practices. Dubisch

(1986, 207), for example, writes of seeing a mother on a beach in Tinos pursue her son into the ocean brandishing a bowl and spoon. I have witnessed (and sometimes participated in) similar scenes in Rhodes involving a hard-boiled egg and a meatball. Yet, arguably, one hears the exhortation *"Disou!"* ("Dress warmly!" literally, "Dress yourself!") almost as often from mothers as *"Fae!"* ("Eat!"). This was certainly the case in my own childhood, although I hadn't fully appreciated the logic behind my mother's and grandmother's seemingly endless pleading and nagging (*"Disou kala! Ghimni ise!"*) until I did fieldwork in Rhodes. Their voices unexpectedly echoed in my mind whenever I heard Rhodian women earnestly urging me to dress my daughter more warmly. Listening to them also unexpectedly conjured the exhilarating sense of freedom I had felt many years ago when I left for college and was finally able to go out at night without being forced to wear a sweater.

When a womb suffers from a cold, it is said to "close" (*klini i mitra*). A closed womb is implicated in infertility in two ways. First, and most mechanically, a closed womb presented a physical barrier that blocked entry of a man's sperm into a woman's body. But a closed womb was also injurious to a woman's fertility because it prevented the elimination of menstrual blood and other bodily impurities. Pent-up impurities festering in a closed womb caused illness that could eventually result in sterility. Coaxing a closed womb to open was therefore one of the main objectives of all the ethnogynecological therapies for infertility.

A diagnosis of womb cold was a retrospective process that reconstructed a woman's recent history of vulnerability and exposure to specific environmental insults. Deducing the etiology of the illness and making a diagnosis, in turn, pointed to the appropriate course of therapy through the application of the Hippocratic principle of opposites: illness caused by cold is treated with hot therapies, and vice versa (Foster 1994). As with any cold illness, treatment of a womb cold involved either external application of heat or its internal generation by means of substances with an inherent heat-producing ability. In the latter category were the medicinal herbs known as the *pirotika*, a local word derived from the root *pir* (fire). Herbs classified as *pirotika* have the inherent ability to generate *piradha*, a local word denoting intense heat, which caused the body, or specific parts or organs of the body, to heat up. Whether internally or externally applied, hot medicines worked by counteracting the cold illness, thereby allowing a closed womb to salubriously open once again.

Therapies administered to open a closed womb almost always combined the double punch of heat and aroma. Within the local taxonomy of healing substances, all the *pirotika* herbs used to treat a womb cold also belonged to the category known as the *mirodhika*, aromatic or fragrant, herbs (from *mirodhia*, fragrance). The hot, aromatic herbs most frequently mentioned as treatments for a womb cold by Rhodian women were sage (*alisfakia*) and the concentrated oil of sage (*alisfakoladho*), cumin (*kimino*), nutmeg (*moskhokarido*), cloves (*gharifalo*), cinnamon (*kanela*), and dittany (*dhiktamo*).[20] Many of these herbs were also indicated as treatments for ammenorhea in the *Materia Medica* compiled by Dioscorides of Anazarbos in the second century AD (Riddle 1985). Also known as *The Greek Herbal*, this popular reference book exerted a profound influence on Byzantine, Arabic, and Western pharmacology that endured well into the seventeenth century (Jochle 1974). In the *Materia*, Dioscorides also categorized medicines by classes and by their drug properties, notably including in the former category the "*aromatika*," aromatic plants and drugs, and in the latter the "*thermantika*," or heat-generating substances—by far the most frequently mentioned pharmacological property (Riddle 1985, 21). Besides this correspondence in classifying therapies, the ways Dioscorides and Rhodian women categorize specific herbs also coincide. To take one example, cinnamon, which figured prominently in the management of women's procreative health, was classified as *pirotiko* and *mirodhiko* in Rhodes, and as *thermantiko* and *aromatiko* in the *Materia* (Gunther 1934).

While the *pirotika* herbs cured according to the familiar Hippocratic logic of opposites, the *mirodhika* worked along an altogether different route. Their efficacy was due to their appeal to the womb's sense of smell. Kiria Sofia described this therapeutic process to me: "The womb breathes, it inhales and sucks up, *roufai*, the fragrance." Taking a deep breath to illustrate, she continued, "It smells the sweet fragrance of the herbs, and it's pleased, *efkharistiete*, and that makes it open." Or, in Kiria Voula's words, "That essence, *ousia*, women have inside them, the womb, as they say, it has a sense of smell, *ekhi osfrisi*. It smells the fragrance and it opens." Rhodian women had little to say about how and why the womb was endowed with this olfactory capability— but then, neither did the Galeno-Hippocratic corpus, in which this belief is also featured. What was not in doubt was that the *mirodhika* herbs enticed the womb to open by appealing to its sense of smell and responsiveness to pleasing aromas.

Hot aromatic herbal therapies were administered in a variety of ways. Boiled to make teas and infusions, they could be taken by mouth. They could also be inserted into the vagina via pessaries, suppositories made by soaking gauze or cotton in the herbal brew and squeezing it to form a small wad "the size and shape of a hazelnut," as one woman described it. A string was tied to one end of the pessary for easy removal, and a fresh one was inserted daily. Poultices were also made from cloths soaked in aromatic preparations and worn like sanitary pads. Finally, steamy sitz baths were prepared by boiling the herbs in large pots or basins over which a woman squatted, the lower part of her body naked, tenting herself over with a large towel or blanket to keep the cold out and the fragrant vapors in. All these therapies were repeated, usually for three consecutive days (or nights, in the case of the sitz baths). The ultimate objective of these combinations of heat and fragrance was the same: to coax the womb to open so that it could expel its accumulated "dirt" in the form of clogged up discharges and corrupted menstrual blood, which were the proximate causes of a woman's inability to conceive. Women who had undergone a course of hot aromatic treatments described shedding dark sheets of blood (*petses*) or abundant liquids (*igra*). To improve their chances of conceiving a child, women should have sex with their husbands as soon as possible after completing the therapy to take advantage of the womb's openness, and afterward keep their legs elevated above their heads.

Fertility Control: Emmenagogues, Abortifacients, and Therapies in Between

The same humoral regimes of the body that underpinned fertility enhancement informed the use of emmenagogues. Emmenagogues are menstrual regulators, that is, therapies designed to "bring down" the menses when there is a perceived delay. An artifact of medical history today, emmenagogues have played a major role in humoral variants of women's medicine since antiquity. By one count, Dioscorides identified 132 different emmenagogues, comprising 14 percent of all the drugs listed in his influential *Materia Medica* (Jochle 1974, 425). If within the humoral model, regular menstrual cycles functioned to cleanse women, refreshing and renewing their bodies through the elimination of dirty blood, then delays in this salubrious "order" of things, in a woman's *taksi*, were potentially cause for concern. Of course, a delay could also signify a pregnancy. In the absence of medical tests, however, early pregnancy was an often ambiguous and uncertain bodily state. A menstrual delay could just as easily be read as the harbinger of a serious internal health problem such as a womb cold. Because of this inherent ambiguity, a woman was able at her discretion to interpret a delay as either blocked menstruation or early pregnancy. Since women often could not be certain for several weeks, or perhaps even longer, which was the case, interpretation and intervention were up to them.[21]

When I asked women of the oldest generation about techniques to induce abortions, my questions were most often met with denial or silence. The oldest women I spoke with roundly condemned abortion as a sin, and more emphatically, as "a big sin" (*meghali amartia*) and a "big crime" (*meghalo englima*), a reference to the Greek Orthodox Church's equation of abortion with murder. In rural Rhodes, as elsewhere in rural Greece, women are closely associated with the spiritual well-being of their families. It is they who perform the family religious rituals, and who attend church and confess more frequently than men. Generally speaking, it is women who are more concerned with sin in the ecclesiastical sense (Herzfeld 1985; Danforth 1989; Dubisch 1991). It is therefore not surprising that women of the oldest generation were reluctant to talk about abortion. When, however, I rephrased my questions and asked instead about menstrual regulation, I found that women who were silent about abortifacients had much to say about emmenagogues.

Women's silence should not be taken to mean that emmenagogues were nothing more than covert or disguised abortifacients, however. In the past and still today, infertility was dreaded, and it represented a very serious problem for some women. All women greatly feared womb colds, which always demanded immediate attention. It has recently been argued, most notably by the historian John Riddle (1997), that after Christianity became hegemonic, women throughout Europe used the knowledge of emmenagogues inherited from antiquity to disguise their intentions and perform "undercover" abortions, as it were. Hidden agendas or bad faith, however, cannot simply be imputed or assumed. Just as oral contraceptives today are used *both* to prevent pregnancy and to treat infertility by correcting irregular menstrual cycles, so too with emmenagogues in the past (Green 1999). In fact, one middle-aged woman told me that when, some years ago, her doctor prescribed birth-control pills to make her erratic cycles more regular, she opted instead to use an emmenagogue she prepared herself each month by boiling onion skins, to avoid having to ingest hormones daily (see Chapter 7 for a detailed discussion of Rhodian women's anxieties over the health risks posed by hormones). Intention is clearly of critical significance. But sometimes, as will become apparent here, it might not be possible neatly or conclusively to decipher intention, even for the woman herself.

Emmenagogues almost always consisted of the same *pirotika* and *aromatika* herbs that were used to enhance fertility. Two additional therapies mentioned exclusively as emmenagogues were infusions made from rue (*Ruta graveolens*) and from the hard outer skins of onions, boiled with or without sticks of cinnamon.[22] While women in their seventies and eighties always characterized these therapies as emmenagogic, women in their sixties and fifties might also acknowledge their abortifacient quality. There is little doubt, though, that even the oldest generation of women knew of their use to induce abortion. This was confirmed by a friend from Ermia, a woman who was born and raised in the

United States but who had permanently emigrated to Rhodes when she married a man from the village. Like many migrants, her family often spent their summers on the island, in part because they hoped their children would eventually fall in love with and marry a co-villager, as my friend in fact had. At one point during her long engagement, she told me, an old aunt took her aside and advised her, should she become pregnant, how to boil and drink a tea made of onion skins. Very likely because my friend was an insider, a kinswoman, and a co-villager, this elderly woman openly divulged the abortifacient quality of onion skins to her but not to me.

Kiria Soula, a grandmother in her early sixties, provided a description of emmenagogue use that is suggestive of how women might have reconciled, if not resolved, their potential moral contradictions:

> When we were delayed, *kathisterimeni*, and we might be pregnant, but we didn't want it, after a few days we boiled onion skins or cinnamon, and we'd drink it on an empty stomach every morning for two or three days so that the blood would come. If you drink the onion skins, you'll see a period. But if it were a child, though, the blood wouldn't come.

Here, in an apparent contradiction, Kiria Soula seems to imply that in the very early stages of pregnancy, also the window of opportunity for emmenagogue efficacy, a child does not yet exist. This position contradicts that of the Greek Orthodox Church, which, long before the scientific "facts of life" were discovered, understood "the sacred gift" of human life to begin with conception (Breck 1998). By the Church's logic, with which women were intimately familiar, the use of emmenagogues to flush out a possible pregnancy was as much a sin as abortion. Kiria Soula, however, appears to adhere to a view that it is possible for a woman to be a little bit pregnant, and that pregnancies and fetuses, rather than being either-or states, evolve and change categories along the way. Such a view is also consistent with the processual and gradualist understanding of personhood outlined at the beginning of this chapter. Finally, it is consistent with a woman's (lack of) embodied experience of conception. If an emmenagogue caused a woman's period to resume, then this could be construed as a posteriori proof that no "child" had been present. At the same time, Kiria Soula does not discount the possibility that the woman might have been pregnant. But then again, she might have been suffering from a womb cold. In the absence of medical tests and a woman's own bodily signs and symptoms of pregnancy, there was simply no way to be sure. Like the women Carole Browner (1980, 1985) studied in Cali, Colombia, who recognize an ambiguous state intermediate between being pregnant and not pregnant, this processual view offered Kiria Soula and others like her some relief from the heavy moral burden of abortion.

Rue (*apiano*), known since antiquity as a powerful abortifacient, was also identified by the oldest women as an emmenagogue, and by others as an effective way to induce an abortion. Rue was also called *vromoapiano*, that is, "stinking rue," a reference to the foul odor and noxious taste that kept more than a few women from being able to use it at all. In both popular and scholarly literature on "women's medicine" and "ancient" herbal knowledge, one occasionally finds a romantic tendency to celebrate the use of rue as a means by which women were able to exert control over their reproduction independent of men and of the medical profession. Familiar and, I admit, sympathetic with this literature, I was excited when I first heard stories of its use on Rhodes.[23] My initial enthusiasm was brought up short, however, when several women recounted their experiences with the herb. Kiria Khariklia, a grandmother in her sixties, provided a vivid description of her attempt to use rue to cause an abortion. Amid the grinding poverty that followed the war, as she struggled just to feed and clothe the four young children she already had, she discovered to her deep dismay that she was pregnant yet again:

> I caught children [got pregnant] very easily, just with the scent, *mono me ti mirodhia*, as they say. When I got pregnant again, I boiled the plant called rue, which many people grew in their gardens. I poured it into the cup I used to drink my milk, but when I raised it to my lips and smelled it, the cup fell out of my hands and smashed on the floor. I started vomiting—it was that awful. I couldn't drink it. It stinks! *A pa pa*, a very ugly smell. But it gives results, *ine apotelesmatiko*. If I could have, I would have drunk it, and perhaps I would have had results too.

After that, she tried the milder onion-skin brew, but to no avail. "I know other women for whom it worked, but me, when I caught a child, it didn't come out with anything." After her failed attempt with the rue, and although desperately short of money, she visited a doctor in Rhodes Town who was well known for performing abortions. In a quiet, flat tone that gave no indication of the heavy irony of the situation, she explained that since she had no cash, she gave the doctor her gold cross to keep as collateral until she could manage to pay his fee.

Kiria Evanthia, in her sixties and a native of Rhodes Town, also used rue to cause an abortion. After the birth of her second daughter in 1955, Kiria Evanthia wanted no more children, but her husband wanted to keep trying for a son. When she discovered that she was pregnant again, she desperately wanted an abortion, but had no way to pay for it without her husband's knowledge. Her neighbor, a Karpathian woman who had recently moved to Rhodes and who knew many herbal remedies, offered to prepare an infusion of rue for her. Unlike Kiria Khariklia, she managed to drink it down. Soon afterward, however, Kiria Evanthia began to hemorrhage. Her husband rushed her to the hospital, where she was diagnosed as having suffered a miscarriage and given a dilation and curettage. Neither her husband nor her doctor ever learned about the rue.[24]

Selective Neglect:
Dealing with Intractable Dilemmas

In the previous section, we saw that even in a context dominated by the Church's position on abortion and by local ideals of large families, other discourses and practices, namely the humoral model of health maintenance and illness prevention, and the local knowledge for pursuing these valued ends were at hand and could be called upon to regulate childbearing. The inherent ambiguity of pregnancy within this cultural system permitted a woman at her discretion to interpret a delay as blocked menstruation or as an early pregnancy, in light of her circumstances and without the difficult, and for some women, intolerable moral burden of abortion. In this premedicalized context, it could be argued, with Foucault, that although silence and secrecy can offer a shelter for power, "they also loosen its holds and provide for relatively obscure areas of tolerance" (1978 [1990], 101).

But one final method of "birth" control that I wish to mention, the selective neglect of infants, allowed no such moral shelter for women. Only one woman confided this practice to me, but her story suggests that others were aware of it as well. Married right after the war to a man she had loved since adolescence, Kiria Katina had two sons within three years. Several years passed before she conceived again. At first, she was pleased to be pregnant, but toward the end of her term she began to be troubled by the sensation of "many arms and legs in my belly." Kiria Katina feared that the child might turn out "anomalous" in some way. When her time came, Kiria Katina gave birth first to one tiny girl, and then, a few minutes later, to another, even tinier one. After the second baby emerged, the women who had gathered to help Kiria Katina with the birth began to wail and lament: "*Dhio kores, dhio spitia!* Two daughters, two houses!" Her husband, Kirios Stamatis, angrily ordered them to be quiet, but a pall continued to hang over the entire family.

A day or two after the birth, a neighbor dropped by to offer Kiria Katina advice on how to remedy her misfortune: "'This is what you will do,' she told me. 'Nurse one of the girls, and give the other only water to drink,'" Kiria Katina recalled. "And so I listened to her, and the child would cry and cry but I wouldn't nurse her." Following the Rhodian naming custom, Kiria Katina planned to name one twin after her mother, Maria, and the other after her husband's mother, Efrosini. Calling herself "*poniri*"—sly, cunning—Kiria Katina explained that she decided to nurse only Efrosini, because no one in the village would suspect her of starving Maria, the daughter who commemorated her own mother. "So I gave Maria only a pacifier with sugar and some chamomile tea"—the latter to fool her husband, who attributed the infant's constant crying to colic. Three nights later, Kiria Katina had a dream:

> There was a knock at the door, and I asked, "Who is it?" "Maria, your neighbor," a woman answered. [Kiria Katina's house was right next to the village church.] I let her in, and it was a beautiful woman, dressed all in white, glowing with a light that lit up the whole house. She was furious, completely beside herself with anger. "Take care of the little angels that I gave you," she told me. "Don't do anything to hurt them! Pay attention to what I'm telling you, or I will cause great harm to your house, *tha kano meghalo kako sto spiti sou!*"

As she finished telling me this story, Kiria Katina began to weep softly. Maria, the woman in white, was, of course, the Panaghia, the All Holy One and Mother of God to whom Ermia's church was dedicated. Kiria Katina interpreted the Panaghia's threat to destroy her "house" to mean that she would cause her other children to die as punishment for her sinful actions. Stricken by fear and full of remorse, she immediately began nursing the neglected twin. Years later, Kiria Katina told me, when her daughter Maria was a grown woman, she confessed to her what she had attempted to do and asked for her forgiveness.

In moments of anxiety and uncertainty, manifestations of the divine in the form of the Panaghia or a saint often appear to Greek women in dreams to communicate important messages and help them resolve difficult situations (Stewart 1997). As Stewart (1997, 888) explains, significant dreams "work on, represent and sometimes heal a distressed relation to the intractable." In this case, the intractable with which Kiria Katina grappled arose from the multiple contradictions in her existential predicament: a devout, dedicated, and loving Greek Orthodox mother who was deliberately abetting the death of her daughter—a gift from God—on the one hand; and on the other, a mother with heavy moral obligations to her living children, which in the economic hardship of the postwar years she perceived as nearly impossible to fulfill. A resolution to Kiria Katina's intractable bind is offered by the Panaghia's combined command and threat. The Panaghia's wrathful demeanor and the color of her dress further underscore the dream's message: white is a conventional symbol of life in the code of Greek dream interpretation (884). In the end, Kiria Katina's narrative poignantly illustrates the difficulty, the impossibility even, of ascertaining a woman's intention in such intractably difficult existential moments.

Infertility and Religious Healing

The Panaghia, as Kiria Katina's dream intimates, is closely associated with women's procreative concerns, and in particular with the problem of infertility. From a woman's perspective, religious healing practices were an integral part of the broader system of ethnogynecological health care available to them in their quest for a child. Women who had difficulty conceiving typically pursued a variety of practices, pragmatically combining the secular, even mechanical, logic of midwives' manipulations and their own self-administered humoral therapies with the very different logic of religious healing. A woman's quest for a child eventually enmeshed her in a multiplicity of therapeutic approaches, each premised in its own epistemological assumptions and each characterized by distinctive sets of practices. Although these various approaches could be drawn upon in combination or serially, the general outlines of what medical anthropologists refer to as a "hierarchy of resort" are discernible from women's conception stories (Romanucci-Ross 1969). This hierarchy comprised a roughly ordered series of therapeutic steps that women followed to address the inability to conceive a child. Usually, after consulting the village midwife and trying a variety of herbal therapies, women turned to the informal religious healing rituals associated with Greek Orthodoxy. A few, particularly those who lived in town, also consulted medical doctors who offered therapies derived from the continental European tradition of biomedicine that remained influential in Greece until replaced by the American variety at the end of the war (Dr. Gherasimos Rigatos, personal communication).

In the ethnography of Greece, religious healing has in fact received a good deal of attention. Up to this point, I have described secular approaches to women's health in considerable detail because, despite their great importance to women, they have been largely ignored by anthropologists. If my narration suggests compartmentalization of the two approaches, however, this would be a misreading. In Greece, as in many other parts of the world, multiple approaches to healing are often used simultaneously. Nonetheless, there persists, as Emiko Ohnuki-Tierney has pointed out, a common tendency in studies of healing to compartmentalize the religious and the secular:

> Healing at religious institutions is accorded a separate category, sometimes with the implication that it is a second-class practice whose medical efficacy must be proved before it can be admitted into the ranks of legitimate medical systems. At the other extreme, romanticism on the part of anthropologists has made religious healing the most powerful healing method. In either case, this separate treatment [of different therapeutic modalities] is unfortunate, because people use these various systems of medicine simultaneously. (1984, 123)

Ohnuki-Tierney's point, made within the context of her study of medical pluralism in Japan, is also highly pertinent to Rhodes. This chapter would thus not be complete without a discussion, however brief, of the role of religious healing in women's quest for therapy. In this concluding section, I describe various modalities of religious healing that, despite the way I present them, were in practice integrally interwoven with other approaches as women sought effective therapies for their inability to bear children.

Religious healing in Greece encompasses a wide variety of practices, ranging from supplications and promises in the form of vows made privately to holy personages, such as saints or the Panaghia, to dramatic public displays of self-sacrifice performed during pilgrimages to specialized shrines (Dubisch 1995a). Women tend to dominate the arena of religious healing, but men and women alike participate in healing rituals for the gamut of illnesses, from mouth sores to cancer (Stewart 1991, 93; 1997). Some holy personages specialize in particular conditions or body parts (St. Eleftherios for childbirth, for instance), while others, especially the Panaghia, have more general capabilities and may be called upon for all sorts of ailments. In addition, the Panaghia has her local manifestations, some of which may be specialists in particular illnesses (Dubisch 1991, 1995a).

The tiny whitewashed shrine of the Panaghia Tsambika, located atop a steep hill overlooking a stunning stretch of Rhodes's eastern coastline, is the most celebrated local example of such specialization. Built on the site of the discovery of a miraculous icon, this shrine is known to be of particular assistance to women who cannot conceive a child. Women also visited the shrine for other gynecological and obstetrical problems, such as spotting or cramping during a pregnancy. Some women went specifically to request the birth of a boy or a girl.

The shrine of the Panaghia Tsambika derives its name from the way in which its icon was discovered. In the most popular folk etymology, the name "Tsambika" comes from *tsamba*, meaning "small light" or "spark."[25] *Tsamba* is a local word whose initial *ts* sound indexes its Turkish derivation. In one variant of the story of the icon's discovery, a shepherd grazing his herd on the hill one night noticed a small light flickering in the top of a cypress tree. Afraid that it might be thieves who were preparing to rob the village below, he ran down the hill to notify the men. The next morning, the village's *palikaria*, the stalwart young men responsible for its defense, grabbed their guns and went up the hill to investigate. There, in the cypress tree, they found a small icon of the Panaghia with a light burning before it. They took the icon back to the village, but the next morning it was gone. That night, they again saw the small light in the cypress tree at the top of the hill. They went back and retrieved the icon, but the following morning the icon had disappeared and once more returned to the hill. This process was repeated a third time, until finally the villagers realized that the icon's behavior was a sign to them to build a church on the hill.

The story of the founding of the shrine to the Panaghia Tsambika belongs to a characteristically Greek genre of stories in which icons figure as protagonists. In this genre, "icons are active participants in their own discovery and in the building of the churches to house them" (Dubisch 1995a, 69). As in the Rhodian version, icons often signal their preferred location by means of a light of some sort. Characteristically, too, they are forced to clarify their intent by actively defying the alternative decisions that humans make about their destination. Often, an icon must assert itself three times before the obdurate and obtuse mortals finally grasp its true desire. In effect, the icon is the medium through which the divine personage, in this case the Panaghia, actively asserts her will. If her desires are not carried out, if the building of a church is not undertaken or if it is left incomplete, the Panaghia may mete out severe punishment in the form of illness or other calamities.[26]

As Jill Dubisch explains, shrines and churches that house such powerful icons "may embody past events . . . and mark earthly places where the power of the divine once was, in one way or another, made manifest. In this manner the sacred is localized and individualized" (1995a, 64). Because of their association with divine power, such sacralized sites become the focus and destination for supplicants who desire to petition favors of the Panaghia or the saints. In the Greek Orthodox Church, divine grace is transmitted to supplicants through the medium of icons. According to Kenna (1985, 359), the relationship between the devotee and the icon is a reciprocal one: "If the onlooker does not look at the icon and respond as a devotee, with veneration, the icon cannot act as a sacrament. Correct behavior toward an icon not only taps its power and keeps it flowing but even seems to call forth that power initially." Women who visited the Panaghia Tsambika's shrine to ask for a child, like all supplicants, venerated the icon by kissing it, lighting a candle, and making the sign of the cross. After performing this public ritual, they then made their requests in the form of a private vow. This vow, called a *tama*, encompasses the request for a desired outcome as well as the offering that will be made if, and only if, the request is granted (Dubisch 1995a, 88).

The following story told to me by Kiria Marika, a widow in her sixties, illustrates how religious healing was woven into the pursuit of a plurality of approaches to dealing with infertility.

Five years after she got married in 1951, Kiria Marika still had not conceived a child. After trying various herbal therapies, she traveled to Rhodes Town to consult the town's gynecologist, the late Dr. K., who over his half-century of practice had treated perhaps the majority of the oldest women I spoke with at some point in their lives. On her first visit, Dr. K. advised Kiria Marika to lie in the sun with her belly exposed for a half-hour each day. Sun therapy, promoted by the renowned Swiss physician Auguste Rollier in his book *Heliotherapy*, was a popular component of European biomedical therapy and "hygiene" from the 1920s onward (Littlewood 2001, 198). In fact, recreational sunbathing is still called *heliotherapia* in Greek today. After conscientiously baking her abdomen for several months with no results, Kiria Marika went back to see Dr. K. As Kiria Marika recalled that visit: "Dr. K. told me that although I might someday have a child, it was also possible that I might not." He advised her to see a specialist in Athens. Kiria Marika kept postponing the trip, however, because she was afraid the news would be bad and she would be bitterly disappointed. Finally, after more than a year and much urging from her relatives both in Rhodes and Athens, she decided to make the journey to see the specialist. Before she left, though, a woman friend persuaded her to visit the shrine of the Panaghia Tsambika and make a vow.

Accompanied by her friend for moral support, she slowly made her way up the steep hill to the tiny shrine to pay her respects to the Panaghia's miraculous icon. Like most supplicants, Kiria Marika made the climb barefoot over a path that, although today smoothly paved over with concrete, was then studded with pebbles and thorns. On her shoulders she carried a rock that she described as "twice the size of a woman's purse." As she climbed, Kiria Marika explained, "I prayed inside, *mesa mou*, to the Panaghia: 'This year I carry a rock, next year I'll carry my child.'" When she reached the shrine, Kiria Marika venerated (*proskinise*) the Panaghia's icon, as is the custom, by kissing it and making the sign of the cross. Then, as her friend had instructed her beforehand, she snipped off a piece of the wick from the oil lamp in front of the icon and swallowed it.

I was familiar with the wick-swallowing ritual, because several older women had already recommended it to me. When women learned that I had only one child, they frequently offered me practical advice, ranging from the names of fertility specialists in Athens (or, in one case, Switzerland) to directions on how to perform a proper supplication to the Panaghia Tsambika. In addition to swallowing the lamp wick, I had been advised to take a length of blue string, measure the perimeter of the Panaghia's icon with it, and wear the string around my waist until I became pregnant. When Kiria Marika also advised me to visit the shrine of Tsambika and, like her, swallow the lamp wick, I asked her how I should go about making my *tama*. "Each woman vows that which she feels," Kiria Marika explained. "A woman's desire, *lakhtara*, is very strong [for a child], but if you make the vow, you must fulfill it! If not, there might be an accident later on." Kiria Marika's voice trailed off as she obliquely, but unmistakably, warned me of the punishing wrath that the Panaghia would visit upon me if I failed to honor my vow to her.

Despite the latitude Kiria Marika gave me in deciding what to promise, the range of vows women actually made was fairly limited, and the offerings promised to the Panaghia usually touchingly humble: a name, some flowers, an inexpensive votive made of pressed tin, a candle molded into the shape of an infant. Clearly, the Panaghia does not demand extravagant offerings, only the heartfelt devotion, faith, and compliance of her votaries. Kiria Marika's vow was one of the most common made by Rhodian women: if she got pregnant, she promised the Panaghia that she would name her child after her, and that she would have the child's baptism performed at her shrine. As Kiria Marika warned me, it was essential to keep one's promise to the Panaghia exactly as it was made.

Soon after undertaking her pilgrimage to the Panaghia Tsambika, Kiria Marika was finally prepared to go to Athens to see the specialist. But before buying her ferry ticket, she waited for her period to come, because, she explained, "I didn't want to be in a strange house, washing my [menstrual] cloths—it wasn't like now with sanitary napkins!" She spent the next four months waiting, all the while afraid to go to the doctor lest she hear him say she wasn't pregnant. Only after she felt the child move inside her did she finally revisit Dr. K. As she recalled their conversation, he said to her, "*Vre* Marika, hey Marika, you're pregnant! Go make a liturgy [of thanks] to the Panaghia Faneromeni [the Madonna Revealed, a shrine on the island dedicated to another manifestation of the Panaghia]!" Kiria Marika told him she'd already made her vow to Tsambika [so her *tama* could be fulfilled only at the Panaghia Tsambika's shrine]. Then she reminded the doctor, "Remember when you told me I wouldn't get pregnant?" "Eh," he replied, "we're not gods." "No, you're not gods," she retorted, "but you shouldn't discourage people. You should say to a woman, 'You'll get pregnant,' even though she may not."

When Kiria Marika's daughter was born, she duly named her Tsambika in accordance with her vow and hired a bus to take the baptismal party to the Panaghia's church for the ceremony. Kiria Marika's name vow to the Panaghia Tsambika is such common practice that "Tsambika" for a girl and "Tsambiko" for a boy are generally recognized in Greece as Dodecanese, and more specifically, Rhodian names. Unfortunately for Rhodians, the initial *ts* sound of the name indexes its probable Turkish origin and, like other such words, it is associated with rural, substandard, and stigmatized forms of speech (Joseph 1992). For instance, one woman told me that when her young son visited relatives in Athens for the first time, a stranger, on learning that his name was Tsambiko, asked him if he was Turkish, whereupon her son became so upset he burst into tears. Because of these associations, the name is also available to outsiders for crafting some creatively Orientalizing insults. Rival sports teams visiting Rhodes for soccer matches may disparage the local team by calling them Tsambikes (the plural of Tsambiko/a), and ridicule them by saying that they are coming to play Tsambiki-stan. Such taunts are gallingly effective because they commingle and play on the name's Oriental associations, the island's eastern location, and, above all, its close proximity to Turkey.

Returning to Kiria Marika's narrative, we see reflected several aspects of ritual healing that play important roles in women's "quest for conception" (Inhorn 1994). First, as Dubisch (1991) has demonstrated in detail, pilgrimage and its associated rituals of religious healing are highly gendered practices. The overwhelming presence of women at the shrines and churches with reputations for healing infertility provides a female community of support for the supplicant. Furthermore, the rituals women perform at these specialized shrines often lie well outside the perimeter of male-dominated official church doctrine and practice, although they may be passively tolerated.[27] Swallowing wicks and tying string around one's waist are ritual practices devised by women themselves to directly access divine power in order to effect healing. Knowledge of these practices is spread among women friends and kin, who also provide emotional support by encouraging women to try them and by going along on the pilgrimage. They belong to what Anna Caraveli (1986, 170) has described more generally as a "symbolic female universe that affects in many ways female activity outside it." As importantly, as Inhorn concludes of the pursuit of ritual healing for infertility in Egypt (1994, 220; her emphasis): "The *empowering* effects of pilgrimage stand in stark contrast to women's *disempowering* encounters with physicians and hospitals." Fear and ambivalence toward physicians and the medical system are evident in Kiria Marika's story. In this case, her relationship with Dr. K. was an amiable one of long standing. In her recollection, he addressed her with the highly informal *vre*, and she also felt enough at ease to reprimand him for not offering her more hope and to advise him on how he should speak to women in the future. That Kiria Marika feared worse from the anonymous specialists with whom she had no personal relationship is apparent from her avoiding going to Athens for more than a year. Resisting Dr. K.'s advice, Kiria Marika intentionally insulated herself from the despair and hopelessness that were sure to follow a specialist's potential diagnosis of infertility. In contrast, her direct and personal appeal to the Panaghia and the rituals she decided to perform herself offered Kiria Marika a sense not only of hope, but also of active participation in her own therapy, unmediated by medical experts and their unpredictable, but potentially devastating, diagnoses.

Visits to specialized shrines are perhaps the most widely available way women unable to conceive attempted to gain access to the divine power that flows through icons, but they are not the only means of doing so. On particular religious festivals, icons were removed from their churches and loaned out to people who had petitioned to take them into their homes. With the priest's permission (rewarded with a donation), a family with a special request to make could keep the icon in their house overnight (see also Kenna 1985, 365). Such vigils in Rhodes were occasions for festive social gatherings, akin to name-day celebrations, in which hosts opened their house to all those wishing to venerate the icon, serving them tea and coffee, sweets, and *koulourakia* biscuits well into the night. Kiria Irini, another woman who had been unable to conceive a child, remembered the night some twenty years earlier when her mother hosted the icon of the Panaghia Skiadheni, another local manifestation of the Panaghia whose home was in the church of the village of Skiadhi. As word spread that this much-beloved icon was to spend the night in their house, a large number of women began to gather. Although the reason Kiria Irini's mother was hosting the icon was not made public, friends of the family could easily guess. So, at one point during the evening, Kiria Irini's friend Maryo stood to recite a *matinadha*, a rhyming couplet improvised according to certain conventional patterns (Caraveli 1985), which Kiria Irini still recalled some thirty years later:

[Panaghia Skiadheni, you who are full of grace
Give Irini two children, a girl and a boy!]

Panaghia Skiadheni, pou 'khis meghali khari,
Dhos tin Irini dhio pedhia, kori ke palikari!

Hearing this, the people in the room applauded and cheered, "Bravo, Maryo!" A skillfully composed *matinadha* is always admired and appreciated for its esthetic achievement. But a truly successful composition must also carry meaning that is relevant to the situation at hand (Caraveli 1985, 265). As Kiria Irini explained, everyone present that evening knew why her family was hosting the icon, and they cheered to second the sentiment behind the couplet as much as to celebrate Maryo's verbal agility.

Communication with the divine can also take place through dreams, as Kiria Katina's story so forcefully illustrated. The night that her family hosted the icon, Kiria Irini had such a dream. In her dream, she remembered:

> I looked at the icon of the Panaghia, and she looked back at me. "What do you want?" the icon asked me. "I want you to give me a child," I answered. The Panaghia didn't say a word, but she made a sign with two fingers, and then I awoke.

At the time, Kiria Irini interpreted the dream to mean that she would have two children. It was only when she gave birth to her son almost exactly two years later that she reinterpreted the dream and discovered its true message.

Finally, in Kiria Marika's story we also see evidence that religious healing was acknowledged and even informally integrated to some extent into Greek biomedical practice. After all, Dr. K. advised Kiria Marika to offer a liturgy to the Panaghia in thanks for her pregnancy, and she did not hesitate to disclose her vow to him. Throughout Greece, icons of the Panaghia as well as of Saint Eleftherios, the patron saint of labor and childbirth, hang on the walls of maternity hospitals. In the ob-gyn department of the Rhodes Hospital, a silver-encrusted icon of the Panaghia hangs just above the door leading from the labor room into the delivery room. Nonetheless, although the two approaches are integrated to some degree, they differed not only in their obviously distinct therapeutic logics and practices, but also, perhaps most importantly, in their locus of authority and control.

In this chapter, I have attempted to reconstruct the range of corporeal understandings and therapeutic knowledge and practices related to procreation that were available to Rhodian women in the prewar period. In doing so, I have dwelt on the secular and mechanical humoral perspective at considerable length. I hope to have also made clear that, however significant, the humoral perspective was one body of knowledge and practice among several that women had at their disposal. Religious rituals improvised and performed within the context of the Greek Orthodox Church offered additional avenues to healing, especially for the problem of infertility. And even the oldest generation of rural women had occasional contact with biomedicine, although of a continental European variety distinct in many important ways from the American-influenced model that would definitively replace it after the war. Humoral and religious (and occasionally biomedical) approaches were used serially or simultaneously, but whatever their combination, their disparate components were not regarded as problematically contradictory or dissonant. Although separate and distinct, they often drew on common themes and symbols (blood, clean/pure v. dirty/impure) while imbuing them with divergent meanings and valences. Both were part of a highly valued repertoire of healing modalities controlled largely by women, and both represented critical resources in their quests to protect or restore their health in general, and their fertility in particular. In the following chapter, I describe how these bodies of secular and religious knowledges and practices were also integral to protecting and assisting women during childbirth and the postpartum period.

Chapter 4

Pregnancy, Birth, and Postpartum Care in Prewar Rhodes

In this chapter, I describe the body of ethno-obstetrical knowledge that prevailed in rural Rhodes through the first half of the twentieth century. I devote particular attention to the figure of the village midwife, the only specialized occupation then performed exclusively by women. Although largely neglected by anthropologists and folklorists, midwives were important members of the "universe of female activity outside the realm of men" described in the previous chapter (Caraveli 1986, 169–70). Embedded in the broader village system of values and understandings, this realm also exhibited "its own variants of these, while many of the tasks, social roles, and expressive genres were gender-specific, limited only to women." Her discovery of this universe led Anna Caraveli to conclude that "narratives about female 'heroes' (worthy mothers or wives, skilled midwives or healers, talented storytellers, or craftswomen) constituted a female history of the village, a body of women's expressive genres, and a female line of transmission" (170).

Like Caraveli, other ethnographers of rural Greece (especially Danforth 1982; Seremetakis 1991) have attended to the mobilization of this "female universe" around the events and rituals of death. Women's role as gatekeepers at the cultural boundary marking the end of earthly life has thus been richly documented. But women, and midwives in particular, also commanded a specialized and culturally valued body of knowledge, also transmitted from woman to woman (usually from mother to daughter), that enabled human beings to cross the threshold into life in the first place. What is more, the midwife, in addition to being an obstetrical expert, was a specialist in the postpartum rituals that initiated the gradual incorporation of the newborn into the larger human community. Midwives were for this reason respected figures in their communities, and children "whose navel had been cut" by the midwife treated her with deference all their lives (Rigatos 1992, 31, my translation).[1]

Pregnancy: Protecting the Open Body

From both official and popular Greek Orthodox perspectives, children were seen as "sacred gifts from God." Because she bore this gift of new life, a pregnant woman was herself infused with a kind of sacred valence. She acquired this special quality, as Kiria Melpomeni explained to me, by virtue of the fact that "she is bringing a person, a soul, *mia psikhi*, into the world. Only God and woman can do this." Through her unique collaboration with the divine, a pregnant woman entered into a prolonged phase of liminality, that transitional state of suspension "betwixt and between" everyday realms of experience that was marked by its own distinctive qualities, behaviors, and expectations (V. Turner 1979). Intensifying the charged valence of a woman's liminality were the dangers inherent in the progressive "opening" of her body that was essential to the process of procreation. This "openness," triggered by pregnancy, culminating with childbirth, and requiring a full forty days afterward to reverse, increased her vulnerability to a host of hazards, both physical and spiritual. Reducing or counteracting the dangers threatening her and the new life she was bringing into being required the vigilance and cooperation of her family and kin, and ideally of the larger collectivity of which she was a part. From the moment her pregnancy was revealed, she became the object of everyday acts of solicitude that expressed a collective desire to protect her, prevent misfortune, and ensure a good outcome.

Despite its charged aura, and unlike childbirth and the postpartum period, pregnancy was not a condition that demanded the care, advice, and esoteric knowledge of specialists. It was, however, associated with an array of special behaviors on the part of the pregnant woman and those around her. Pregnant women, for example, could demand and expect special foods to satisfy their cravings. After their fifth month or so, they could sit comfortably with their legs apart (*havdha*), an immodest posture that otherwise would have provoked criticism and gossip. Conversely, if a nonpregnant woman indulged in such behavior, she might be chastised for inappropriately acting "like a pregnant woman, *kani san gastromeni*" (Chrysssanthopoulou 1984, 27–28).

From the time a woman interpreted certain bodily signs and symptoms, such as nausea, food cravings, and, above all, quickening, as pregnancy, she entered a state of liminality that made her susceptible to penetration by a host of harmful physical and spiritual forces. Like other transitional phases of the life course, pregnancy acted like a magnet for the devil and other vectors of disorder and chaos (Chrysssanthopoulou 1984, 29; Stewart 1991, 173). And like other highly desirable states and qualities, such as youth and beauty, pregnancy provoked the devil's envy and rage (Stewart 1991, 174). Kiria Melpomeni struggled to describe the spiritually charged and endangered nature of pregnancy to me:

> How can I explain it? The devil, *o exopodhotis*, is very drawn to the [pregnant] woman, *tin enkolai poli*. He's very jealous of her, all of nature is jealous, even the four walls of the house, as they say, are jealous of her, because she is bringing a person, a soul, into the world. Only God and woman can do this.

Like the devil, the malignant and capricious spirits known as the *xotika*, the "things outside," were also envious and eager to destroy the new life within the pregnant woman's body. Lurking in the liminal spaces of the community—the woods, streams, and crossroads—they waited to pounce on the weak and vulnerable. Their attacks could cause serious misfortune and horrible calamities, including miscarriage, illness, paralysis, insanity, and death. Among the *xotika* most threatening to pregnant women and infants were the neraides, called *(a)neraes* in rural Rhodes, demons that took the form of beautiful women seductively dressed in flowing white robes who destroyed their victims by dancing them to death. Less frequently mentioned, but still feared, were the *aerika*, or *iskiomata*, devious shadowlike spirits that infested the air; and the *ghelloudes*, female demons who destroyed infants and children by sucking their blood or strangling them (Hondrou 1984; see also Stewart 1991, 252).

The same desirable qualities that attracted demons also made pregnant women particularly vulnerable to the evil eye (*to kako mati*). The evil eye is a harmful force emanating from the eyes and transmitted by the gaze. It may be consciously or unconsciously triggered in a person who covets or envies the good fortune of another—her wealth, beauty, children, or material possessions (Stewart 1991, 232–34; Herzfeld 1986b). It may also be inadvertently caused by benign admiration, even on the part of those persons closest to a woman who sincerely wish her well (Campbell 1964, 339–40). A pregnant woman's exceptional susceptibility to attack may also be associated with the fact that, as Veikou (1998) found in her study of a village in northern Greece, the evil eye tends to be associated with conditions that disturb collective norms and expectations, as much by exceeding and surpassing them as by failing to meet them. Although a pregnant woman is obviously upholding the pronatalist values of her community, her condition can still be interpreted as a kind of bodily excess that clearly marks her as unusual and beyond the ordinary, and it may be for this reason too that she is especially prone to attract the evil eye.

Even if its origins are inadvertent and one's intentions benign, the harmful consequences of the evil eye are the same. Once struck, the person envied or admired may become listless and take sick; if the coveted object is inanimate—a car, for instance—it may begin to malfunction (Stewart 1991, 232). Such attacks are officially "recognized by the Church as one of the devil's weapons," and to give the evil eye is considered a sin (Campbell 1964, 337; see also Veikou 1998, 447). Victims may be treated by locally knowledgeable curers (often family members) or by the recitation of special prayers by the priest.

To forestall the harmful effects of the evil eye, and to avert blame for causing another's misfortune, people should avoid paying compliments, especially to pregnant women, babies, and children, who are known to be particularly vulnerable to attack. Or, if expressed, their admiration and praise should be thoughtfully bracketed with an apotropaic gesture. Standard prophylactic measures include formulaic spitting or making the sound of spitting ("*ftou*") three times, and uttering the ritual phrase "*na min vaskathi*" (may it not be subject to the evil eye) (Stewart 1991, 233). In Rhodes, women of the oldest generation also repeated the phrase "*pou, mashalla*" three times: *pou* in imitation of spitting, and *mashalla* from the Arabic *ma sha Allah*, literally, "whatever God wants." The pungent smell of garlic or even uttering the word "garlic" (*skordho*) also protected against the evil eye.[2] By means of such gestures, co-villagers publicly performed and actively affirmed their concern for the well-being of the person or thing admired, as they deflected suspicions of the sin of envy and of the intent to cause harm.

Another prophylactic strategy against the evil eye is concealment. Mary Lefkarites (1992, 392), who studied pregnancy and birth in rural Rhodes in the mid-1980s, reports that in the past pregnancies were routinely hidden. Given the physically compact and socially dense environment of Rhodian villages, however, concealment usually could not be maintained for very long. Even before she began to show, inquisitive co-villagers living in tight quarters were often able to read the signs of pregnancy from a woman's facial expressions and from the changes in her behavior, nausea and vomiting in particular, as in the village saying:

Na pantreftis, na gastrothis, na stravomoutsouniasis.
[You get married, you get pregnant, and your face screws up in a grimace.]

But some women told me they had never attempted to conceal their pregnancies. "Why hide it?" Kiria Toula wanted to know when I asked her. "The pregnant woman is very happy and proud. So why should she try to hide it?"

Whether or not she attempted to conceal her condition, a conscientious woman observed a host of precautions to avoid spiritual harm during pregnancy. The devil, as Greeks evocatively put it, "has many feet" (*o dhiavolos ekhi pola podhia*). In other words, demonic forces are devious and ingenious, capable of assuming many shapes and devising many ruses to tempt Christians and achieve their nefarious goals (Campbell 1964, 332–33). Fortunately, if the devil can manifest in many forms, the countervailing benevolent power of God can be accessed through an equally various array of means. At the very least, pregnant women in Rhodes protected themselves against the evil eye by always wearing objects associated with the power of Christ and the Panaghia. Most importantly, these included crosses and the phylacteries or amulets known as *filakhta*, little packets containing shards of holy relics and holy substances such as incense (see Dubisch 1995a, 94). They also pinned to their clothing a special triangular phylactery known as the Panaghia containing a verse from the Bible, some wheat, and five black sesame seeds.[3] If, in spite of all her precautions, a woman was still attacked by demonic forces, she could ask the priest to perform a kind of exorcism by reading a special blessing over her, *na tin dhiavasi*, and anointing her with holy oil (Chryssanthoupoulou 1984, 31).

In addition, women could request protection from holy personages such as the Panaghia, as well as from particular saints who were associated with good pregnancy outcomes. The Panaghia, as already noted, is intimately associated with procreation across a woman's life cycle. Accessible through prayer and certain rituals, the Panaghia could be supplicated to cure infertility, help a woman overcome problems with her pregnancy, and guide her through difficult moments in childbirth. The Orthodox saint most closed associated with pregnancy and birth is St. Eleftherios. The only private maternity in Rhodes, for example, is named for this saint. This association derives not from any thaumaturgical events of the saint's life, but from the folk etymological linkage made between his name and a woman's "liberation," *eleftheria*, from the spiritual and physical dangers of pregnancy. Pregnant women in Greece are routinely wished "*kali eleftheria*," meaning a good or easy and, above all, safe birth. Among its many names, the placenta in Rhodes was known as the *lefteri*, because it punctuated the birthing woman's final "liberation" from these life-threatening dangers. Birthing women sometimes clutched an icon of Saint Eleftherios as they labored. If the birth was a difficult one, the midwife and others present at the birth would direct their prayers to him: "*Ay' Lefteri, lefterose tin*! Saint Lefteri, liberate her!"

Associating a saint with a particular specialty on the basis of such folk, and technically false, etymology is a common Greek practice (Chryssanthopoulou 1984, 32). Thus, St. Fanourios is the patron saint of lost objects, because he reveals (*faneroni*) that which is concealed. For similar reasons, pregnant women might pray to Saint Evsthathios, to secure (*stathein*) their pregnancies, "*ghia na stathi to pei*," that is, not to miscarry. Or, they might pray to St. Simeon so that the baby would be born without blemishes (from *simion*, mark). The Forty Saints are also considered the special protectors of pregnant women, in particular from the threat of miscarriage. Their name evokes the auspicious completion of the forty-day postpartum period, the *sarantisma* (from *saranta*, forty). Pregnant women should take care to venerate all these saints and not provoke their anger by neglecting to observe their feast days (33). Through this array of intermediaries, a pregnant woman had multiple channels for accessing the sacred power of God, the ultimate benevolent force, upon which she could call for protection, support, and spiritual comfort during her time of heightened vulnerability to the equally numerous forces of harm and calamity.

Food, the Open Body, and the Social Body

Few foods were specifically prescribed or proscribed during pregnancy, and for the most part pregnant women continued to eat as they always had. The single most important dietary rule had to do with the aroma of cooking food. If a pregnant woman happened to smell food as it was being prepared (*na pari ti mirodhia*), she was strictly obligated to eat at least a bite. Failure to do so could cause something to go seriously wrong with the pregnancy. In the worst case, a miscarriage could result—a heavy enough responsibility that a pregnant woman, however reluctantly, usually felt obliged to ask, and other women duty bound to insist, that she at least sample the dish she happened to smell. Otherwise, as Kiria Toula cautioned in ominous terms that conveyed some sense of what was at stake, "*bori na pialothi i ghineka*," a woman might be swamped or overcome (a local form of the word *pelaghosi*, to be lost, as at sea). In the best of outcomes, the baby would bear a birthmark in the shape of the food not eaten (a bean or a fish, for example) on the precise spot that its mother happened to scratch after smelling it. For example, Kiria Marina, a woman from a village in western Rhodes, was born with a dark patch on one of her cheeks. This birthmark was attributed to the pancakes (*tighanites*) the next-door neighbor was frying when her mother was pregnant. Their intense aroma had aroused Kiria Marina's mother's desire, but her sense of shame, I was told, kept her from approaching her neighbor to ask for one. Even today in the villages of Rhodes, and occasionally in the city too, a pregnant women who passes by someone's kitchen, perhaps even a stranger's taverna, might be offered a bite of whatever food happens to be cooking on the stove. "*Sou mirise?* Did you smell it?" she might be asked. If she refuses, the cook will try to coax or admonish her. "If not for your self, then eat a spoonful for the baby." Tenia, a friend in her thirties, recalled her elderly neighbor's alarmed reaction when she repeatedly turned down her offer of a plate of food during her pregnancy: "*Panaghia mou, my child, kore mou! Na ekho egho tin amartia!* That I should be burdened with this sin [of the consequences]!" her neighbor implored her. Although Tenia herself considered the belief absurd, seeing the old woman so upset, she relented and took a bite.

Because the aroma of food readily escaped the confines of the kitchen and could waft through the village, a cook often felt a responsibility to seek out a pregnant woman and give her a taste of the meal she was preparing. Even if she weren't certain that a pregnant woman had actually "caught the scent," a conscientious cook took no chances and sent a small plate over to her house as a precaution. Sometimes, I was told, women returned from their chores to find several helpings of food waiting for them by the hearth. Not sharing could result in discord and gossip, but pregnant women too had to be careful not to appear to be taking advantage of the solicitude of co-villagers and abusing the system, so to speak. A woman from a village in western Rhodes described a co-villager so notorious for her habit of wandering about at mealtime, sniffing out the choicest foods, that other women began to gossip about her. To this day, now decades later, her name remains attached to this and similar ruses. "Just like Pelaghia," villagers joke, if someone is suspected of taking advantage of the system. Even though they might joke about excesses such as Pelaghia's, women expressed a strong sense of duty to offer food freely and earnestly in order to avoid the blame, even the sin (*amartia*), in the words of Tenia's neighbor, of jeopardizing this sacred gift from God.

It should be obvious by now that pregnancy activated a collective sense of responsibility for the woman and the new life she carried within. This "ethos of care," moreover, ran against the grain of the more competitive and agonistic expectations that characterized many ordinary social relations, most notably exemplified by the logic of the evil eye.[4] Seremetakis has also described what she calls "an ethic of care" thematic of the death laments sung by women in Inner Mani. As she observes, there are many precise parallels in the symbolism and practices associated with birth and death in rural Greece. Both, she suggests, can be symmetrically conceived of as passages, the first from "the outside to the inside," and the second from "the inside to the outside" (1991, 68). In their laments, Maniat women deploy the imagery of shared substance (blood, food) to create and prolong a sense of affective community of the dead with the living. As Seremetakis also observes, this nonagonistic female ethic runs counter to and complements the competitive, hierarchical male modes of exchange that dominate the larger society (88). Whether due to the matrifocal and endogamous nature of rural Rhodian society, which usually ensured that a woman was surrounded by her close male and female kin, or to the specific, highly positive valences of pregnancy and birth, the ethos of care in Ermia and other villages did not appear to be confined exclusively to women. Women's food sharing was perhaps the most concrete manifestation of the ethos of care activated by pregnancy, but everyday gestures of support and protection were also expected of men, and particularly of husbands.

Underlying all these gestures was an implicit understanding of the pregnant body as one whose boundaries were diffuse, permeable, and thus exquisitely responsive to the thoughts and actions of others. From this point of view, one that anthropologists usually label a "sociocentric" or "relational" model of the person, the pregnant body can be seen as representing "a locus of shared relationships" (Lieber 1990, 74). The example of rural Rhodes reveals that certain bodies may also fluctuate and vary in their degree of relationality over the course of the life cycle. As we have seen, a healthy woman's body regularly alternated between open and closed states. During pregnancy and childbirth, a woman's openness, and hence her permeability and responsiveness to the actions and intentions of both human and supernatural others, reached its peak. For this reason, villagers also stepped up their performance of protective behaviors and gestures at such times, both to indicate their support and to forestall suspicion of harmful desires.

In rural Rhodes, the sensory modalities of taste, smell, hearing, and vision were the most salient vectors connecting the pregnant woman to others in the community. They were vehicles that could transmit and trigger positive or negative effects, and thus could work either to safeguard or jeopardize her pregnancy. For this reason, they required continuous, self-conscious monitoring on the part of others. As a woman's bodily openness and permeability increased over the course of pregnancy, she became ever more susceptible to penetration by the evil eye that emanated from an admiring or covetous gaze. And she became extremely vulnerable to the aromas that issued from their kitchens. Co-villagers gave ongoing demonstrations of their concern for, and solidarity with, a woman and the new life she carried by assiduously uttering apotropaic formulas in her presence and by conscientiously sharing their food. In short, they joined with her in a collective responsibility for the well-being of her body and the outcome of her pregnancy.

Miðwifery anð Birth

Into the middle of the twentieth century, every village on the island and every neighborhood in Rhodes Town had at least one practical midwife, the mammi. Some of the larger villages such as Ermia might even have had two or three at any given moment from which a woman could choose. The mammi represented a critical cultural resource for women on a number of counts. First, she commanded a corpus of specialized knowledge and technical practices that equipped her to deal with both normal and potentially life-threatening difficult births (*dhiskoles ghenes*), such as breech presentations. Second, she was a specialist in postpartum care, visiting the new mother and her infant every day for a week or so after the birth. During these visits, she examined the mother, bathed and changed the infant, inspected its navel, washed its soiled clothes, and sometimes washed the dishes and cleaned the house as well. Finally, she played an integral role in the cascade of postpartum rituals that incrementally incorporated the infant into the community of Orthodox Christian persons. Clearly, the mammi performed a much broader array of services than those associated today with the professionally trained midwife. Thus, glossing the word "mammi" as "midwife," as I have done until now, is somewhat misleading. Modern Greek in fact clearly discriminates between the two. In Greek, the homely demotic word "mammi," which is almost identical to the colloquial word for "grandmother," is used to refer to the practical or unschooled midwife, while "*maia*," derived from the more prestigious Ancient Greek, refers to the professionally trained and certified midwife.

Kiria Vaso, the daughter of the late Kiria Arghiro, one of Ermia's most highly respected mammis, recalled how, day or night, if called to attend a birth, her mother would drop her chores, or leave her bed and her children, hasten to the woman's house, and not return for hours. Witnessing these sacrifices, Kiria Vaso told me that, although she had learned a great deal about birth from her mother, she herself had never wanted to follow in her footsteps. Nonetheless, as she described her mother's life, it was also obvious that she was proud of her work and of the esteem in which she was held in the community. Like most mammis, Kiria Arghiro had learned midwifery from her mother. However, she herself did not begin to practice until her husband was killed in an accident at work and she was left a widow with four young children to raise. Eventually, she also became Ermia's only bonesetter, learning on her own how to mend broken bones with splints made of bamboo and casts molded from the pine resin paste she ground herself in her stone mortar and pestle. Her skills at both midwifery and bone setting were widely appreciated not only in Ermia—attested by the fact that hers is the only photograph on display in Ermia's museum—but in neighboring villages as well. All the while, Kiria Arghiro continued to work in her fields, vineyards, and olive groves to meet the subsistence needs of her family.

Given her intimate role in helping to bring forth God's "gift of life," the mammi's work was considered sacred. It was a vocation undertaken, as Kiria Vaso explained of her mother, *ghia tin psikhi tis*, as a good deed and act of charity "for the sake of her soul," not a job to be done in exchange for money (as was the case generally in Greece [Chyssanthopoulou 1984, 41; Rigatos 1992]). A mammi's services were thus never directly compensated with cash, which was in scarce supply in any event—in Ermia, eggs often served as the unit of currency until after the war. Women and their families showed their gratitude by giving the mammi a sack of wheat or some produce from the family's garden. "You gave whatever you had," people explained. The mammi did receive a few small coins, but always in the context of certain postpartum rituals, described later. During her visits in the week after the birth, she was honored with special meals prepared from the choicest foods a family could afford—meat, normally eaten but once a month and on feast days, or perhaps some fish brought up from Lindos a few kilometers down the coast. These meals would be especially lavish if the baby turned out to be a firstborn boy or, if a family already had a couple of sons, an earnestly desired daughter. A few months later, at the baby's baptism, the family gave the mammi a special gift, usually a dress or a pair of shoes.

A pregnant woman typically worked in the fields or at home until the moment she was "caught by the pains" (*tin epiasan i poni*), that is, until she began to feel her contractions. When called for, the mammi made her way to the woman's house as soon as she could and stayed with her throughout the birth. Which mammi was sent for depended on the networks of relatedness linking the families of the midwife and the birthing woman. Not all mammis were remembered with equal respect and warmth. One, in particular, was said to yell and swear and blaspheme when encountering difficulties with the birth, behaviors that, even decades later, some women remembered as distasteful and even frightening. Nevertheless, if a woman were closely related to this particular midwife, she had little choice but to call for her assistance.

The first thing the mammi did when she arrived at a birthing woman's house was say a prayer and make the sign of the cross. Kiria Maria, a mammi from another village, described how, after praying, she washed her hands with alcohol, a practice she had learned from an Italian professional midwife and had afterward always insisted on: "*Kathariotita*, cleanliness, above all!" Next, she proceeded to examine the woman by palpating her abdomen and inserting her middle finger into the woman's vagina to help her determine the extent of dilation and the position of the baby. A woman from another village remembered with a chuckle how, after examining her in this way, the mammi decided that she had been called too early. "'You're not ready,' she told me. 'Go whitewash your house, and when you're done, I'll be back to help you.'" If the mammi determined that a woman's time was in fact near, she set to work, lighting the fire and putting water on to boil to have ready to wash both infant and mother after the birth.

If her examination revealed that the baby was not presenting in the normal headfirst position, the mammi tried both internal and external techniques to turn it. Kiria Maria told me the story one of these "difficult births," *dhiskoles ghenes*, as she called them:

> I remember one birth: it was night and they didn't call me early. I came and I felt her stomach with my hands, and then I put my middle finger inside: the baby was not in its position, *sti thesi tou* [that is, headfirst]. Nor could I find its feet. So, I took her and I put her on a blanket, and I told her husband and her mother to hold onto the edges. And then we tossed her in the air several times. And this turned the baby just enough. I wrapped my finger in a corner of the white apron I always wore—I wrapped it because the baby is slippery and it would slip out of my grip— and I put my finger in again. And this time I found a little leg, and I put in another finger, and found another little leg. And then slowly, and little by little, *sigha-sigha*, I turned the baby, and brought the bottom around first. And I kept my two fingers inside, on either side, to keep the vagina [*colpo*] open wide, so that the child wouldn't suffocate. . . . Birth is a big responsibility! *I ghena ine meghali efthini!*

In this birth, Kiria Maria used the technique of blanket tossing to turn the infant just enough so that she could find a foot to grasp and maneuver it into a bottom-first position. Shaking or tossing, a technique advocated in the Hippocratic corpus and practiced in ancient Greece, persisted as a method for turning babies in parts of Western Europe well into the nineteenth century.[5] In another instance, an Ermiot woman related how her mammi, after feeling her abdomen and determining that the baby was not in position, had her lie on a blanket and told her relatives to shake her gently and repeatedly. In this case, the shaking was enough to fully turn the baby, and it was born headfirst. In the "difficult birth" Kiria Maria described, it was necessary to further turn the baby by its feet, a technique known as "internal podalic version." Described by some physicians today as "a lost art" (it has been largely replaced by the caesarean section), internal podalic version was a technique first advocated (in print) by Soranus in his enduringly influential *Gynecology* (Porter 1997, 72), the classic second-century obstetrical text that was copied, plagiarized, and poached by countless authors throughout Europe and elsewhere well into the early modern period.[6]

One of the mammi's major goals during labor and birth was to promote the "opening" of the woman's body. As Kiria Maria explained:

> The womb has elasticity, and it opens. If it opens even more, the child comes along slowly, *sigha-sigha*, and it comes just fine that way, *erkhete mia khara etsi.*

Mammis used techniques such as massaging the perineum with olive oil to soothe the birthing woman, as well as to help her achieve an optimal state of "openness" essential for a successful birth. Openness was also sympathetically invoked by always leaving the windows and doors of the house slightly open during the birth. On her part, the birthing woman also symbolically unfettered herself by taking off her earrings and rings. In other regions of Greece, husbands removed their clothes, unbuttoned their shirts, loosened their belts, or took off their shoes for the same purpose (Chryssanthopoulou 1984, 38).

Kiria Maria's tools, she told me, were her hands and a pair of scissors. The scissors, she pointedly informed me, were strictly for cutting the umbilical cord. They were never used to cut the woman's perineum, although Kiria Maria was well aware that such cutting was common practice among doctors. Clearly and self-consciously distinguishing her approach from theirs, she explained that when she assisted a birthing woman, she was determined

> not to tear her up, *na min tin kseskiso*, the way the doctors did. The doctors, they cut with the scissors right away. No. When the pain was strong, when the baby was crowning, I would use my two middle fingers to help (you can't do it all just with your hands) to widen it [the vagina].

Saying this, Kiria Maria held up her two middle fingers, now thickened and permanently bent in their arthritic joints. Making slow, deliberate circles in the air, she showed me how she had once used them to stretch the vaginal opening by massaging the vulva. Also to prevent tearing, she rubbed the woman's perineum with a little olive oil. By means of these techniques, Kiria Maria claimed that the women she attended had never torn when giving birth.

Mary Lefkarites, who was able to interview several Rhodian mammis in the 1980s, corroborates Kiria Maria's claims—as well as her attitude:

> Tearing was rare among the women I interviewed. In fact, midwives took pride in relating to me their skill in assisting births without tearing. The practices of using soap or oil around the perineum, pinching the perineum at the time of birth as well as being patient during labor were viewed as measures for preventing the tearing of the tissue. (1992, 394)

Avoidance of tearing was confirmed too by the many birth stories told to me by Ermiot women. Describing her own births some thirty years ago, Kiria Sterghoula recalled her mammi using procedures identical to those described by Kiria Maria:

> She put a little olive oil on her hands, and she massaged my belly, which was a comfort. Then she massaged me down below [indicating a circular motion with her middle fingers exactly like the gesture Kiria Maria had made]. It felt like honey, honey, *meli, meli*, when she did that; you felt such a relief![7]

If a woman's womb was opening too slowly despite all her efforts, the mammi turned to the flower known as *tis Panaghias to louloudhi*. A species of germander (Teucrium polium), the Panaghia's flower was also called *tis Panaghias to kheri*, the Panaghia's hand. This flower, it was said, was brought to the island from the Holy Land by pilgrims returning from Jerusalem. In a practice found in other parts of Greece, and elsewhere in Europe (Chryssanthopoulou 1984, 42; Gelis 1991, 117; Rigatos 1999, 60), the mammi put the Panaghia's flower in a glass of water and gave it to the woman to hold. Even if the flower was very dry, its desiccated petals would gradually revive and unfurl, until finally, fully extended, it resembled an open hand. As the Panaghia's flower gradually opened, so too would the woman's womb sympathetically follow and eventually "open."[8]

Women gave birth in the corner of the house known as the *ghonia*, which according to the uniform Rhodian plan was always located on the right-hand side as one faced the door. The hub of the family's daytime activities, the *ghonia* consisted of the fireplace and hearth and the built-in storage platform, called the *panga*, that enclosed both. Raised about a foot and a half above the ground, the *panga* was the warmest spot in the house, made more snug and inviting still by the bright woolen rugs, woven by the women of the family, that draped and cushioned its hard surface (Fig. 6). Birth never took place

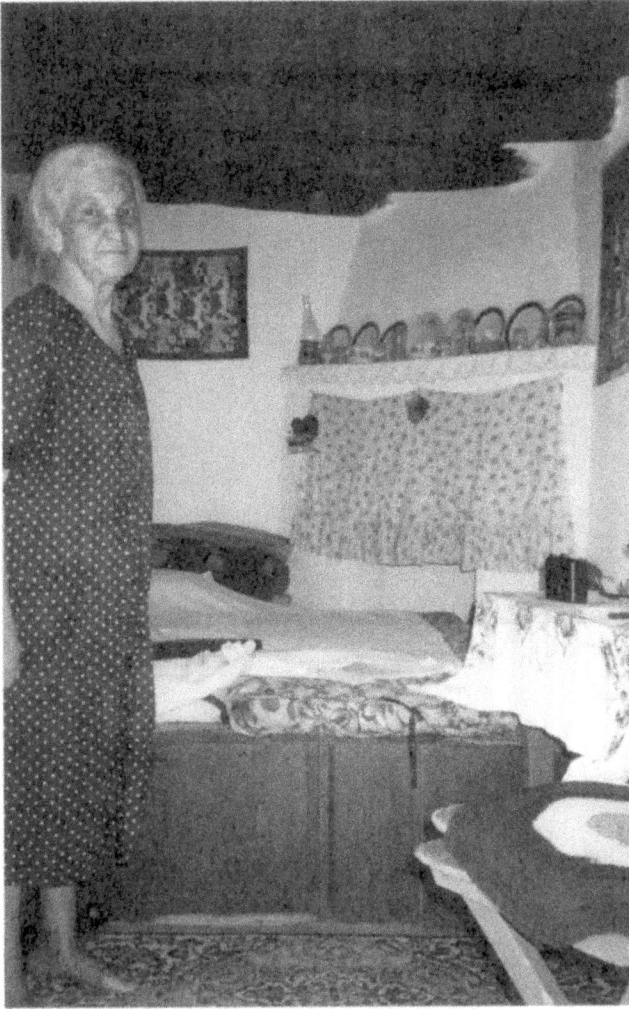

6. *Panga* and corner hearth in Kiria Vaso's house.

on the couple's bed, which was located in the rear half of the house. Because the marital bed was considered sacred (*iero*), contamination through contact with the bloody lochia and other ritually unclean fluids of birth was strictly avoided.

A woman usually gave birth in a sitting or semi-reclining position, her legs sometimes draped over the edge of the *panga*. She was always held and supported from behind, usually by another woman, who was formally known as the *nefrou* (from *nefro*, kidney). Occasionally, her husband filled this role. Some mammis carried birthing stools with them. These *seli*, as they were called, looked like regular chairs without the woven straw seat.[9] In rural Rhodian houses, the raised *panga* automatically conferred the advantages of height, the assistance of gravity, and greater visibility for the mammi. Occasionally, a woman might kneel while giving birth. Kiria Maria, though, told me that she

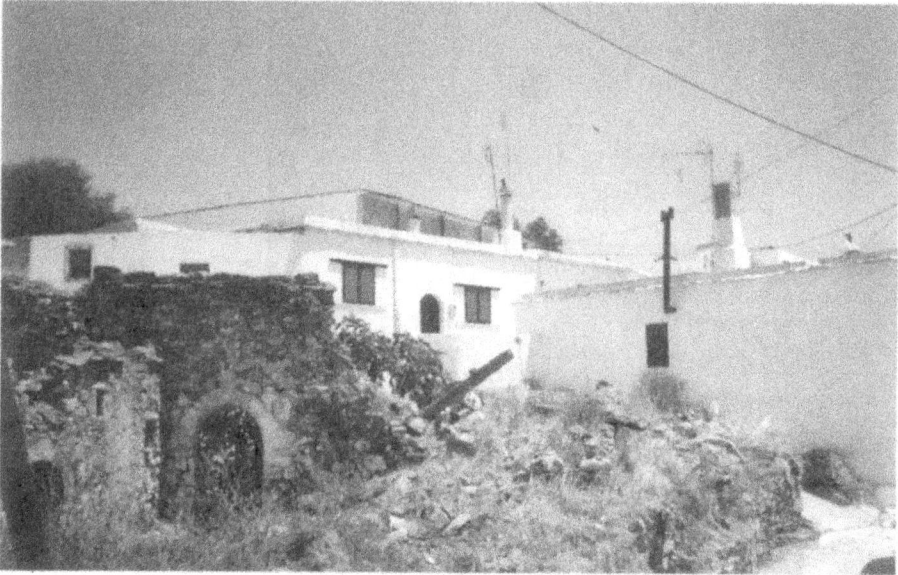

7. Ruin of an old Ermiot house, featuring typical entrance arch.

discouraged women from kneeling because she believed this position made tearing of the perineum more likely.

When the time came to push the baby out, a rope was tied to one of the iron bars that used to protect the windows of every village house. Now obsolete, these bars can still be seen on the ruined houses that lie in crumpled heaps throughout Ermia (Fig. 7). In the past, they were indispensable for keeping out thieves and other intruders while people were away working in their fields all day, or even for weeks during the wheat harvest. "*Nangase!* Bear down!" the mammi would order when it was time to push, and the birthing woman pulled on the rope to help her exert more pressure. If, as her labor wore on, a woman became too exhausted to push, the mammi cajoled her, massaged her back, or put some of her hair in her mouth to make her gag and thereby cause her to automatically contract her abdominal muscles. Sometimes, she might even give her a slap.

Although birth always occurred within the protected enclosure of a woman's house, it was not a particularly private event. Those present varied according to circumstances and the desires of the woman but always included her mother, if she were alive, and possibly her mother-in-law and other close female relatives. In some Rhodian villages, women who had given birth easily in the past were invited to attend, while those who had experienced difficult births were excluded. If word spread that the birthing woman was having difficulties, other women from the village gathered in front of the door of her house and prayed, led by a literate woman (*gramatizoumeni*) who read verses from the Bible (Hondrou 1984, 5).

A birthing woman's husband might also be present if she so desired, a fact that surprised some of the young Rhodians I knew who had sometimes had to struggle to convince their doctors to allow their husbands into the delivery room.[10] Unlike these younger women, for whom a husband's presence was usually appreciated and desired, older women's preferences varied considerably. For some, like Kiria Athena, it was largely a matter of indifference. Her husband, Kirios Ghianis, an Ermiot man now in his eighties, had stayed with her throughout the births of their first two children. He recalled the anxiety and concern he had felt at the time. "When she suffered, we suffered too, we worried about the birth, why it was taking so long." Touched by his comments, I turned to his wife, Kiria Athena, and asked how she had felt about having him with her. Did that comfort her? "Having him there, not having him there, it didn't make any difference, *to idhio itane*," she said, laughing heartily. "*We* were hurting! They don't give birth, they don't hurt, *we* hurt! The comfort you feel comes *after* you give birth; when the child falls, slides from your womb, such a sweetness, *mia ghlika*, you feel when the child comes, you can't imagine."

Kiria Fotini, in contrast, recounted how having her husband with her all through her long and difficult labor had helped her when she most needed encouragement. At one point, when her strength was seriously flagging, he even began to recite *matinadhes*, the rhymed couplets described in the previous chapter, in an effort to revive and support her. I mentioned this story to Kiria Maria and asked if she had ever heard a man compose a *matinadha* for his wife during birth. "No, never," she snapped in her characteristically curt way. A moment later, though, a slight smile twisted the corners of her lips. "Eh," she added in a softer tone, "he must have loved her very much."

One Ermiot woman, Kiria Sofia, could still recite by heart the *matinadhes* her late husband Ghiorghos had written to her when she was pregnant some forty years earlier. Working at the time as a guest worker in a Swiss factory, Ghiorghos was unable to return to the village in time for the birth. In a letter he sent his wife in her last month of pregnancy, Ghiorghos composed these verses to humorously complain:

Sofia mou, kamia fora sto grama sou,
mou 'vales ke traghoudhia
    Tora vlepo, Sofia mou,
pou khathikansi oula.

[Sofia dear, in your letters
you used to write me poems.
        Now I see, Sofia dear,
all that is lost and gone.]

To which his wife responded with her own verse,

Kamia fora sto grama mou,
sou 'vaza ke traghoudhia
        A' tora m'epiase, Ghiorgho mou,
tis ghenas i afouria.

[Once, in my letter
I did send you some poems.
        But now I'm full, dear Ghiorgho,
of fear and worry over birth.]

Picking up on his wife's fears in his next letter, Ghiorghos offered her encouragement with this reference to Queen Frederika, wife of King Paul, who reigned over Greece at that time:

Ti ghena min tin fovithis,
k'ekhe kardhia Sofia.
        Ghiati ke i Vasilisa
ekane pedhia tria!

[Don't be afraid of birth,
and take courage, Sofia.
        Because even the Queen
gave birth to children three!]

When I asked the oldest Ermiot women to recall the role that the mammi had played in their births, the first thing they usually mentioned was the encouragement and support she provided. A woman who had birthed her first child at home with the mammi and her second in the hospital in Rhodes explained why she decided to return to the mammi for her third: "She stayed with us, she helped us, she encouraged us." And another woman remembered appreciatively, "'Soon, soon,' the mammi would say to me, 'it's coming soon, it won't be long now before you're liberated,' and that helped me a lot." Clearly, the encouragement and continuous support she provided were deeply valued dimensions of the mammi's services.

Individual midwives had their own personal styles, however, and not all were equally appreciated. Ermiot women who had been assisted by Kiria Arghiro warmly recalled her kindness and support. But another mammi was less fondly remembered. One woman in her seventies recalled how this mammi had given her a hard slap on the back to get her to push when all her strength seemed to be gone. Another remembered how this same midwife had thrown a slipper at her when she told her that she could no longer push. If all mammis were remembered with gratitude, it is nonetheless also true that each had her individual style that was variously appreciated, even if sometimes a woman's social ties bound her to a particular mammi when she would have preferred another. I make this rather obvious observation because the figure of the village midwife has perhaps been idealized in some of its recent representations. To avoid such "undue romancing" (Jolly 1998, 15) and to respect the messy variability of women's experiences, it is worth pointing out that, like biomedical practitioners, practical midwives might vary not only in the level of their skills and knowledge, but also in their bedside manner.

Along with their continuous presence and support during birth, mammis also were respected and appreciated for their skill and knowledge. Rhodian women of the oldest generation often favorably compared them to doctors. Of course, before the war, most women in rural areas simply did not have the option of giving birth in the hospital in Rhodes, which was mainly used by those who lived in the city and by a few of the wealthiest villagers. In any event, at that time the hospital was typically regarded as a place of death rather than an appropriate place to give birth. Doctors were summoned only if something went horribly wrong with a birth; by that time, a bad outcome was usually a foregone conclusion. A woman interviewed by Mary Lefkarites explained why she refused to give birth in the hospital in 1939:

> Some were going [to the hospital]. I was afraid to go because I thought that I would die [there]. If you heard the word "hospital," you would say to yourself that you would die [there]. You preferred your home. (1992, 394)

But even if a doctor was locally available, women generally preferred to give birth in their houses with the mammi's help. On occasion, this situation led to friction and conflict between doctors and midwives, as in the following story told to me by Kiria Maria. Toward the end of Kiria Maria's long career as a mammi, a young pathologist was stationed in her village to complete his obligatory rural service. When Kiria Maria helped deliver a severely malformed infant that died a few hours later, the doctor filed a formal complaint against her. Despite the support she received from the baby's parents, who refused involvement in the case, she was punished with a large fine for practicing without a license. Her son paid the fine, and Kiria Maria retired soon thereafter.

The variety of women's encounters with midwives may help account for their subsequent preferences with respect to where, and with whom, to give birth. Most women who had given birth to one child with a doctor and to another with the village mammi said they preferred the latter. When some of these women had a third child, they usually chose to stay in the village and birth with the midwife. Mary Lefkarites (1992, 399) found that the majority (eight out of eleven) of the women she interviewed who had experienced both settings also preferred birthing at home. But not all women felt this way. For instance, Kiria Athena, who had birthed her first child with a doctor in Rhodes and her other two with the slipper-throwing mammi in Ermia had no preference: "*To idhio itane,* the pains are the same," she said. In such instances, it may be that a woman's problematic experience with the mammi influenced her decision to subsequently give birth with a doctor, just as the opposite could, and often did, occur.

The old women with whom I spoke in Ermia could not recall a single mother or baby who had died in childbirth. Although such a perfect record is unlikely, it is no doubt the case that most births did have successful outcomes. Kiria Maria claimed that she herself had never lost a mother, and only a single infant (the one that was born severely malformed), although she did know of *other* mammis who had lost both. Almost certainly, there is an element of selective recall, along with perhaps a measure of "undue romancing" of the past, in the villagers' recollections. Almost as certainly, I believe, they also point to the practical skills of the mammi and of the high esteem in which she was held.[11]

Afterbirth

Delivery of the placenta was generally regarded as the most dangerous part of birth. The placenta was known by a number of names. It was called the *istero* or *akoloutho,* the "after" [birth]; the *lefteri,* because it marked the final "liberation" of the woman; as well as the *dhefteri,* or "second," because it was considered a "second birth" (as in the obsolete English and French word "secundine"). To help expel the placenta, the mammi massaged the umbilical cord between her thumb and forefinger, often to the accompaniment of prayers uttered softly to the Panaghia, Saint Eleftherios, and perhaps her own personal patron saint as well. Once delivered, the placenta was closely inspected and its spots counted to prognosticate the total number of children the couple would eventually have.[12] It was then disposed of with care, although without particular ceremony, in an out-of-the-way place where no one was likely to tread, usually buried in a corner of the village ossuary. Careful disposal was also important to prevent animals, especially dogs, who were associated with the devil, from finding and devouring it—an evil omen indeed (as Chyssanthopoulou [1984, 46] reports for other parts of Greece as well; see also Delaney 1991, 64, for rural Turkey; and Gelis 1991, 167, for France).

The umbilical cord was never severed before the placenta had been fully expelled. After the cord stopped pulsating, the mammi cut it with her scissors or a knife about two or three inches from the navel, then snugly tied the stump with sewing thread seven times with seven knots, using ordinary cotton thread for most families, silk thread for the richest. Kiria Maria, for whom cleanliness was a point of pride, told me that she always sterilized her scissors with alcohol. Other mammis used ouzo or the locally distilled spirit, *tsipouro*. The baby's end of the cord was washed in wine and smeared with a paste made from soot or burnt grain mixed with oil.[13] The naked baby was placed on the ground for a few minutes so that its body would become strong (*gherokomo*) and its flesh firm (*na sfiksi to kreas tou*). If the baby needed resuscitating, the mammi vigorously massaged its body with a brush or placed it alternately in hot and cold water (Lefkarites 1992, 395). An Ermiot man in his eighties recalled how, when his last son was "born in a faint," the mammi plunged him back and forth between the pots of hot and cold water and "the baby woke with a start and began to cry."

Once the infant was taken care of, the mammi turned her attention to the woman. After washing her off, the mammi wrapped her abdomen with a long cloth made from two kerchiefs knotted together. This binding, worn throughout the postpartum period, was intended to help a woman's womb return to its former shape and place. Although Rhodian women did not describe it as such, this abdominal encircling can also be interpreted as promoting the process of uterine closure.

Finally, the birth concluded with the ritual known as "the salting of the baby" (*to alatisma tou morou*). After the mammi wiped the infant clean, she rubbed salt all over its body. The salt-encrusted baby was then ceremoniously given its first bath, called the *loutro* or the *lousimo*, in a new ceramic basin that had been exclusively reserved for this purpose. In nineteenth-century Rhodes, warm wine scented with bay leaves was used instead of soap and water (Rodd

1892, 107). The close relatives who had gathered for the salting ritual then took turns throwing coins into the basin. When the bath was finished, the salted water (*to apolousma tou pei*) was disposed of with the same care that had been shown to the placenta. The mammi usually tossed it into a corner of the ossuary or another out-of-the-way place. The coins were hers to keep.

The salting ritual was practiced throughout Greece, though elsewhere it often took place on the first or third day after the birth.[14] Salting was a practice advocated by Soranus in the section of his *Gynecology* entitled "On the Care of Infants" to ensure that "the surface [of the baby's body] be hardened and rendered immune to the development of rashes" (Temkin 1991, 83). Following a similar logic, in rural Rhodes too, salt was said to "cure" the baby's skin, in the manner of meat cured with salt for preservation, and thus helped prevent rashes and other skin disorders. But the salting ritual had other objectives as well: it ensured the development of good sense and a logical mind, and the apotropaic qualities of salt repelled the devil and other demonic forces (Campbell 1964, 334). As the folklorist Vassiliki Chryssanthopoulou explains, salt has highly positive meanings and powers across many domains of Greek culture:

> If added to food, salt improves taste; food without salt is considered not tasty and judged negatively. Applying a culinary metaphor, Greek people characterize the behavior of individuals in terms of the positive associations of salt. A reasonable or clever person is said to "say tasty things" (*leei nostima pragmata*), while a foolish person is described as "not tasty" (*anostos*) . . . [and] "without salt" (*analatos*). Phrases such as "You are completely untasty, you have not got any salt on you" (*Mpit analatos eisai*), or the question "Has the midwife not salted you?" (*Then s'alatise y mammi?*), are applied to people who are considered to be rather foolish. (1984, 69)

Salt is also a symbol of community and social solidarity. "Sharing salt" implies a common bond between individuals, and close friends are said to "share bread and salt" (*faghane psomi ke alati*) (70). By salting the infant, the mammi played a crucial role in setting it on its trajectory toward its domestication and social incorporation. In short, salting simultaneously protected the child from spiritual harm, toughened its tender body, and instilled its mind with good sense, and ultimately drew it into the circle of human sociality.[15]

After concluding the ritual of salting and the baby's first bath, the mammi turned to the more mundane care of the infant's body. She squeezed a few drops of lemon juice into its eyes to cleanse them and prevent the formation of mucus and mucus crusts. Then, using three layers of cloth, she began wrapping and swaddling the infant. The first cloth was a small triangle that covered the baby's loins in the manner of a diaper. Poor families made these from scraps of old clothes; the wealthiest used soft cotton embroidered with blue thread to protect against the evil eye. For boys, the inner cloth was also important in firmly binding the scrotum, which was typically enlarged after birth, to help reduce it to a more appropriate size and also to prevent a hernia if the baby bore down too hard when crying. Two other cloths wrapped the infant's entire body, except for the head. Finally, the infant was swaddled in the *pentaria*, a strip of narrow cloth about a meter in length. The *pentaria* was so called, I was told, because it was the width of five (*pente*) fingers.[16] The spiraling coil of cloth wrapped first the baby's upper torso, then its arms, and finally its legs. The *pentaria* ended in an even narrower strip about an inch in width, which was bound around the infant's feet to complete the swaddling process (*faski-oma*). Finally, a specially embroidered cloth cap, the *peretthitsa*, was snugly pulled over the baby's head and ears. This done, the mammi handed the compact and immobilized little bundle to its mother. The birth then formally concluded with the *sarantonia*, a purification ritual that was exclusively the mammi's. The mammi took a glass of water given to her by one of the women who had been present at the birth and used it to slowly wash her hands, reciting the Kyrie Eleison prayer forty times as she did so. When she finished, she thanked God for allowing her to receive a new life in her hands and finally went home.

Care of the New Infant

The mother's role in shaping and giving substance to the infant's body did not end at birth. Mothers followed a rigorous regime of daily practices that were regarded as necessary to the proper physical and esthetic formation of their children. From its ears to its feet, the infant's body was the focus of minute attention and intense concern. To promote the straight growth of her baby's nose, a mother massaged it frequently between her thumb and index finger in a downward motion. To prevent furrows, she regularly smoothed the baby's brow. To keep one side of its head from becoming flatter than the other, she turned her infant, who was essentially immobilized by swaddling, at least twice a day and after each nighttime feeding. To strengthen the baby's neck, the new mother regularly drank a special soup made from roosters. Swaddling was supposed to help develop straight legs, although more than one woman skeptically observed that her child had turned out bowlegged, nonetheless. For a well-shaped head (*na kami to pei kalo kefali*), as well as to prevent colds, the baby wore the *peretthitsa* cap continuously for at least the first two months. The baby's ears were always tucked securely under the cap to prevent them from sticking out later on. Whenever the baby was undressed or given a bath, its limbs were always tugged and stretched according to a standard formula to help them develop properly. Each leg or arm was first vigorously pulled and then crossed over to touch the opposite leg or arm. A similar regime of stretches has been described by Delaney for rural Turkey, and detailed instructions can also be found in Soranus's "On the Care of the Newborn." For example, Soranus advised that the infant's limbs be stretched to touch the opposite side of the body, and that its nose be massaged each day to make it "comely" (Temkin 1991, 105–7).

To treat or prevent rashes, babies were dusted with a powder made from roasted white bay leaves that had been pounded to a fine, silky consistency. Sprinkled on a baby's genitals, underarms, and neck, this made for a redolent infant whose recollection often brought a smile to the faces of old women when they described the practice. "*Ke moskovolouse to pei*! And the baby smelled wonderful!"[17]

Infants were not nursed immediately after birth. The colostrum (*tsiro*), the clear, nutritious fluid that precedes the first flow of milk, was always expressed and discarded. Perhaps because of its transitional status or its anomalous color and appearance, colostrum had an ambiguous valence that led to its avoidance. According to Soranus, it was an unwholesome substance produced by "bodies which are in a bad state" after the agitation of birth (Temkin 1991, 89). He advised that it be discarded, and avoidance of colostrum is still common in many parts of the world influenced by Greco-Islamic medicine (Delaney 2000; Dixon 1992; Laderman 1983; Manderson 1998; Van Hollen 2003). Like the other bodily products of birth, the colostrum was carefully deposited in the ossuary or another out-of-the-way place. Breast milk, in contrast, was regarded as a pure and even quasi-sacred substance. Throughout rural Greece, for example, it was until recently used to cure eye ailments of all sorts (Blum and Blum 1965, 87). Until its mother's milk came in, the infant was spoon-fed chamomile tea. Chamomile also helped the baby expel the meconium (*pises*), its first dark, sticky stools, and clear the phlegm from its throat. Although the infant was a highly desirable, even quasi-sacred presence, these effluvia were regarded as dirty. Their complete elimination was necessary to cleanse the infant before nursing could begin (Chryssanthopoulou 1984, 60). Chamomile tea also occasionally was fed to the baby afterward as well, especially if it had a stomach problem.

Infants drank only their mothers' milk for the first five or six months. At that time, mothers introduced the weaning food known as *alevria*, a pap made from toasted wheat flour, butter, sugar, and water. Infants also were given pacifiers consisting of a cloth bundle into which a bit of sugar had been folded. They were nursed for at least a year, often for two, and some continued until they went to school. The connection between nursing and sterility was widely known, even if it was also acknowledged to provide a not entirely reliable method of avoiding pregnancy.

Postpartum Care of the Lekhona

The postpartum was the most richly elaborated period of a woman's procreative experience. From the moment she gave birth, and for next forty days, the new mother existed in a highly charged and vulnerable state of liminality. During this time, she was known as the *lekhona*—or *lekhousa*, in village parlance—a term derived from the ancient Greek word for bed, *lekhos*.[18] This term is still routinely used by Greek doctors today to refer to a woman over the course of the puerperium. Puerperium is the biomedical term for the six-week period during which the uterus returns (more or less) to its pre-pregnancy size that, interestingly enough, overlaps almost precisely with the forty-day postpartum period of the past.

In this section, I describe the physical care of the lekhona and her infant, and the ethnomedical practices that were observed to prevent illness, regain health, and promote healing after birth. In the following section, I describe the ritual practices that were equally integral to the safe negotiation of this highly charged phase of the life cycle. In practice, many of the central and most distinctive symbols, metaphors, and practices associated with the postpartum period were notably hybrid, simultaneously combining secular and ritual meanings. For instance, the lekhona's "open" state referred to the anatomical openness of her womb, which made her exquisitely vulnerable to cold insults, and at the same time to her existential state of openness and hence her susceptibility to the various demonic forces that swirled around her. Similarly, the fire that was kept burning day and night to provide physical warmth and restore thermal balance to the lekhona's body, dangerously chilled by the loss of blood during childbirth, was also an apotropaic force essential in warding off these same demonic forces. Salt offered protection from the devil, as it toughened the infant's body and instilled common sense. Finally, the lochia associated with birth were simultaneously a sign of the woman's ritually unclean state and the vehicle for the elimination of bodily "dirt" that had to be expelled to restore her health. The hybridity of these core symbols and metaphors is all the more notable in that they appear to seamlessly condense and braid multivocal meanings and practices associated with the secular traditions of Galeno-Hippocratic and Soranic medicine on the one hand, and with the spiritual belief system based on the distinct tradition of Greek Orthodox Christianity on the other.

Ideally, the lekhona should remain confined to her house for the duration of the postpartum period. *Na sarantiso*, roughly translated as "to complete forty," is the verb that signifies the completion of the postpartum period and subsequent ritual purification of lekhona and infant by the priest. Confinement offered protection from the many dangers, both spiritual and physical, that now literally threatened the lives of the new mother and her infant. Indeed, for forty days after giving birth, the lekhona was said to live with "one foot in the grave" (*m'ena podhi sto lako*).[19] Because of her heightened vulnerability, the lekhona was never left alone. Usually, her mother or another female relative moved in to take care of her, perform the household chores, and ensure that she rested and regained her strength after the exhausting ordeal of birth. In practice, however, only women from the wealthiest families could afford to neglect their work outside the house and remain in confinement for the full postpartum period. No matter how poor a woman was, though, it seems that most observed at least a couple of weeks of seclusion after giving birth. Tucked away in the house, whose every means of entry was guarded by layers of protective devices, lekhona and infant were also buffered from attack by the demons whose jealousy and malevolent designs, activated by her pregnancy, were now driven into high gear with the arrival of new life. At the same time, the lekhona herself was considered polluting or unclean and her isolation and confinement were necessary to avoid endangering others as well. Only at the conclusion of the forty-day postpartum period, marked by the special ritual of "churching," would both woman and child become incorporated into the social and religious life of the village

For about a week following the birth, the mammi came by each day to check on the lekhona and her infant. She palpated her abdomen, checked for bleeding, and offered advice as needed. If a woman's breasts were engorged and painful, the mammi prepared hot compresses and counseled her on how to breastfeed. She also examined the infant, unwinding the swaddling cloth to inspect its navel for signs of infection and make sure it was drying out properly. Kiria Maria told me that she always examined the infant's mouth for signs of thrush as well. When the stump of the umbilical cord dried out and fell off after the third or fourth day, it was the mammi who presented it to the father to retain as keepsake and blessing all his life (*ghia evloghia*), as also occurred elsewhere in Greece (Rigatos 1992, 31).[20] The mammi vigorously massaged the infant's arms and legs, gave it a bath, rubbed the remnant of its umbilical cord with olive oil, and then snugly wrapped it anew. Depending on the mammi, she might also sweep the house, wash the dishes, and do the baby's laundry.

The focal point of the lekhona's postpartum recovery was her womb. From the humoral perspective described in the previous chapter, the postpartum was a critical period on at least two counts. First, a woman's thermal balance was profoundly disrupted by the loss of "hot" blood during birth. Compounded by the continuing flow of lochia afterward, this blood loss left the lekhona in a vulnerably chilled state. To regain her health and strength, the heat lost during birth had to be restored to her body as quickly as possible. By the same logic, the lekhona should strictly avoid cold substances; she was never given cold water to drink, for instance. (Explaining these practices to me, Kiria Eleftheria paused to marvel, "Now, from the very first day after birth I see women eating ice cream!"). Second, the womb's exaggerated state of openness, so essential for a successful birth, had to be reversed to prevent cold currents from freely penetrating the lekhona's body. A cold assault on her vulnerably open womb could affect a woman's health and compromise her fertility for the rest of her life. Thus, it was vitally important that she carefully follow procedures to avoid cold, restore lost heat, and promote the closure of her womb.

One of the most important means of restoring bodily heat was the drinking of a special infusion known as *to thermo tis lekhonas*, the "lekhona's heating substance."[21] Almost as soon as the birth was concluded, the mammi prepared the first pot of this tea. For the next forty days, a special ceramic pot of the lekhona's tea was kept continually ready and warm by the fireplace. The tea was made from a variety of herbs and spices, all of which were classified as *pirotika* therapeutic substances; that is, they possessed inherent heat-generating qualities. Recipes for the tea varied slightly from woman to woman but invariably featured cinnamon, and might also include cloves, sage, and nutmeg. Always sweetened with honey, another symbolically "hot" substance, this aromatic tea was by all accounts quite delicious. Permeating the house for forty days, and inevitably escaping outside, the pungent aroma of warm cinnamon tea announced to any passerby that a lekhona was secluded within. In addition to the lekhona, who sipped her tea throughout the day, relatives and neighbors, men and women alike, were invited to drink a cup. The tea was always offered to any visitors who dropped by to offer their blessing and wish the family a congratulatory *kalo riziko* (may it have a good destiny or fate) on the new birth. Children especially were drawn to the lekhona's house and clustered about in the hope of being treated to a cup of the sweet, fragrant brew.

The lekhona's tea was important in restoring and protecting health in a variety of ways. The warming properties of its ingredients helped replenish much-needed heat to the new mother's depleted body and counteract her susceptibility to cold insults. As will be recalled from the previous chapter, all of the tea's ingredients also were used in the preparation of emmenagogues. The same heating properties that enabled cinnamon, sage, and cloves to loosen and liquefy retained menses when a woman suffered a womb cold also promoted the flow and expulsion of the lochia during the postpartum period (*katevazi to ema*). Like menstrual blood, lochia were regarded as both physically dirty and ritually unclean. It was therefore vital to a woman's future health, as well as her future fertility, that she be thoroughly cleansed of this "dirty" blood. By promoting the flow of lochia, the tea helped restore the lekhona's body to a "clean" state, desirable from both a physiological and ritual perspective. Further, for reasons that no woman could adequately explain to me, the tea was also beneficial because it helped the lekhona produce an ample supply of breast milk. A clue to understanding the implicit logic underlying this otherwise obscure connection may be found, once again, in Galen. In Galenic medicine, blood, semen, and milk were regarded as "fungible fluids" (Laqueur 1990). On this view, a woman's breasts functioned as organs of "transmutation" that turned blood into milk. Achieving this process of "concoction," however, required heat (Hobby 1999, xxxiii). Although milk did not figure prominently in local Rhodian ethnophysiology, the prescription to drink heating substances such as the lekhona's tea to produce milk would appear to be in accord with this Galenic line of reasoning.

Critical to the process of recovery was keeping the lechona warm and rested. A fire was kept constantly burning in the house, except for the hottest summer months, to help restore the heat that had been lost during childbirth. Rest and avoidance of physical exertion were also important. The mammi's considerable help with the newborn and around the house for the first week after the birth has already been mentioned. Whenever possible, a woman's mother moved in with her to take over the household chores and attend to the other children. As an Ermiot woman in her early sixties from one of the wealthier families in the village, Kiria Tasoula, described her seclusion, she left the house only briefly and rarely; her mother took charge of most of her household chores for the full forty days after each of her four births. "*Me ikhe kalomathimene*, my mother spoiled me," she explained. "I was her only daughter, and she wouldn't let me do anything. . . . She didn't want me to get tired, to catch cold."

To preserve and restore the lekhona's strength, the mammi also advised her to wait a certain amount of time before having sex with her husband. Ideally, couples should abstain for the full forty-day postpartum period. Both local

beliefs and the Orthodox Church regarded the postpartum period as a ritually unclean state, akin to menstruation, during which sexual intercourse was
proscribed. Equally important, abstention prevented the lekhona from sapping
her energy, every shred of which should be directed toward her recovery. Additionally, sexual intercourse always caused the womb to open and so interfered with the slow process of its returning to its former condition. Among
the many reasons a woman's mother moved in with her during the postpartum
period was that her presence in the one-room house acted as a sort of "barrier
method." Having her mother sleeping in a bed only a few feet away, I was told,
diminished the possibility that a lekhona's husband would try to have sex with
her too soon after she gave birth. In short, every effort was made to keep the
lekhona warm, rested, and undisturbed to prevent her from chilling and sapping her strength and to promote the gradual closure of her womb.

To ensure an abundant supply of breast milk in the days immediately following birth, in addition to the lekhona's tea, a woman should drink lots of
soup. A special soup was made from roosters that her husband or her mother
butchered for the occasion. The lekhona regularly drank rooster soup not only
to regain her strength and promote the production of milk, but also to insure
that the baby would develop a strong neck.[22]

Postpartum Rituals of Incorporation

The Greek Orthodox Church, like other religions deriving from Abrahamic
tradition (Delaney 1991), recognizes the postpartum as a forty-day period of
seclusion and segregation from the everyday social and religious life of the
community. Suspended between important markers along the trajectory of
Orthodox personhood, lekhona and infant existed in an endangered, liminal
state that was officially marked off at both ends by the rituals of the Church.
On the first day after the birth, the priest visited the lekhona to read a special
prayer and bless the house with holy water (*aghiasmos*). This prayer recognized
"the uncleanliness of [her] body" and called upon God to "forgive" her and
"those who have touched her." At the same time, the priest called on God to
"protect and guard her from every attack of the Devil . . . from jealousy and
the evil eye" (quoted in Chryssanthopoulou 1984, 52). Before he left, the priest
always left behind some holy water for the lekhona to use to purify herself, her
infant, and anyone who crossed the threshold of the house during the postpartum period.

Forty days later, lekhona and infant went to church for the Sarantisma, the ritual that formally concluded her seclusion and marked her complete reintegration into the social and religious life of the community. The priest again read a special blessing, and if the infant were male, the priest carried it into the sanctuary, where they circled the altar three times. If it were a girl, the priest took it only as far as the steps of the sanctuary to pay its respects to the icon of the Panaghia. When this brief ritual was concluded, woman and infant, who had entered the church through the *atsalos tholos*, the disorderly dome (the entrance reserved for menstruating women and lekhones, as discussed in Chapter 3), departed through the central male door. Afterward, she and her infant were free to enter the church, and she was once again permitted to take communion (the infant's first communion took place at baptism). Sarantisma and its blessing also marked the end of a woman's heightened vulnerability to the threats posed by the forces of evil.

Between the brackets of these official Orthodox rituals, the lekhona and her infant existed in a highly charged "open" state. Openness, as discussed earlier, is generally valued as auspicious (Hirschon 1978). Postpartum openness is ambiguous, however. It is auspicious because it has enabled the creation of new life, but dangerous because it exposes the woman—and by extension, her infant—to penetration and attack by a variety of malignant forces. In addition, like a menstruous woman, the lekhona herself is thought to be endangering. But the lekhona's ability to cause harm is far more potent. It was as if the awesome power unleashed in the process of giving birth overflowed the boundaries of her body to provoke all manner of disorder in her immediate environment. In various regions of Greece, for instance, it was believed that her presence in another person's house could cause the crockery to spontaneously shatter or provoke an infestation of mice. Those with whom she conversed would be plagued by headaches. Vegetation withered and died after she passed by and had to be sprinkled with holy water as a countermeasure. Even the mountains could start to tremble when she faced them (Chryssanthopoulou 1984, 52–53).

The list of ritual behaviors, precautions, and apotropaic devices and practices related to the postpartum seclusion is exhaustingly long and diverse. Vigilance against the forces of evil—a panoply of xotika, the devil in his multifarious guises, and the evil eye of other humans stirred by admiration or provoked by envy—took multiple forms and was deployed in ever more proximate spirals and overlapping layers of protection. Enclosure within the space of the house was the foremost measure taken to protect the vulnerable mother and infant. The ritually open and liminal state of the lekhona and infant were counteracted by confinement to the sanctified space of the house, whose every possible means of entry was guarded against the intruding forces of harm. To maintain its sanctity, all of the house's boundaries and interfaces with the exterior first had to be purified and then symbolically fortified to prevent penetration by the forces of evil. Not only doors and windows, but also bodily borders, such as clothing and swaddling cloths, represented such boundaries. All were heavily and redundantly guarded.

Among the most potent prophylactics against evil and the devil were the sacred objects and symbols of Greek Orthodoxy, in particular crosses, icons, oil, bread, and holy water (*aghiasmos*). Both threshold and door of the house were purified by the priest with a sprinkling of holy water. Window ledges were protected by small palm frond crosses plaited by school children and sanctified by the priest during the Palm Sunday service. The mammi tucked one of these palm crosses inside the infant's swaddling cloth on the first day of its birth. A special wheat biscuit (*koulouri*) baked in the shape of a cross was also placed in the infant's *kounia*, its cradle. Another cross-shaped biscuit was hung from the *kamara*, the archway that separated the *ghonia* from the interior of the house. Small gold crosses and icons of the Panaghia, as well as little phylactery bundles, were pinned to the exterior of the infant's clothes. Their protective power was considered foolproof, as demonstrated in the following story I was told about Kiria Melpomeni's sister-in-law. One night during her postpartum seclusion, she began to worry about her flock of sheep. Because the moon was full and the sky was lit with as much light as at dusk, she decided it would be safe to go outside to check up on them. As she walked along the path to the sheepfold, *aneraes* dressed in flowing white robes emerged from a nearby river and started to dance around her in a circle. With each revolution of their dance, the circle became tighter, and just as the *aneraes* were about to close in on the terrified woman, they caught sight of the palm leaf cross she had pinned to her baby's carrying bag. Immediately, they began to scream, took flight, and disappeared.

Concentric circles of defense also protected the lekhona herself. Even within the safety of her house, she was further secluded under a sheet that was draped over her bed in the manner of a tent. Over this sheet were hung various apotropaic objects, such as a palm leaf cross, a needle with a broken point, a head of garlic, and an iron spindle. The sheet both kept her warm and protected her from any marauding spirits that might manage to penetrate the house's ritual fortifications. As a further precaution, the lekhona always wore something made of gold, usually a piece of her bridal jewelry. A woman's marriage was a highly auspicious event and objects associated with it conferred spiritual protection throughout her life. Gold earrings or pendants made from

Turkish pounds (*lires*) of various denominations were given to a bride on her wedding day—pentolires, "five lires," if her family could afford them; lires of lesser value denominations if they could not. After the wedding, her bridal jewelry was hidden away and taken out only on ritual and festive occasions, such as the annual village saint's day celebration (*panighiri*) or another wedding. Throughout the postpartum seclusion, a lekhona always wore some of her gold lires or other articles of her bridal jewelry as protection against the xotika demons.

Fire also offered important protection to both mother and infant from the xotika. "The fire, the light, didn't allow the evil, *to kako*, to come inside," as one Ermiot woman explained. The fire that J. K. Campbell (1964, 154) observed "burning day and night" in the house of the Sarakatsani lekhona even in the intense heat of summer was intended not only to restore heat to her body, but also to protect her and her infant from malignant spirits. Mothers also sometimes placed a smudge of soot from the fireplace on the infant's forehead or, more discreetly, behind its ear to ward off evil. The color black, strongly associated with death, is another common apotropaic device. It is possible that the entailments of fire, such as the black soot used to mark the infant, acquired their apotropaic powers from this potent symbol of protection. The flame of the olive oil lamp on the icon shelf, the *iconostasi*, also was kept lit throughout the postpartum confinement.

The xotika, who were the prime targets of these precautions (and others too numerous to mention), were especially prone to wandering abroad at night, looking for someone to attack. As one woman explained, "Daytime is for people, the night is for evil, *to kako*." Because of this danger, come nightfall the house was always tightly shut. In J. K. Campbell's (1964, 154) memorable description of the Sarakatsani, "for the first forty days after the birth, the hut or house after dusk is like a city under siege, with windows boarded, the door barred, and salt and incense at strategic points, such as the threshold and window cracks, to repel an invasion of the devil." If the lekhona absolutely had to leave her house for some reason, she made every effort to return before dark. She was never to leave the house after sunset. Even inside the house, she should never be left alone. Ideally, her mother should always be at her side, not only to do her chores and prevent her husband's sexual approach, as mentioned earlier, but also, and equally important, to be on the alert for intruding demons.

Given the family's high state of alert, the xotika were forced to adopt deviously clever tactics if they were to get close enough to attack the lekhona and her infant. One well-known way the xotika attempted to penetrate the barricaded house was to conceal themselves on the clothing or shoes of visitors. Because of this danger, after an initial flurry of visits from well-wishers, people stayed away from the lekhona's house. Those who did enter, usually only close family members, were always purified first with a sprinkling of holy water. Similarly, a newborn's clothes were never left outside to dry overnight. If someone forgot to bring them in before dark, they were placed by the fire to drive out any concealed spirits. To be truly safe, the baby's laundry should be dried inside the house by the hearth fire.

Ideally, an infant that had not completed the forty-day seclusion period, known as an *asarantisto* (literally, "un-fortied") baby, should also remain within the protected confines of the house. An Ermiot woman told me a cautionary story to illustrate what might happen if this prohibition were violated. It was the time of the wheat harvest, when the work of cutting and gathering the grain had to be completed in time or a family might face starvation. Because of this urgency, her grandmother's cousin, a lekhona who had spent barely two weeks in seclusion, had little choice but to leave for the fields with her infant. That night, the *aneraes* grabbed the baby and hauled it to a nearby lake where they drowned it. In another version of the same story, I was told that the *aneraes* exchanged the infant for another that was paralyzed. Shortly after that, the baby died. Another woman told me that sometimes the *aneraes* might spare a baby, if they found it attractive and took a liking to it. More often, they destroyed it.

Fathers also had to take special precautions. To avoid encountering the xotika, they were expected to return home before sunset instead of staying in the coffee shop until late in the evening as they otherwise might have done. When they reached the threshold of their house, they could not enter straightaway. They had to remove their shoes and, in winter, their coat and other outer garments as well, and leave them outside the door. Then, they had to hop over a burning stick that was taken from the fireplace and placed in front of the entrance to the house. Only then, and after making the sign of the cross, could a father enter his house. These precautions were necessary, as one man put it, so that he would be "clean" (*katharos*) when he returned to his house from the outside. Otherwise, he might inadvertently become the vehicle for an evil spirit bent on entering and harming mother and infant.

The forty-day seclusion period, during which the lekhona lived "with one foot in the grave," also represented a kind of symbolic death and entombment after the act of physiological birth. Rebirth and full social recognition of mother and infant would take place only after the official Orthodox ritual of churching that formally marked the conclusion of this period. In the meantime, the postpartum itself was punctuated by a series of rituals that enacted the gradual and progressive purification and domestication of the infant. Some were minor, but two were more elaborate, and in both the mammi played a central role.[23] The first, which I have already discussed, was the salting of the baby. The second was the ritual known as *i efta [meres] tou morou*, or simply, *i efta*, "the seven [days]." Both definitively disappeared along with the midwifery tradition I have described in this chapter, although the salting ritual appears to have persisted a while longer than the considerably more complex ritual of the seven days.

The ritual of the seven days was so called because it took place a week after the birth. Elsewhere in Greece, this ritual usually occurred on the third or fifth day after birth; only in the Dodecanese Islands was it was typically held on the seventh (Rodd 1892). The seven days marked the occasion when the three Fates, *I Tris Moires*, visited the newborn to mete out its life's fortune. *Moira* is derived from the word denoting "the lot or rightful portion of the individual" and in modern Greek refers to the destiny of a person (Krikos-Davis 1982, 106, 108). The Moires are three quarrelsome sisters, each of whom has her special task to perform. The Fate known as the Kalomoira allotted the child's portion of good luck (as discussed in Chapter 3). The Fate called Kakomoira doled out misfortune, illness, and hardship. The third sister, by the number of times she turned her spindle, ordained how long the thread of the child's life would run (128). For the ritual of the seven days, the new parents prepared a lavish evening meal to which they invited their closest relatives, friends, and the mammi in anticipation of the Fates' visit. The lekhona, who otherwise stayed carefully covered in her bed high in the back of the house, came down for the occasion to join her guests, who sat in a circle around the baby. The infant was placed in a wooden trough used for washing called the *skafi* into which various objects had been placed: books, pencils, or a shovel for boys, for example, and needlework and spindles for girls.[24] The mammi then took the infant from the trough and pretended to leave the house with it. Three times she said good night to everyone and got as far as the threshold, which she purified by censing it with incense. As she did so, the mammi softly recited a blessing, which might take the form of a *matinadha*. "*Sta chrisa na pesi to moro ke i tikhi tou na to kalomirasi*. May the child fall into gold and its fate be full of good fortune."[25] After the mammi returned from the threshold for the third time, the infant's mother quizzed her as to what she had seen on her journey. The mammi then recounted the blessings that were bestowed on the child: "I saw Christ, the Panaghia, and the Three Moires," the midwife replied. "And what did they say to you?" asked the infant's mother. "The child is blessed by Christ and Panaghia, and is given good fortune, *kalomoiro*, by the Fates," answered the mammi (Papchristodoulou 1964, 206). The mother, taking back her infant and placing it in the cradle again, rewarded the mammi with the small gift of a loaf of bread, a cup of sugar, and a bar of soap.

After this, the mammi proceeded to the next ritual, which took place around the trough. She gave candles to each of the guests, who lit them and stuck them to the rim of the trough. As they did so, each guest softly muttered the name of the particular saint to which they dedicated the candle (*onomatizete*), offering a wish and a blessing for the infant: "May St. Irini coddle it!" "May the Panaghia raise it!" Wishes could also be made for the child's future professional success or particular physical attributes, such as strength or beauty. If later in its life, the child grew into an accomplished adult, villagers might comment that "*sta efta tou ta valasi*, this [fate] was given to the child at its Seven Days." As the guests offered their good wishes for the child's future, each placed a gold or silver coin in the cradle and another, smaller coin, according to their means, into the hand of the mammi. The first candle to melt down indicated the saint who would become the child's patron. When all the candles had melted, the mammi extinguished the stubs in a cup filled with honey and walnuts that she passed around to all the guests. All dipped in a finger and, dabbing a little of the honey on their lips, offered the child a blessing: "Just as the honey is sweet, so too may the child's fate be sweet. *Opos ine to meli gliko na'n etsi i moira tou.*" The candle stubs were then stuck onto the archway that divided the house, next to the cruciform biscuit, to ensure the future fertility of the family and the blessing of God. This concluded, the guests sat down to feast and drink, all the while making toasts and wishing the newborn a good fate. After the meal, the leftovers, along with three additional small plates laden with sweets and other delicacies, were left out for the three Moires who would arrive later in the night to mete out the child's fate.[26]

Like the rituals performed by infertile women described in the previous chapter, those of the salting of the baby and of the seven days lay outside the bounds of male-dominated official church doctrine and practice, although, like them, they were passively tolerated. All formed part of the female universe of activities that clustered prominently at the thresholds of life and death. In this chapter, I have shown the dual roles performed by the mammi as an obstetrical specialist commanding a unique and critically important array of secular knowledge, and as a mediator with divine and quasi-divine forces on behalf of the newborn infant. When the mammi rubbed the newborn with salt during the ritual of salting, she initiated the gradual expulsion of the demonic from the body of the infant that would be completed upon the formal rite of baptism. In the seven days ritual, she supplicated on behalf of the infant with Christian deities and Fates alike to ensure blessings for its future. Returning three times from the threshold to act as a kind of Kalomoira herself, she inevitably brought tidings of the blessings that awaited the child: good fortune, wealth, and the protection of Christ and Panaghia. By offering honey and walnuts to all who attend the ritual, she officiated over a kind of secular communion that symbolized the sweetness and fecundity in store for the child in the future. Ultimately, the mammi in her person embodied the inextricably entwined sacred and secular dimensions of Rhodian ethno-obstetrics in the prewar period.

Chapter 5

Medicalization and Modernity:
New Reproductive Technologies,
New Maternal Bodies

On a typically cloudless morning in June, I went to visit Katerina in one of the gleaming new neighborhoods that in recent years have pushed the border of Rhodes Town relentlessly southward. I had first met Katerina, an outstanding athlete who had occasionally competed outside Greece, when she was in her early twenties and still unmarried. By the time I interviewed her a few years later, Katerina was in the middle of a yearlong maternity leave from her secretarial job in the Rhodian office of an international company. As we chatted about her recent pregnancy, I brought up the practice of offering tidbits of food to pregnant women, which, in its display of collective concern for their well-being and for the outcome of their pregnancies, admittedly had captivated me. "*Vlakies*! Stupidities!" Katerina responded, impatiently shaking her head, causing the highlights in her thick ponytail to glint and shine in the bright morning light. Like all Rhodian women today, she gave birth in the hospital, and like nearly all the young women I spoke with, she found the option of birthing at home unthinkable. Her pregnancy was carefully scrutinized over a dozen prenatal visits and monitored by five ultrasounds. Polaroids of these fetal images launched her daughter's baby album, which rested before us on her glass-and-chrome coffee table. To educate herself about her pregnancy, Katerina had attended childbirth classes, watched videos loaned to her by friends, and consulted several books. She was the first Rhodian woman I encountered who had a copy of the best-selling U.S. pregnancy guide *What to Expect When You're Expecting*, just translated into Greek the year before (1998). But most helpful to her, she told me, was the Greek guide *Birth Is Love*, to which she often turned for reassurance and information during her pregnancy.

This too lay on the coffee table, next to the baby album and a Greek translation of Penelope Leach's *Your Baby and Child: From Birth to Age Five.*[1]

As Katerina's reaction hints, the ethno-obstetrical system that once shaped women's understandings and everyday practices concerning pregnancy and birth, described in the previous chapter, has either vanished altogether or been demoted by many younger Rhodians like Katerina to the category of *vlakies*. Summarily dismissed as stupidities, they have come to be regarded as the irrational traces of an earlier, benighted time. In her 1997 ethnography *From Duty to Desire*, Jane Collier describes strikingly similar reactions in the village in southern Spain she first visited in the 1960s and returned to study again in the 1980s. There, too, the younger generation might refer to the traditions central to the social identity of their parents—in this case, the long courtships and protracted mourning rituals—as "*tonterías del pueblo*, village stupidities." Comparing her two moments in the field, Collier identifies a significant generational transformation in subjectivities and self-presentations— from a "traditional" past in which people's behavior was represented as motivated by social obligation and unreflexive adherence to social conventions, to the "modern" present, in which younger people see themselves as free "to think for themselves" and make (rational) choices accordingly (6). As Collier insightfully observes, such constructions of "tradition" and "modernity" reflect the Enlightenment view of tradition as "modernity's devalued opposite" (13). On this view, the traditions of the past come to be seen as constraints on the individual's freedom to make rational choices from an ever-expanding field of options. In Greece and Spain (both of which have long occupied an ambivalently marginal location in the Northern European imagination), labeling the knowledge and practices of the recent past "stupidities" can also be interpreted as a means to rhetorically distance the speaker from (and elevate her above?) that past. For Collier, the transformations in subjectivity she found are ultimately linked to the shift in the foundations of social inequality, specifically, from inherited land as a source of status, power, and wealth in the older agrarian political economy to occupational achievement and income in the new industrial context. As we saw in Chapters 2 and 3, Rhodes has undergone a similar shift, although to an economy based on tourism rather than industry. As importantly, I would add, in Spain in the 1980s, as in Rhodes in the 1990s, the discourse of tradition versus modernity was also closely bound up with the issue of Europeanization and hegemonic symbolic constructions that associated the rational and the modern with stylized understandings of Europe.[2]

Rhodian women of the youngest generation also use the loan words "*tabou*," "taboo," and, equally tellingly, "*folklor*" when describing the beliefs

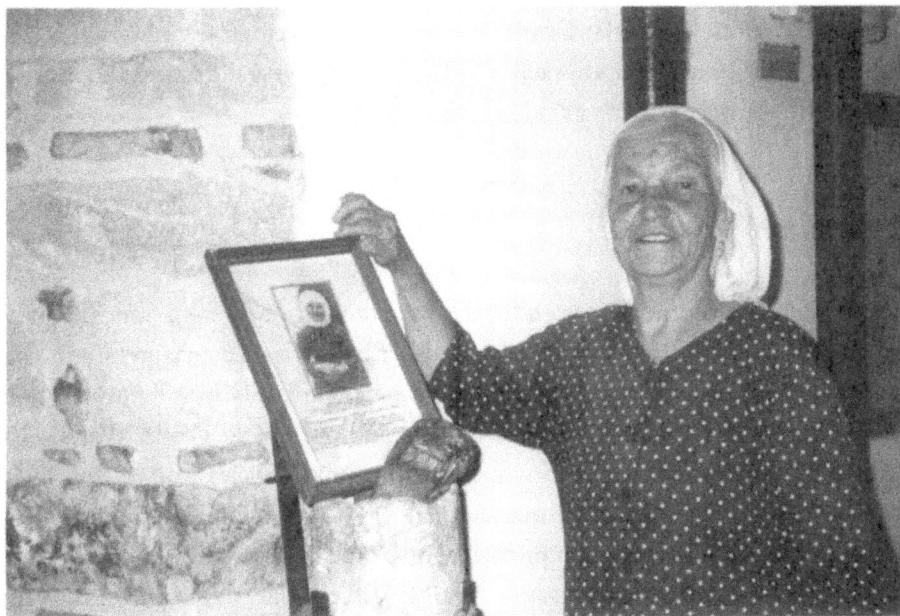

8. Kiria Vaso posing in front of her mother's photograph in Ermia's museum.

and practices their mothers and grandmothers held about the body. If the use of "*tonterías*" in Spain, like "*vlakies*" in Greece, evokes a dichotomy between a rational present and an irrational past, in Rhodes, terms like "tabou" and "folklor," with their quasi-ethnological overtones, also suggest an acutely self-conscious sense of living in a present in which the past has been objectified and assigned to the realm of anthropology and folklore. In an apparent paradox, though, once successfully undermined, the past can acquire a new kind of aura and value. From the safety of distance, the past (or, at any rate, selective aspects of the past) becomes grist for a quintessentially modern sense of nostalgia for a lost authenticity (D. Miller 1994, 205; Herzfeld 1991; Ivy 1995). In Rhodes, this nostalgic anthropologizing of the past is increasingly evident in the local ethnographies and village museums that have proliferated over the last decade or so. Of course, the museum boom is partly a response to the predilections of tourists, who pay a small fee to enter and gaze at the artifacts of "traditional Greek culture." Just as importantly, however, the village museum is regarded by the contemporary ex-villagers who built it as a way to preserve the material culture of the community's past, recently recouped from its refuse piles and storage bins, so that it will not be lost to future generations. And so, amid the dusty looms, discarded wooden plows, and time-darkened icons on folkloric display at Ermia's museum, one can find the photo of Kiria Arghiro, the last mammi to practice in the village, propped behind the mortar and pestle she once used to grind her remedies (Fig. 8).

Transition

In Rhodes, the rupture between local understandings of health and the body premised on the ethnomedical models described in earlier chapters and the postwar model grounded in biology and biomedicine to which I turn in this chapter, took place largely over the two decades following World War II. In urban areas such as Rhodes Town, Italian colonial policies caused this shift to begin somewhat earlier. A major objective of the colonial civilizing mission in Rhodes had been the provision of biomedical services and the delegitimation and eventual elimination of all lay practitioners, known collectively as the *praktiki*. Thus, by 1925, just two years after the Treaty of Lausanne officially handed the Dodecanese Islands to Italy, the new General Hospital of Rhodes had been completed. This impressive building was an apt symbol of Italy's determination to prove its capacity as a modern imperial power, and to distinguish itself from the despotic, Oriental variety of imperialists it replaced (N. Doumanis 1997, 41). As if to underscore this point, the sprawling new building was erected on the site of the old Ottoman hospital, which was tiny by comparison and had ministered mainly to the extremely sick and the dying. When a maternity wing was added in 1938, some of the town's wealthiest women began to give birth there, attended by Italian nuns, midwives, and doctors. Around this time, the colonial government promulgated a decree that prohibited anyone from practicing a profession without a degree from an Italian institution. This new policy was most devastating to Greek teachers, the largest group of professionals, but the handful of Greek doctors practicing at that time was also hurt. Some Rhodian women were selected to study midwifery in Italy; others received training under Italian practitioners living in Rhodes Town.

Still, most women in Rhodes Town continued to rely on the mammis, and on the few medically trained midwives, until well into the 1950s. Each neighborhood had its own mammi to which a woman could turn. For example, in Niokhori, where I returned to live each year, most births were attended by the mammi known affectionately by all as To Fotinaki, "Little Fotini" (Vratsalis 1990, 248). A few mammis enjoyed wider reputations. Kiria Khrisanthi, a seventy-one-year-old native of Rhodes Town, was born at home, as were all of her seven siblings, with the assistance of Kiria Anoula (remarkably for that time, all eight siblings survived to adulthood). Highly regarded beyond the confines of her neighborhood, this mammi, in Kiria Khrisanthi's words, "helped half of Rhodes give birth." After the war, the large influx of migrants from the smaller Dodecanese islands replenished the supply of midwives to Rhodes Town. In those lean years, midwives from Halki, Symi, Karpathos, and elsewhere offered an inexpensive alternative to Dr. K., the town's sole obstetrician. In rural areas, the mammis, along with the other *praktiki*, served as the major providers of health care for at least a decade longer. Nor were access and cost the only factors preserving practical midwifery. Even into the 1960s, some village women continued to regard the hospital as a "place of death" rather than as a fitting place to give birth (Lefkarites 1992).

At the time of liberation and incorporation of the Dodecanese Islands into the Greek nation, only a handful of doctors of any kind practiced on Rhodes. In 1950, the late Dr. K., whom I introduced in Chapter 3, opened a private maternity clinic in Rhodes Town that for the next fifty years provided the only private maternity services available in the region. Some of the smaller towns on the island had a resident general practitioner (*pathologhos*) that might be called on if serious complications arose during a birth. Lindos, for instance, the island's second-largest city and a regional center (*komopolis*), had such a *pathologhos*, but older Lindians told me that he never attended births unless something went badly wrong. By the 1960s, however, the local midwifery tradition was rapidly disappearing. Many of the mammis had died and the rest had stopped practicing. Kiria Arghiro of Ermia, for example, died in 1963, a year after she helped her daughter Vaso give birth to her last child. Like the other mammis throughout Rhodes, she left no replacement. Kiria Vaso, who had learned a great deal about midwifery from her mother, emigrated the year after her mother died to join her husband in Germany, where she worked for the next eight years in a nursing home. In any case, as she told me, she had little interest in becoming a mammi and facing the hard work, unpredictable hours, and heavy moral responsibility her mother had shouldered. Kiria Eleftheria's mother and grandmother had practiced as mammis in a village in central Rhodes. But like Kiria Vaso, she had no desire to follow her foremothers' example. "No, no, we didn't believe in that any more," she explained when I asked her why. "We were the younger [ones], the more modern [ones], *imaste ke pia i pio nei, i pio moderni*." By the early 1970s, even village women had little alternative but to travel to Rhodes Town to give birth either in the private clinic or in the public hospital. By this time, though, as Kiria Eleftheria's comment hints, encompassing changes in the cultural logic of Rhodian society had made birth in a biomedical setting increasingly desirable for many women and their husbands.

Distinctive Knowledge

As in Kiria Vaso's case, migration was one important force that eroded the continuity of local midwifery and ethno-obstetrics. After the war, large numbers of Rhodians left the island to find jobs as guest workers in the nations of the European core, welcomed temporarily as a source of labor crucial to rebuilding their postwar economies. Others streamed farther abroad. Many others moved to Athens, joining villagers from all over Greece who were feeding the city's explosive growth. Migration was not a new phenomenon, to be sure. But the postwar wave differed from that of the early 1900s both in its intensity and in the fact that women were now nearly as likely to migrate as men.

Although migration contributed to the erosion of local knowledge and practices, the most influential transformation was undoubtedly the dramatic increase in the levels of literacy and formal education. A movement to expand education had begun in the latter part of the nineteenth century and had achieved some notable successes. But it was only in the fluid social environment of the postwar period that schooling was embraced by broad sectors of Rhodian society. During this time, too, access to higher education expanded as several new universities were founded throughout the country. Recognizing formal education as perhaps the most important means to mobility and security in the new social environment that was taking shape after the war, Rhodians—urban, rural, and migrants alike—were prepared to make monumental sacrifices to educate their children. If in the prewar rural context the enduring "central motto and imperative" of parents had been "to augment and multiply what is passed on from one generation to the next," (Vlahoutsikou 1997, 295), in the postwar period the nature of that "more" shifted wholesale from land, animals, and other forms of agrarian wealth to credentials and education. Parents toiled in the hope that their labor and sacrifices would enable their educated children to acquire a job in the city, ideally as professionals or civil servants, and avoid the hardships and insecurities they had endured. The massive wave of postwar migration certainly amplified this trend, as remittances from family members living abroad injected important streams of cash that helped underwrite the educational project of those who stayed behind. As a result of the strong motivation of parents, children, and sometimes other family members, more Greek high school students go on to university than in any other country of the European Union (Delighiani-Kwimsi 1993b; Tsoukalas 1976). More impressive still was the unusual degree of democratization that characterized Greek higher education in the postwar period, as evidenced by the fact that fully one quarter of university students through the late 1970s and beyond came from peasant backgrounds (Frangoudaki 2003, 207).

Initially, girls were less likely to attend school than boys were, particularly in the rural areas. However, by the 1970s, education was increasingly appreciated as the securest route to social mobility for both boys *and* girls. Tsambika, a teacher in her midthirties, described the new sense of priorities in her village in the early 1980s when she finished high school: "Boy or girl, that was the goal, *o stokhos*, to go to university. If a girl passed [the entrance exams], the feeling was "bravo, you succeeded," *ta kataferes*; if you didn't pass, you didn't succeed, *dhen ta kataferes*, so go get married." By that time, girls throughout Greece were as likely as boys to attend school at all levels, including university. By 2000, women students outnumbered men in many university departments; after graduation, they outperformed them in the competition for coveted public sector jobs (Close 2002, 217; Delighiani-Kwimsi 1993b, 314).

Besides representing one of the surest bets for obtaining a stake in the emergent social and economic order, education was highly valued as a sign of distinction. Education, especially at the university level, represented, in Bourdieu's sense, cultural capital, a potent symbol of social status. Particularly in rural areas and among the working class, the distinction conferred by formal education was often reified and fetishized in the material object of the diploma, *to ptikhio*. Older Rhodians also sometimes referred to education as "the golden bracelet" (*to khriso vrakhioli*), a gendered metaphor that evokes the distinction endowed in the past by the opulence of a bride's dowry jewelry. This is an image richly saturated with entailments that link a woman's education to her destiny to marry, preferably to marry *well*, and implicitly, to her destiny to procreate. At least initially, higher education for women was seen as a symbol of, and a means to, elevated social status through a good marriage. After the 1970s, however, a woman's education was also valued as a means to establishing a career of her own, *na kano kariera* (Delighiani-Kwimsi 1993b). While of obvious economic consequence, a *kariera* was in addition increasingly important as a sign and vehicle of becoming a modern Greek woman.

Achieving the goal of higher education often necessitated the combined efforts and sacrifices of mothers, fathers, and at times of older siblings. The payoff, however, conferred a reflected prestige on the entire family. This point is forcefully conveyed in the following story I was told by Stella, a middle-aged woman living in Rhodes Town who was married to a doctor, the profession that claimed one of the highest rungs on the local ladder of distinction. Not long after her marriage, Stella went to visit her mother-in-law, who still lived in the village where Stella's husband was born. There, as was customary in the past, Stella was addressed by a neighboring woman who came to welcome her as *iatrina*, a feminized version of *iatros*, doctor, and a courtesy honorific that paid homage to her status. Hearing this, Stella recalled, her mother-in-law became irate and began to scold her neighbor: "Why do you call her *iatrina?* I made him a doctor!"[3] In the past, as today, a good portion of parents' sense of self-worth and their social reputation was shaped by how successful they were in establishing their children in society. Once educated, however, these children rarely stayed in the village. Inevitably, they settled in Rhodes Town, Athens, and other cities where they participated in the new middle-class way of life. Unfortunately for their parents, this was a way of life that, now as in the preceding century, denigrated and marginalized the practices of village culture. Vassos Argyrou (1996, 37), analyzing the dynamics of this process in Cyprus, found that one of the most profoundly poignant of the "unintended consequences" of parental hard work and sacrifice was a shift in knowledge and power from "from father to son." As we shall see, on Rhodes this process entailed an equally profound (and often equally painful) shift from mother to daughter. To grasp more fully how this shift came about, it is helpful to take a closer look at the concept of distinction.

As elaborated by Bourdieu (1984), distinction is deeply relational. That is, the ability to convey social meaning—specifically, to communicate social position within a hierarchy—is always premised on contrast and difference, and thus requires an implicit or explicit Other. Anthropologists have importantly qualified and added to this concept by emphasizing that, although this semiotic process may be common to contemporary class-stratified societies, any account of distinction must also "embrace a more specific and cultural set of motivations" (LiPuma 1993, 31). Historically, higher education has figured prominently in the culturally specific hierarchy of symbolic capital in Greece (Tsoukalas 1976). From the founding of the Greek nation, education was assigned a privileged role in the creation of a cultural image of modern Greece (Faubion 1993, 59; Gourgouris 1996, 87). Charles Stewart has usefully drawn on this significant dimension of formal education in Greece to make sense of the eclipse of the xotika and, by implication, of local knowledge more broadly on the island of Naxos. His argument is also pertinent to the rapid demise of ethnomedical knowledge in Rhodes (which accorded a featured role to the xotika):

> In the nineteenth century, the educated sector of Greek society labeled
> the peasantry "ignorant," a condition that explained their preservation of
> and constant traffic in "traditions" regarding supernatural powers among
> other things. But categories such as the "supernatural" or "superstition"
> could never have been conceptualized, let alone defined, except by another
> group possessing distinct notions of the "natural" and the religiously
> proper. *Education founds such a difference; it establishes (constructs) standard*

as opposed to substandard types of knowledge. . . . In this regard the will to knowledge reveals an aggressive and even violent aspect precisely because it raises one to a dominant position over those who remain ignorant. (1991, 127–128, my emphasis)

As Stewart (116) argues, belief in the xotika and other forms of local knowledge on Naxos has been suppressed not so much by the application of logic and rational contemplation as by the mockery and embarrassment of the younger generations now authoritatively in possession of standard knowledge. Others have observed similar reactions to the heart-wrenching death laments sung by women in rural Greece. Seremetakis (1991, 162) notes that urban Maniats reacted to the mourning rituals of village women with "abhorrence," dismissing them as "irrational and even barbaric event[s], indicative of rural backwardness." And Caraveli (1986, 170) records the embarrassment that these laments provoked among "the rising village middle class" elsewhere in Greece. I would add that although the difference founded by education is fundamentally a class difference, in the fluid social environment of postwar Greece it was almost everywhere equally profoundly a generational difference. Of course, the two often overlapped, just as education and urbanization were also closely intertwined (Argyrou 1996). Thus the reversal in power relations between parents and children was intimately associated with the shift in knowledge and cultural capital precipitated by the massive expansion of education in the postwar period. Especially for those of rural origins, acquisition of standard knowledge, standard language (as opposed to the distinctive Rhodian village dialect), and urban savoir-faire elevated them to a (class) position of authority over their parents.

The contradictions inherent in this novel situation were not lost on the women in the youngest generations with whom I spoke. Many experienced as awkward and uncomfortable the reversal of power between them and their mothers. It was a subject that some found difficult to discuss with me. An exception was Sofia, a primary school teacher with a degree in political science, with whom I developed a close friendship over the years. Sofia offered in lively detail her perspective on what it was like to come of age in a village in Rhodes in the late 1970s:

> Our village was more "open" than some of the others, and in some
> ways, even more so than Rhodes Town. This was because ours
> was a politicized, *politikopiimeno*, village, and we had a progressive
> mentality. But we weren't the only one—there were many other
> villages like ours, too. . . . In the *metapolitefsi* [the restoration of

democracy in the postjunta years] we had several students who went to the Politechnical University [in Athens, and an epicenter of the Greek student movement of the time], and so the KKE [Communist Party of Greece] had a strong presence in our village. These students came back on vacations, they talked with us, and they helped us a lot. The elders used to say that all the young people in the village were revolutionaries, communists. And there was a terrible clash, *mia foveri singrousi*, with the older generation. They complained that the youth were rebellious, that they provoked their parents, and the villagers gossiped about them.

EG: What did they say?

Sofia: They said, "The girls are smoking, the girls are keeping company with the boys, the girls go to the *kafenion*, the coffee shop, and sit with the boys and drink beer!" [Laughs]. Parents would get upset with us, and sometimes we'd fight, but we were determined that change had to occur. . . . We read a lot, discussed a lot among ourselves, listened to rock music. We dressed differently, too—in flowing Indian skirts—and we wore no makeup.

EG: Why not?

Sofia: Because we were politicized, because of the women's movement. We were very restless.

EG: There appears to be a large gap between you and your parents. How has that affected you, psychologically?

Sofia: There's a chasm, *ena khasma*, between us. This is common in Greece. There was a huge development [*ekseliksi*] from one generation to another.

EG: How did you handle it?

Sofia: Look, let me tell you, I didn't have a lot of contact with my parents. I did my own thing. I lived, I went on with my life without waiting for my parents' approval, . . . from a young age I was like that. I wasn't tied to them, I was independent. I took it for granted—all my [women] friends did at that age. We said, "*Vre,* hey, let's go forward, we're not looking back."

EG: How did your parents react?

Sofia: They felt insecure. They reacted, especially my mother, but I just went forward; . . . there was lots of conflict. But now they've adapted to everything. It wasn't just me, I've seen it with all my friends. There was a huge difference between us and our parents, especially in the rural areas. . . . In Greece, you see, we don't have class differences the same way they do in other countries. In Greece, a large percentage went from farmers to the university in one generation.

At this point in our discussion, I brought up another woman I'd interviewed, a doctor around Sofia's age who, like her, was born and raised in one of the more remote Rhodian villages. This woman had told me that whenever she visited Athens, she went to see a psychiatrist and that one of the recurring issues she discussed in therapy was her strained relationship with her mother, who still lived and farmed in the village:

> Look, me too; . . . don't think that it was easy. Sometimes, I felt, I would have wanted parents who understood me. Then, at the time, it was very hard for me, *me kostize emena poli*, that in my house I didn't have this understanding. At sixteen, seventeen, eighteen, you felt a constant conflict in the family—all my friends did and we talked about it together all the time. I never went to a psychiatrist, but I felt this conflict.

Sofia's narrative gives an intimate glimpse into her lived experience of the fault lines that distanced many (though certainly not all) Rhodian women of her generation and class background from their mothers. Noteworthy, too, is the way that Sofia firmly situates these fault lines within the political and social ferment that followed upon the demise of the junta, a symbolic watershed in the recent history of the Greek nation (Papagaroufali and Georges 1993). Sofia clearly credits higher education as well as self-education through reading and lively discussions with her (politicized) age cohort as important agents of confrontation and rupture between the generations. But her narrative also hints at the extent to which this generational rupture was legitimized, and made perhaps even more vehemently oppositional, for the rejection it implied of the conservative "traditional" values associated with, and touted by, the discredited right-wing junta regime. Against this historical context, Sofia's insistence on "going forward" and "not looking back" can also be seen as expressing her engaged commitment to the good fight toward Greek social and political modernity.

Local knowledge about the body in Rhodes thus came to be suppressed and displaced from one generation to the next through much the same aggressive and often confrontational process that accounts for the demise of the xotika beliefs on Naxos. As local knowledge was demoted to the realm of the irrational (*vlakies*) or, only marginally better, to the quaintly ethnological (*tabou*, *folklor*) and as science and biomedicine became the progressive and modern ways of thinking about health, illness, and the body, the oldest generation of women by and large stopped passing on their ethnogynecological and ethnoobstetrical knowledge to their daughters. Just as importantly, daughters no longer turned to their mothers for information and advice. Like Sofia, many "did their own thing," that is, they fashioned themselves in dialogue with other, more valued sources of information and knowledge. Indeed, in an unprecedented development, daughters now began to instruct their mothers in the new biomedical knowledge (for example, urging them to get Pap smears). The degree of rupture between the generations was perhaps best indexed by the fact that almost no woman born after 1960 was aware of the core ethnogynecological principle that the womb had a sense of smell. One day early in my research I interviewed a woman in her seventies who was born on the small neighboring island of Tilos and had moved to Rhodes as a young girl. A young Rhodian acquaintance recently graduated from an Athenian university knew her family well and introduced her to me as someone especially knowledgeable about iatrosophia, the old remedies. Sitting in on the interview, she heard about the womb's olfactory capacity for the first time (although her own mother, in her midfifties, knew about it, I later found out). After the interview, she privately insisted to me that this belief must be peculiar to Tilos, marginal and backward as she imagined the island to be, and emphatically denied that *any* Rhodian woman believed such a thing.

When I asked women of the oldest generation why they didn't talk about these matters with their daughters, I seldom got a verbal answer. Typically, women responded with a shrug and usually met with silence my efforts to get them to elaborate. Sometimes, if a woman's daughter happened to be present during an interview, an arched eyebrow or an exclamation of "Mama!" delivered in a shocked, amused, or impatient tone in reaction to her mother's explanations provided additional insight. A final vignette illustrates these reactions. One Sunday evening in August, I sat with a group of women in the *platia*, the square, of a village in Eastern Rhodes, in point of fact a shapeless broadening of the main asphalt road anchored by a single dusty plane tree. Grandmothers and mothers had gathered to enjoy the *meltemi*, the stiff summer breeze that blew in from the Turkish mainland to cool the sweltering summer night. As we settled as comfortably as we could on a concrete bench to eat our ice cream on a stick, chatting and idly minding children of all ages who were riding their bikes and playing in the *platia*, I started talking to the oldest women about my research. Eventually, a lively discussion of bygone practices developed. It was evident from many of the younger women's surprised reactions that they had never heard many of these stories. Soon they were breaking into peals of laughter ("They held you by the waist and shook you?!") and prodding their mothers for more. In short order, my attempt to conduct scholarly research was hijacked by the younger women for their evening's entertainment.[4]

Schools, Literacy, and Authoritative Knowledge

After the war, the classroom became a central site for the wholesale diffusion of the anatomic model of health and bodily functioning and for the displacement, once and for all, of the long-standing ethnomedical model. Routing this local knowledge (and its practitioners) represented the triumphant culmination of a century-long crusade (*stavroforia*) waged by prominent Greek doctors and other social reformers (Korasidou 2002, 198). Almost as soon as the Greek nation began to recover from the devastation and disarray caused by the lengthy War of Independence from the Ottoman Empire, women's education became a topic of intense national concern and debate. From the outset, women's education was intimately linked to the issue of national health. Prominent doctors of the day were instrumental in highlighting health in general, and children's health in particular, as a fundamental national resource which, to be attained, demanded disciplined allegiance to the principles of modern hygiene. The family was identified as the primary locus of hygienic practice, and within it, women were targeted as those bearing primary responsibility for the health and well-being of its members. As the leading doctors of the day maintained, it was only when women's "ignorance" (*aghnia*), "destructive superstition" (*olethria prolipsis*), and "mistaken and distorted ideas" (*sfaleras ke strevlas idees*) were extirpated and replaced by new rules predicated on scientific knowledge that the national population could increase and its health and vigor improve, goals that were essential to meet if the nascent Greek economy and society were to progress (Korasidou 2002, 195–97).

The content of women's education was one of the most important fronts on which this crusade was waged. In the prescriptive literature of this period, inculcating a sense of responsibility for combating dirt, pollution, and disease was deemed one of the main objectives of women's education (Bakalaki 1994, 91). After 1850, the subject of domestic economy, seen as essential to the achievement of appropriate canons of motherhood and wifehood, became part of the curriculum of the secondary schools for girls.[5] Known as *parthenaghoghia* (schools for the training of virgins), these secondary schools were initially private institutions attended mainly by daughters of the elite (78). Nonelite women, usually on scholarship, were also trained at the *parthena-*

ghoghia to serve as primary schoolteachers (ibid.; Vergotis 1997). After graduation, some of these teachers fanned out into the countryside to work in the primary schools that began to proliferate throughout Greece at the end of the century (Sant Cassia with Bada 1992; Vergotis 1997).

During most of the period of Greek nation building, Rhodes and the other Dodecanese islands remained under Ottoman rule. Nonetheless, elite discourses from the Greek mainland found their way to the island through a variety of routes, including the distribution of Greek publications, the circulation of diaspora elites, and the dissemination of elite discourse through Greek-language educational institutions. Schools in Rhodes were organized and supported by the Greek Orthodox Church, under the local administration of the metropolitan (akin to archbishop), who ultimately answered to the patriarchate in Constantinople. This essentially independent, ethnic-religious Greek school system was possible because of the considerable local autonomy afforded by the *millet* system through which the Ottomans had organized and managed their massive empire (Savaronakis 1991).

By 1880, the education of ethnic Greeks under Ottoman rule had increasingly come to occupy the attention of the Greek government. Prompted by the looming Balkan conflicts, and fed by a renewal of irredentist sentiment that aspired to spread the ideology of Hellenism among the so-called unredeemed, Greece looked forward to the eventual incorporation of the Greek-speaking Ottoman subjects into the national body (Koliopoulos and Veremis 2002, 162). Over time, the government in Athens moved to gain full control of the curriculum of nonnational Greeks by neutralizing the authority of the patriarchate over educational matters. As Greece succeeded in shaping the direction of local community and educational institutions, curricula obligatorily reflected the discourse that flowed from the national center (*ethniko kentro*) of Athens (Savaronakis 1991, 202). By the end of the nineteenth century, local schools in Rhodes were being subsidized by the Greek Ministry of Education, which also provided the textbooks and dictated the curriculum (Vergotis 1997). As a consequence, the values of the Athenian bourgeoisie came to dominate the educational system and the curriculum in Rhodes.

Greek curricula of the turn of the century, like those of Western Europe and the United States at the time, assumed a social world strictly divided by gender. Indeed, after the primary level, this was literally true, as girls and boys attended separate schools. Girls' education focused on domestic economy, increasingly conceptualized as a science according to which the household would be managed by women trained to rationally maximize scarce means to meet the myriad competing demands of their household members (Bakaklaki 1994). On their part, leading physicians of the day regarded the schools as desirably "closed" spaces, protected from the "bad influences" of daily life, in which they could promote their "crusade" to improve the health and vigor of the next generation (Kalafati, cited in Korasidou 2002, 213). In Rhodes, girls attending the *parthenaghoghio* also learned about health and hygiene from the *skholiatros*, an official who kept track of their health status and recorded and reported their illnesses on an annual basis (Vergotis 1997). An ever-expanding number of girls were thus exposed to the idea that the ultimate responsibility for monitoring and maintaining the health and well-being of their family members rested on their shoulders. At least one manual from the early twentieth century explicitly linked a woman's duty to safeguard her family's health to her duty to the nation (Bakalaki and Elegmitou 1987, 298).

As occurred on the mainland, some of the Rhodian girls who graduated from the *parthenaghoghio* went on to serve as primary schoolteachers in the countryside. By the early decades of the twentieth century, primary schools had been built in almost every village on the island, and for the girls who attended, hygiene and domestic arts such as sewing were standard subjects on the curriculum (Vergotis 1997, 49). Little is known about the impact of these classes on the pupils; however, as Bakalaki (1994, 97) has suggested, "it is legitimate to expect that, if nothing else, the employment of urban educated teachers in different parts of the countryside contributed to people's exposure to the ideals of womanhood and femininity endorsed by the educated class." Ultimately, in the words of the Committee for Practical Education that oversaw curricular matters in Rhodes, the objective of girls' education was to produce "*teleie ikodhespine ke kale dhidhaskalise*" (perfect housewives and good schoolteachers). The goal of the boys' curriculum was to mold boys into "*morfomenous polites*" (educated citizens) (Vergotis 1997, 37). Although the wording of these official goals might imply a disjuncture, in fact the two were intimately related in the minds of educational reformers of the time. Women served the nation primarily by reproducing vigorously healthy, rationally educated future (male) citizens.

Universal education in the postwar period disseminated a new cultural logic that helped unravel the secular strands of the iatrosophia tradition. At the same time, the particular narrative of national identity promoted in the curriculum may have unwittingly helped preserve its religious dimensions. Both change and continuity were valued in the official vision of national culture and identity on display in the uniform school texts used throughout Greece. As represented in history texts, for example, change was desirable only "when it is seen as 'progress' or as a 'civilizing process,' that is, as technological and economic growth, which in turn is identified with the higher, 'more civilized' culture of Western Europe" (Avdela 2000, 248). An important pillar of continuity in this official vision was represented by the living tradition of Greek Orthodoxy. Compulsory religious instruction through primary, middle, and high school attempted to promote and reinforce commonsense understandings of a national (Orthodox) identity. If, as noted earlier, "education . . . establishes (constructs) standard as opposed to substandard types of knowledge" (Stewart 1991, 128), then mandatory lessons in Orthodoxy in the national curriculum (however much students may grumble about having to take them) may have played a role in maintaining the continued legitimacy of religious healing. Be this as it may, despite the steady secularization of Greek society and the intensive use medical technologies of all kinds in maternity care, religious healing continues to offer an alternative or complementary health care option that was valued by many women. This was true even for many of the youngest generation, although young women were as likely to attribute the efficacy of a pilgrimage to a shrine or the ritual removal of the evil eye, for example, to the general psychological benefits of belief (akin to the placebo effect) as to divine intervention.[6]

As school attendance became nearly universal in the decades after the war, more and more girls were exposed in the classroom to new ways of understanding health and hygiene. Rarely, however, did they learn specific details about their own bodies. Still today, sex education is noticeably absent from the Rhodian curriculum at any level. It would seem that one of the main lessons imparted by the school curriculum was the general valorization of notions of scientific progress and technological development. To acquire more specific knowledge about their bodies and reproductive health, many women began to educate themselves by reading on their own.

Reading Pregnancy in Greece

In the 1960s and 1970s, women gained greater access to anatomic and biological knowledge via a number of alternative routes. Informal tutoring took place during women's increasingly frequent clinical encounters with the mushrooming number of medical professionals. As prenatal visits began to be seen as part of the routine care of pregnancy, they became important occasions for education as well as surveillance. As a Rhodian doctor succinctly described it to me, one of the obstetrician's primary tasks during these prenatal visits was "to explain to the woman what it means to be pregnant, what's happening inside her." After 1966, when television arrived in Greece, the mass media also became important routes of dissemination of medical information. Not least, women themselves played an active role in acquiring new knowledge. Outside the classroom, they began to buy and read additional texts to educate themselves about their bodies. Especially influential in this project of self-education for the transitional generation were the nearly ubiquitous women's health encyclopedias, sold door-to-door even in the most remote villages of Greece in the postwar period. With titles like *The Doctor Advises* and *Gynecological Encyclopedia*, these books covered in clear and accessible language a remarkably broad array of women's health topics from a biomedical perspective. The next generation of women, those born between 1960 and 1970 who came of reproductive age in the 1980s and 1990s, could choose from a much larger selection of books and guides that focused specifically on pregnancy, childbirth, and the care of infants and children.

Education, self-education, and the privileging of textual knowledge that resulted from universal literacy made possible the emergence of what Barbara Duden (1993) has called the "bibliophile body." Duden's term is apt for the recognition it accords to the role that women themselves play in producing the new forms of self-knowledge through their reading of expert texts. Indeed, talking with young Rhodians like Katerina, I was made aware of the extent to which they, like their North American counterparts, have turned to pregnancy guides and other print and visual media to educate themselves about pregnancy and birth (Rothman 1986, 45). Roughly half the women in my early hospital study (1990–1992) had consulted a pregnancy guide, which could often be spotted on their bed stands. By 2000, nearly every woman I met who had recently given birth had read at least one book or pamphlet over the course of her pregnancy. However variously these texts may be read and interpreted, they undeniably afford women the opportunity, at their will and leisure, to educate themselves about pregnancy and birth. Pregnancy guides thus represent an important, if relatively overlooked, vehicle through which women are able to access biomedical knowledge and, through this pursuit, have the opportunity to become experts of themselves and of their pregnancies.

Rendering scientific concepts of pregnancy and birth into accessible language and visual images, these guides have become important adjuncts to prenatal visits and to the medicalization process in general. In Greece as in the United States, pregnancy guides offer women detailed biological information and instructions on nearly every aspect of their pregnancy. Indeed, the guides are premised on the assumption that "being pregnant" is the necessary, but far from sufficient, grounds for having a baby and becoming a mother. To successfully undertake and complete the project of pregnancy, the guides presume, women need tutoring on how to participate in pregnancy and continuous self-monitoring to make sure they are properly following instructions (Georges and Mitchell 2000, 187). Pregnancy guidebooks can thus be regarded as intimate biopolitical conduits that offer each woman who consults them a set of resources for informing herself and reconfiguring her understanding of the pregnant body and of her responsibilities as a future mother.

Although these guidebooks typically promote themselves as ways for women to acquire the knowledge they desire about their pregnancies and thereby to empower themselves to take more control over their bodies, they also do more. Their aura of scientific objectivity notwithstanding, pregnancy guides inevitably reflect the cultural and political contexts of the society in which they are produced. In particular, they participate in and reinforce historically and culturally specific public conversations about "the obligations of the maternal body to the larger social body" (Blum 1999, 3). Thus, at the same time that they offer "universal" biomedical lessons, they implicitly serve as "instruments of acculturation, telling [women] in subtle or not so subtle form what is acceptable and what is not, what it means to be part of the culture that produces the book" (Michie and Cahn 1997, 3). For all these reasons, they deserve careful consideration.

Authorizing Modernity

It is a curious and intriguing fact that in Greece, as in the United States, one guide far outstrips all the others in popularity. In Greece, the preferred text is *Birth Is Love* (*O Toketos Ine Aghapi*). In the United States, it is *What to Expect When You're Expecting*. Each in its own way, *What to Expect* and *Birth Is Love* are publishing blockbusters. Some twenty years after it first appeared, *Birth Is Love* remains the only book-length pregnancy guide written by a Greek. Many other guidebooks are available today, but all are translations of texts from other countries, mainly England, France, and the United States, and all lag far behind *Birth Is Love* in popularity. Currently in its ninth edition, *Birth Is Love* has sold tens of thousands of copies (personal communication, Sikaki-Douka). Keeping in mind that Greece is a country of some eleven million people with one of the world's lowest birth rates, this makes *Birth Is Love* a huge bestseller by Greek standards.[7] Its circulation is amplified further still by the fact that, as commonly occurs in the United States as well, countless used copies are passed from woman to woman. What's more, *Birth Is Love* was the guidebook most often preferred by the midwives who offered the private childbirth classes attended by many of the women I interviewed.

In this section, I consider this neglected genre, with a particular focus on how the rhetorical constructions of mothers and pregnancy featured in *Birth Is Love* have been shaped by Greek discourses on gender, maternity, and nation.

The author of *Birth Is Love* is a professional midwife, Aleka Sikaki-Douka, who lived for a while in Canada and England, and practiced and taught midwifery in Athens for many decades. Although retired, she continues to lecture and write popular articles on a variety of topics related to pregnancy, birth, and contraception for national newspapers and women's magazines. Sikaki-Douka's best-selling guide is generously illustrated with dozens of anatomical drawings, electron micrographs, and reprints of Lennart Nilsson's famous fetal photographs, as well as many full-page color pictures of fathers holding babies and women in leotards exercising and in the various phases of hospital birth. Like most North American guides, the style is informal, with the author adopting an intimate, woman-to-woman tone and often addressing the reader as "we." Unlike them, though, women's voices in the form of quotes are almost completely absent, as is the question-and-answer format common to many North American guides. Throughout her text, Sikaki-Douka speaks with the authoritative voice of a member of a medical profession whose beneficently paternalistic and directive model of relations with the patient remains largely intact.

Stylistic differences aside, *Birth Is Love* appears to have much in common with the most popular U.S. pregnancy guides—from the full-page captioned reprints of Nilsson's photographs of the developing fetus that launch the text, to their shared objectives of increasing women's participation in their pregnancies. On closer reading, however, *Birth Is Love* is grounded in strikingly different cultural understandings and deploys distinctive symbolic codes, idioms, and rhetorical strategies to often divergent ends. Elsewhere, Lisa Mitchell and I have examined in detail the thematic differences and commonalities between *Birth Is Love* and some of the most popular North American pregnancy guides (see Georges and Mitchell 2000). Here I focus specifically on the ways in which pregnancy and maternal subjects are rhetorically constructed in *Birth Is Love*. I begin by examining how the book's sometimes implicit, sometimes explicit, and often imperative, mandate that women become "informed" regarding the physiological functioning of their bodies in medico-scientific terms is inflected by specifically Greek story lines, rhetorical conventions, and historical and cultural understandings.

The author's credentials and authority are established at the outset by the preface, which was written by a well-known professor of obstetrics and gynecology at the University of Athens who was also for many decades the director of the maternity clinic at one of Greece's major public hospitals (his titles follow his byline). As a physician/professor, this doctor occupies the highest rung in his profession's hierarchy and belongs to the category of physician regarded by patients as the most prestigious, authoritative, and desirable. After praising the book and assuring the reader that it will become "an essential aid for every Greek woman," the doctor devotes the remainder of his half-page prologue to a critique of the state of contemporary Greek women's scientific literacy:

> One large part of the problem faced by Greek women who await a child is unfortunately the result of misinterpretations, old superstitions, and mistaken prejudices. It is time for the younger generation of Greeks, properly informed, to face more responsibly and scientifically the subject of pregnancy, birth, postpartum, and also contraception.
>
> Today's Greek woman has no reason to envy other women of the civilized world, and for that reason she is entitled, but also obligated, to follow the spirit of her times, as this is expressed in the up-to-date development of science. To this end, I am sure, this book will contribute. (Sikaki-Douka n.d., 7)[8]

Thus, from the very first page of *Birth Is Love*, the doctor authoritatively sets the terms for discussing a major theme that will recur throughout the text: the need to remedy the problem of Greek women's scientific illiteracy.

Terms such as "civilized," "up-to-date," "superstition," and "science" recur throughout *Birth Is Love* and draw on a network of associations whose historical roots date back to at least the nineteenth century. Each is embedded in the familiar binaries often used to frame debates over the nature of Greek national identity, which continue to be used strategically in daily discourse today. Against this historical and political context, the doctor's exhortation to young Greek women to actively position themselves on the symbolically privileged side of these binaries (progressive, civilized, Western, modern science), an exhortation Sikaki-Douka repeats at many points in the text, can be read as a call to take responsibility for their role in favorably representing themselves and the Greek nation to the "civilized" world, viz., Europe and the West. Thus, in contrast to the most popular North American guides, in which scientific knowledge of the pregnant body is portrayed primarily as a means to reduce risks to the fetus (Georges and Mitchell 2000; Michie and Cahn 1997; Oaks 2001), in *Birth is Love* this knowledge is represented as an essential part of the project of becoming a modern pregnant Greek subject. As Sikaki-Douka asks her readers:

> How is it possible for a person to grow up at ease and correctly without knowing how the body works? (33)

The embryological knowledge [described thus far] offers you the joy and satisfaction of learning, of seeing, and of living, even if only in your imagination, what is occurring in your insides, in your uterus, in the pregnant woman's body (66).

Most women arrive at the clinic in complete ignorance about what is to follow. . . . Pregnancy, birth, and the postpartum period are a time in each woman's life that must be experienced consciously, with active participation, rationally and calmly. Our objective should be to personally inform ourselves about the functioning of our reproductive organs and of the biological processes of the body's systems during pregnancy (11).

The text abounds in such exhortations—"It is essential, yes, essential, for each woman to be informed about her physiological functioning," Sikaki-Douka stresses in her own prologue to the guide (11). However, she seldom explicitly elaborates the specific objectives of acquiring this bioscientific knowledge. When she does, they include such ends as the ability "to actively participate, to control our behavior, our demonstrations, expressions of our feelings," "to plan," "to behave in a conscious, rational and logical manner, and remain controlled," "to be active, logical, calm" (154).

In this respect, the dominant themes and rhetorical constructions found in *Birth Is Love* display some striking parallels and continuities with those characterizing the historic Greek debate over women's education in general discussed earlier. In the nineteenth century, Greek intellectuals argued that women's literacy and education were doubly essential if Greece was to move progressively toward the West/Europe and at the same time to symbolically disassociate from its stigmatized Eastern/Ottoman past (Bakalaki 1994; Herzfeld 1986a). Like women's illiteracy in former times, in *Birth Is Love*, women's *scientific* illiteracy is deployed as a metonym for the more general "backward" and "premodern" features of Greek national identity that must be overcome if Greece is to be identified with a more civilized West and, in particular, with Europe. And in both instances, modernity is unmistakably gendered: it is the Greek woman who functions "as an apt trope for the condition of Greeks generally" (Herzfeld 1986a, 232). In *Birth Is Love*, as in the nineteenth-century debates over pedagogy, Greek women are figured as the opposite of the (male) modern; it is they in particular who must be refashioned by means of formal education and self-education in order to step up to the plate as fully modern subjects. Throughout *Birth Is Love*, scientific knowledge is represented as valuable symbolic capital, and as a means for pregnant women to acquire the qualities long associated with both the ideal and the assertion of modernity: planning, rationality, control, logic.[9]

Using another rhetorical strategy also common to nineteenth-century reformers, Sikaki-Douka invariably buttresses the legitimacy of her claims and recommendations by reference to European authorities and practices (Bakalaki 1994, 78). As she tells the reader in her prologue, she "often refer[s] to how the system works outside of Greece, because," she remarks somewhat cryptically, "this is something that bothers me." These references are most often textual, but on occasion Sikaki-Douka also draws on her firsthand experiences in Canada and England. The guide is in fact studded with references to a large number and variety of European and North American physicians, researchers, and writers, as well as to specific European and North American practices. Within a quarter page on page 134, for instance, Sikaki-Douka mentions Europe twice, in addition to Denmark, Belgium, Finland, and France. Among the scores of references to experts, she cites Greeks only a handful of times.

At several points in the text, Sikaki-Douka also uses these rhetorical strategies and the binaries so familiar to the discourse on Greek national identity to mount a muted and partial—and at times contradictory—critique of the Greek medical system in general and of the delivery of obstetrical care in particular. Although as a professional midwife Sikaki-Douka is part of this privileged system, to some extent she speaks from the margins of a profession that has progressively restricted the scope of her professional practice and authority. Urban midwives, although highly trained, today play a strictly auxiliary role in Greek obstetrics. Thus, Sikaki-Douka tags particular beliefs and practices as European and Western not only to persuade women to adopt them, but also to critique the Greek system and customary practices, most often in an oblique manner. Invariably, when the juxtaposition of "in our country" and some locale abroad appears in the text, it is to rebuke the Greek practice and implicitly recommend an often idealized and essentialized Western model as a replacement. For example, when recommending the participation of fathers-to-be in the labor process, she writes:

> In our country, the father's participation in birth is limited to simply taking his wife to the Maternity Clinic when she is ready to give birth and handing her over with a perfunctory kiss. . . . I remember in England a father warmly and supportively holding a woman's hand the moment of her contractions, trying to breathe with her to help her with the rhythm and to encourage her. Even trying to wipe her perspiring face, to cool her, to relieve her. The woman is calm and relaxed, allowing herself his care, and time rushes by in this warm atmosphere. (57–58)

Here Sikaki-Douka uses the ethnographic authority implicit in her eyewitness account of Western lands in an attempt to persuade her reader of the desirability of allowing men to accompany their wives during labor. This is also one of the rare instances in the text where Sikaki-Douka exhorts women and men to forcefully confront their doctors in order to effect change in standard obstetrical practice. Assuring them that "there exist many doctors with a new mentality, who've studied abroad" and who would concur with this practice, she fires a volley of imperatives:

> Fathers, then, take action, read, inform yourselves, lay claim to your personal right to face birth as a unique event for each of you. (58)

> Women, you would do well to . . . try to cultivate, incite, urge, expect your husband's presence and participation. . . . Don't hide behind unjustified excuses. (59)

No mention is made in the text of a woman's mother, or of other female kin, as appropriate companions during labor. Implicit in Sikaki-Douka's preference for the husband is an idealized paradigm of an egalitarian Western companionate marriage over both a stylized patriarchal Greek model and the extended networks of female kin that usually rally around the birthing woman. There is an irony at work here: under the ethno-obstetric model described in the previous chapter, husbands in rural Rhodes were commonly present at births—if women wanted them there—to offer physical as well as moral support.

Throughout the text, Sikaki-Douka's profuse reliance on the tropes of Europe and the West partakes of a practical rhetorical strategy that has been identified as "Occidentalism." Like the more familiar concept of Orientalism (Said 1978), Occidentalism is a simplified and stylized construction of the West deployed to variable social, political, and economic ends depending on the context (Carrier 1995). Perhaps as a consequence of the contradictions within her own positionality—she is a cosmopolitan member of an elite profession that has increasingly devalued the status of midwives—Sikaki-Douka uses Occidentalist strategies at different places in the text *both* to lay claim to the moral authority instrumental to educating and disciplining modern medicalized pregnant subjects *and* to mount a critique (albeit of a partial and sometimes veiled nature) of selected aspects of Greek obstetrical practice that she deems insufficiently modern. Either way, her appeal to the cultural authority of Europe reflects and reproduces, as it did in its nineteenth-century manifestations, "the importance of the perspective of a dominant other upon the world and the self" (Bakalaki 1994, 103).[10]

The Bibliophile Body and the New Hierarchy of the Senses

The shift from the ethnomedical to the biomedical model obviously entailed a profound epistemological transformation in the ways in which bodily health, illness, structure, and function were understood, as well as in the nature and locus of medical authority. But it also entailed an equally profound transformation in the sensory modalities by which knowledge of the body was acquired. The growing scholarship on the history of the body has yielded the important insight that modes of perception are differently foregrounded in different historical contexts and different social structures (see, e.g., Feher 1989; Howes 2005). Which mode or modes of perception are privileged, furthermore, is intimately associated with what is known and how it is known. Put otherwise, "local epistemologies," ways of knowing rooted in local contexts, are grounded in, and built up from, the historically specific ways in which the senses are hierarchically ranked and valued (Stoller 1997, 3; see also Seremetakis 1994).[11]

A large body of work on modernity has copiously documented the hegemony that vision and visualizing technologies came to assume in medicine as in other domains of culture (Bynum and Porter 1993; Barley 1988; Howes 2005; Reiser 1978). I examine the dominant place occupied by vision in biomedical practice later in this chapter, when I turn to the example of fetal ultrasound imaging. Here, I wish to sketch some of the locally specific dimensions of the transformation in the hierarchy of the senses as it occurred in Rhodes.

Barbara Duden (1993, 91) adapts from Bourdieu the concept of "hexis" to signify the mode of perceptual orientation that predominates in a given historical period. This is not to say that if one modality, for example, the visual, is dominant that other sensory modes are utterly displaced or somehow "lost" (Seremetakis 1994). What the notion of hexis does entail is a hierarchical ordering in the value and authority assigned to the various sensory orientations. Because this rank order is not a timeless given but specific to distinct epochs and configurations of power, it follows that sensory hierarchies will be reshuffled as these configurations change over time. Most students of the modern hexis emphasize the primacy given to vision. There is less agreement, however, on the shape of the hierarchies of the past. Some, like Walter Ong (1982), posit the universal and primordial preeminence of sound. When the habit of literacy becomes widespread, according to Ong, aural and oral interactions are displaced by visual technologies such as script and electronic media. The visual eventually becomes the privileged foundation for evidence and the oral is demoted to "hearsay" or, of direct relevance to this study for the links it posits among gender, generation and illiteracy: "old wives' tales." Barbara Duden, in contrast, argues for the preeminence of what she calls "hapsis." Haptic experience refers to the tactile, in the broadest sense: "touch, taste, the sense of space, the feel for atmosphere" (1993, 91). On Duden's view, hapsis too is demoted when optical technologies of all sorts—from printouts to ultrasound images—become the privileged sites of knowledge production about the body's internal states.

Hearing and hapsis played important roles in the body of ethnomedical knowledge that helped women make sense of bodily signs and symptoms in prewar Rhodes, but other sensory modes were also significant.[12] In particular, scent and olfaction, so often neglected, even denigrated, in the history of the senses (Corbin 1986), occupied a privileged position in the local sensory hierarchy. The previous two chapters have offered several illustrations of this prominence. As we have seen, the womb, the organ central to a woman's health and well-being, was endowed with a sense of smell. Aromatic appeals to the womb's olfactory capacity were therapeutic strategies critical in combating illness and infertility. Women who became pregnant very easily, like Kiria Khariklia, said of themselves that they conceived "just by catching the scent" (*mono me ti mirodhia*). We also saw that the aroma of cooking food could provoke disaster in pregnancy and communal discord if its imperative message to share food were ignored. If heeded, aroma could connect women through the ethos of mutual care and concern for each other's bodies and for those of the future members of the community. Within the local semiotics of scent, it was the fragrance of hot cinnamon tea wafting from the lekhona's house that announced the recent birth to any passerby. Similarly, it was the scent of crushed bay leaves used to powder infants, which old women unfailingly recalled with a smile, that signified a new mother's loving care and attention, and thus her competence.

In contrast to scent and smell, vision was the ambivalent sense. To be sure, under certain circumstances, openness and display were valued for their ability to communicate status and sociability (Hirschon 1978). But vision was also the vector for the malevolent force of the evil eye (*to kako mati*), and an important cause of illness and misfortune. As such, it was to be feared and protected against as exhaustively as possible. Concealment was one means of protection, but one that was not, obviously, always feasible. Formulaic utterances, the power of the spoken word or the imitative sound of spitting ("ftou, ftou, ftou"), were another. Significantly, so too was the penetrating odor of garlic. In the local hierarchy of the senses that prevailed in the prewar period, then, the potentially dangerous charge carried by vision could be trumped and preempted by the power of both the aural/oral and the olfactory.

The waning importance of the olfactory, tactile, and aural sensory modes is a prominent feature of the shift to biomedical understandings of the body and, more broadly, of modernity in general (Lucien Febre, cited in Corbin 1986, 6; Elias 1982; Reiser 1978). Within the modern hierarchy of the senses, smell in particular came to be associated with animal behavior and with savage and "lower" forms of humanity. As Paul Corbin (1986, 7) has shown, beginning in the eighteenth century, "scientific convictions produced a whole array of taboos on the use of the sense of smell," ultimately relegating it to "the bottom of the hierarchy of the senses, along with the sense of touch." The demotion of smell, however characteristic of scientific practice, was not universal, to be sure (its value in the production of certain commodities such as wine and perfume is an obvious exception). Still, it is tempting to speculate that the negative associations that devalued and stigmatized the olfactory sense helped foster the silence of the oldest generation of Rhodian women. For the educated and literate daughters and granddaughters of the women for whom scent and smell had played a privileged role in managing their health and procreation, the "primitive" connotations of this sensory mode would have downgraded and made suspect the knowledge it produced. In this way, the younger generations of Rhodian women helped promote, at times tacitly and at times explicitly, "the historical repression of memory that the cultural periphery can impose on itself" (Seremetakis 1994, 9).

Generating the Transition to Biomedical Hegemony

Against this background, it should not be surprising that the redefinition of women's procreative events and experiences into biomedical categories required the turnover of a generation to complete. Almost twenty years before my research, cultural anthropologist Mary Lefkarites studied the transition from home to hospital birth in Rhodes. Lefkarites's work is extremely valuable for the narratives she collected from village women who still had one foot planted in the ethnomedical model but who were making the leap into biomedical birth with the other. Her research reveals that these women, that is, those giving birth in the 1950s and 1960s, often challenged and resisted biomedicine's bid for exclusive authority over their procreative experiences. Raised within the ethnomedical model, but with new possibilities of biomedical care and hospital birth now widely available for the first time, most of these women (eight out of the eleven who experienced both models of birth) preferred the practical care of the village mammi to the ministrations of the doctors in Rhodes Town. Among the main reasons for this preference was the hospital policy of excluding family members: women sorely missed the attention and support those closest to them provided as they labored and gave birth (1992, 399). Dina, a woman in her forties when Mary Lefkarites interviewed her, had this to say about why she decided to give birth to her second child at home in the village, after having gone to the hospital for her first birth:

> The women were kseni [strangers] to me. I was embarrassed. . . . I experienced great loneliness. I wanted my husband and my mother near me. . . . I gave birth by myself. My husband was in the village. Everyone was in the village. Nobody knew I had given birth. My husband learned two days later because the village was so far away. . . . I gave birth to my first child alone because the nurses, the midwife were all kseni to me. Who could I complain to? (398)

Eleni's grievance was similar:

> My mother and husband were outside the labor room and they [medical staff] would not let them in to take care of me. Was I in a prison or had I gone to give birth? (399)

Kiria Vaso, daughter of the mammi Kiria Arghiro, offers another illustration of this common complaint. She told me the following story on three separate occasions, each time with the same combative, triumphant air. In 1962, when Kiria Vaso was almost forty and her three children nearly grown, she discovered to her dismay that she was pregnant once more. Because the pregnancy was an obvious sign that she was still (inappropriately) sexually active at her age, it caused her to feel ashamed. Considering an abortion, she traveled from her village to Rhodes Town to discuss the procedure with a doctor there. In the end, however, her husband wouldn't hear of her going through with the abortion and she kept the pregnancy. Kiria Vaso had given birth to her first two children at home with her mother's help and had the third in the Rhodes hospital. The experience of hospital birth had left a bad taste:

> There was no one to help me, to give me courage. No one to say, like my mother did, "It's coming soon. Soon now, you will be liberated." No one. The midwife scolded me for yelling. She said it would cause the baby to be sucked back up, high into my belly, if I yelled, and it would take longer to give birth. I struggled to keep quiet and I stayed like that for hours, alone.

When the time came to give birth to her fourth child, she decided to have it at home with her mother's help. After the birth, she went to Rhodes Town again to the same doctor for a postnatal visit. Taken aback at the sight of her holding a healthy infant son, he asked Kiria Vaso who had attended the delivery. "*I mana mou*, my mom," Kiria Vaso replied. "*Who?*" He asked again in disbelief. "*I ma-na-mou!*" she drawled out the syllables for him, more loudly this time. "*Koufos ise?* Are you deaf?" Each time she told me this story, she chuckled with evident satisfaction at her response to the astonished young doctor. Having observed dozens of clinical encounters with this doctor, who is very popular for his bedside manner, I too was astonished: I had never heard any woman talk to him that way. For a woman who came of age in the decades after the war, speaking to her doctor in that fashion (unless seriously provoked) was as unthinkable as giving birth at home would have been.

In marked contrast to the women of this transitional generation, many of the youngest women with whom Lefkarites spoke in the 1970s found the anonymity of the hospital an attractive alternative to what they had come to see as the excessive interference of their extended families in their affairs. As a more companionate model of married life gained currency, young couples saw hospital birth as a way to gain "some control over one aspect of their lives" (Lefkarites 1992, 403). Others valued the antiseptic environment of the hospital, as the home was recast as a less hygienic and therefore unsafe place to give birth. Finally, doctors came to be regarded as the only practitioners who could insure a safe birth. As Popi, who gave birth in 1961, explained:

> I was afraid of giving birth at home. I thought of birth as so dangerous,
> so frightening, that I did not feel anyone [at home] could help me
> except for the physician. [He is] like God. Especially if he gives you
> a little encouragement. You feel that he is the reason [for nothing bad
> happening]. (404)

Clearly, by the mid-1970s or so, the meaning of "home birth" had been dramatically reconfigured. Where formerly the hospital had been seen as a place of death and home a haven of security and support during birth, now home was charged with danger and the hospital became a symbol of safety and reassurance.

Parallel to this shift in meaning was another: in a distinct inversion of the supplanted ethnomedical perspective, pregnancy and the climactic moment of birth now became the focus of elaborate secular rituals and interventions whose objectives were to ensure a healthy baby. Simultaneously, the postpartum underwent a process of deritualization; its symbolic significance as a liminal period fraught with danger for both mother and infant faded and, for many if not all women, completely disappeared.[13] A few women still observed the forty-day postpartum seclusion, while others might stay indoors for a week or two, mainly, as I was told, to avoid exposure to the microbes to which both mother and child were thought to be especially vulnerable after the ordeal of birth. This reversal in perceptions and practices closely mirrors the pragmatic realities of giving birth in contemporary Greece. Today, the death of a baby or a young child is a relatively rare occurrence.[14] Infant mortality has dropped impressively over the last few decades, from 40.1 per 1,000 live births in 1960 to just 5.7 in 1998. As noted in the introduction, Greece's rate is considerably lower than that of the United States (which had an infant mortality rate of 7.2 for the same year).[15] Perhaps the greatest obstetrical achievement of the post-war period has been the sharp decrease in the likelihood that a woman will die as a consequence of pregnancy or birth. At just seven per hundred thousand in 1995, the rate of maternal mortality among Greek women is in fact one of the lowest in the world (Dimitrakakis et al. 2001).[16] Again, by way of contrast, the U.S. rate in that year was twelve per hundred thousand.[17] Clearly, a lekhona in the twenty-first century no longer had one foot in the grave after giving birth. With an average of 1.27 children born to each woman in her prime reproductive years, attention now became intensely focused on the process of pregnancy and on ensuring by all means possible the health of its increasingly scarce final outcome, the newborn baby.

Greek Regimes of Maternity Care: Cultural Inflections and Comparative Perspectives

As medical anthropologists have turned to the study of biomedicine as a cultural system, the extent to which metamedical forces have shaped its central beliefs and practices has become increasingly apparent. A growing body of case studies has demonstrated that biomedical knowledge and clinical practice are far from immune to the effects of the larger society and polity in which they are embedded. This development has led to a rethinking of biomedicine(s) as plural, in recognition of the fact that medical beliefs and practices often reflect and reproduce culturally specific values, interests, and power relations.

In a comparison of medical specialties, obstetrics stands apart for the pronounced cross-national differences in the design of maternity care as well as everyday clinical practice. The quilt of cross-cultural difference in obstetric practices is especially intriguing given that, over the last several decades, a growing body of scientific research has challenged the efficacy of most, if not all, of the procedures commonly used in the biomedical management of birth (Davis-Floyd 2003). In part as a result of the mounting number of these "outcome studies," some obstetrical procedures that were once routine in the United States, Canada, New Zealand, and some parts of Europe, such as enemas and pubic shaves, have been abandoned. Others, such as episiotomies, incisions made into a woman's perineum to enlarge her vaginal opening, are on the decline. Outcome studies have demonstrated that episiotomies, once believed to prevent serious tears in the perineum, in fact *promote* such tears, something that women's health activists have argued for decades. Nevertheless, the use of many other interventions of dubious efficacy, such as electronic fetal monitoring, fetal ultrasound scans, and drug-induced augmentation of labor is on the increase (Davis-Floyd 2003, xiv). Clinical practice has largely ignored the extensive research literature that challenges the effectiveness of these procedures and documents their unwanted and often harmful side effects, such as increased rates of caesarean sections.[18] The result is what has come to be known as the "evidence-practice gap" (xii). That is, in the clinical practice of obstetrics, many procedures whose usefulness has been refuted by a substantial body of scientific research not only continue to be popular but also, in many cases, are used more intensively than ever. As much as anything else, this paradoxical situation underscores the need to scrutinize carefully the "metamedical" factors shaping the contours of contemporary obstetrical regimes.

With this background in mind, in this section I describe contemporary Greek obstetrics from a comparative perspective, in order to foreground its culturally distinctive features. Accounting for the specificities of Greek obstetrical care also requires examining its characteristic technological interventions as these are used in everyday practice. In other words, it requires attention to how locally specific meanings are constructed through the pragmatic negotiation and deployment of these technologies. Looked at from this perspective, technologies may work along a number of dimensions that may have little to do with their medical outcomes (Pfaffenberger 1992, 501). Embedded in specific contexts of social practice, technological artifacts may also be said to work in ways that can best be thought of as expressive and performative. That is to say, they may often be appropriated, consumed, and deployed as a means of constructing and expressing a particular identity and sense of self. In this expanded sense, technologies can be seen as working insofar as they enable actors to fashion the identities they deem valuable or desirable (507). Finally, as Davis-Floyd has shown in her influential study of birth in the United States (1992; 2003), obstetrical interventions may also have important ritual dimensions. Their repetitive and intensive use in the U.S. hospital setting serves to socialize American women into the core values of their society, including, most prominently, how to become a mother who "believes in science, relies on technology and recognizes her inferiority (either consciously or unconsciously) and so at some level accepts the principles of patriarchy" (1992, 339). As I shall argue later in this chapter, both doctors and women in Rhodes desire obstetrical technologies for a variety of reasons, both symbolic and pragmatic, that at times have little or nothing to do with their technical utility or efficacy.

Today in Rhodes, as throughout Greece, pregnancy and birth have become thoroughly and intensely medicalized. That is, they are understood as pathological or potentially pathological conditions and events that require the surveillance and intervention of certified biomedical experts, guided at every turn by technology to ensure a successful outcome. Except for the occasional accident of timing, all births today take place in a hospital or clinic under the supervision of an obstetrician. Planned home births are exceedingly rare and difficult to arrange.[19] For most of the Rhodian women I interviewed, as for Katerina, they were largely unthinkable. *"Ma pos?* But how? This isn't done here." I was often told when I asked if they would have liked to have birthed at home.

Midwives also participate in birth, but almost always in an auxiliary and dependent role. The 3,500 registered Greek midwives are all credentialed, highly educated professionals (Pechlivani and Adam 1999). To become a midwife, a high school graduate must first pass the difficult Panhellenic university entrance examination and then complete three years of coursework plus one year of practical training. In the early years after the war, a fresh cohort of these medically trained midwives provided obstetrical care to rural areas throughout the country. Their brief stint of independent practice was thwarted, however, when the supply of obstetricians began to swell and, as the postwar Greek birth rate plummeted, soon outstripped the falling demand for their services. Today, midwives play a strictly subordinate role in birth. Only under extraordinary circumstances would a midwife be permitted to conduct a birth on her own. Nationally, less than 5 percent of pregnancies and births are attended solely by a professional midwife, and this tends to occur only in the most remote areas of the country. Unlike the purview of midwives elsewhere in Europe, Greek midwives' participation in *prenatal* care is also quite restricted. For instance, in contrast to midwives in many other EU countries, they do not have the right to decide whether to offer ultrasound, serum screening, or folic acid to patients. In general, their functions are limited to assisting obstetricians during birth, much like labor and delivery nurses in the United States, and providing some postpartum care (Kooij et al. 1999). Not surprisingly, a recent national survey of Greek midwives found that only a little over a half felt that their present work made use of their professional knowledge (Pechlivani and Adam 1999).

A distinctive feature of Greek professional midwives is the degree to which they espouse highly favorable attitudes toward technological interventions of all kinds. Dr. F., a Greek obstetrician who had studied medicine and practiced in the United States for many years and now worked in Greece, compared midwifery practice in the two settings for me. Accustomed to the less interventionist philosophy held by most U.S. nurse-midwives, Dr. F. described his surprise at the highly favorable (what he called "aggressive") attitudes toward technology held by their Greek counterparts:

> When I came here I expected that since there were so many midwives working in the hospital that practice would be less aggressive than in the States. But here they [the midwives] are superaggressive. Very different from the States—I didn't expect that. They're very aggressive.

The lack of pluralism in obstetrics contrasts with other domains of Greek health care, where alternatives to biomedicine have multiplied in recent years. Especially in the cities, therapies as diverse as homeopathy, yoga, acupuncture, reiki, and chiropractic coexist with biomedicine, and everywhere, religious healing continues to be popular. Up to the present, however, no oppositional or alternative models have emerged that seriously challenge the hegemony of obstetricians and the rigid protocols of hospital-based care. In the United States, Canada, and elsewhere in Europe, such challenges have often been spearheaded by feminist health activists (DeVries et al. 2001). The Greek feminist movement has been instrumental in effecting profound social and legal changes, particularly at its peak in the 1970s and 1980s (Papagaroufali 1990). However, much of the movement's energies coalesced around the urgent task of revoking Greece's repressively patriarchal family law (the now defunct Family Code). Reforming the reigning obstetrical model was not among the most pressing concerns of the time.

In 1997, an organization called Evtokia (good birth) was founded in Athens to promote a less technologically intensive and interventionist approach to birth. Evtokia sponsors childbirth classes in which a dedicated group of activist midwives alert women to the pitfalls of the technological procedures routinely used in Greece. Since its inception, Evtokia has invited some of the world's leading natural childbirth activists, such as Frederick LeBoyer and Suzanne Arms, to give talks at their center. The creation of Evtokia is a development that promises to open new possibilities for a less medicalized model of birth, but its impact so far on expanding women's options has been fairly small. Sometimes, attending the center's classes could even result in frustration, as one Athenian friend complained to me. Having diligently attended

Evtokia's weekly lectures and support group in the last few months of her pregnancy and learned in great detail about the risks and disadvantages of the most common obstetrical interventions, she nevertheless experienced all of them (including a caesarean section) once she entered the hospital to give birth. (Some Rhodian women voiced similar complaints about the pregnancy guides from Western Europe or the United States that they had read in preparation for birth. Illustrations of women birthing in water or reclining comfortably on capacious birthing bags tantalized them with appealing alternatives that were locally unattainable.) Still, in 2000, a graduate student in Athens happily wrote to tell me that she had managed to achieve her goal of giving birth at home with the help of an Evtokia-affiliated professional midwife.

As should by now be obvious, biomedical obstetrics has a privileged status in the provision of care to pregnant women largely unfettered by challenges from alternative practices or oppositional discourses. This privileged position rests on two main foundations that underpin all of Greek biomedicine. First, biomedicine is firmly supported by the state and enjoys preferential access to state resources. All Greece's medical schools are public and funded by the state, and about 85 percent of Greek doctors work for the public National Health Service (ESY) in some capacity (Colombotos and Fakiolas 1993). Second, biomedicine in Greece, as in so many other parts of the world, enjoys a symbolic dominance grounded in social respect and prestige. In large part, biomedicine's symbolic value derives from the prevailing modernist narrative that closely associates science and technology with progress and, concurrently, stigmatizes and demotes other bodies of knowledge as backward-looking examples of ignorance, irrationality, and quackery (Jordan 1978 [1993], 201; Davis-Floyd, Pigg, and Cosminsky 2001), a narrative that in Greece has been subtly promoted through the educational system and reinforced by the media. These advantages ultimately endow biomedicine with a powerful "structural superiority" that firmly, if sometimes invisibly, reinforces its authority over all aspects of health care (Lee 1982, cited in Jordan 1993, 201). Although biomedicine enjoys these advantages almost universally, for numerous and complex reasons, Greek obstetrics evinces a particularly amplified version of this symbolic dominance.

At first blush, obstetrical practice in Greece looks very familiar to anyone who has given birth in a U.S. hospital. In fact, North American attempts to influence Greek health care date from the interwar period, with the arrival of the Rockefellar Foundation in 1929 and its initiatives to reform the public health system. These efforts had mixed results, however, and were effectively halted by the outbreak of the Second World War (Giannuli 1998). Later on, in the bipolar world that took shape after the war, American influence was

was more effectively exerted through the Truman Doctrine, which identified Greece as a crucial "domino" in the emergent cold war, poured in large amounts of foreign aid, and for the next several decades turned it into a client state of the United States (Gallant 2001, 179–180). In the subsequent restoration and restructuring of Greek health care, the U.S. biomedical model that was introduced along with other reforms soon overshadowed the prestige and influence formerly exerted by German and French biomedicine (Dr. Gherasimos Righatos, personal communication). At the Rhodes Maternity Clinic where I did my research, for example, the director at the time (and for many years before and after) had trained in the United States in the 1960s. Of the five Rhodian obstetricians Mary Lefkarites interviewed (1992), one had completed his residency in the United States and another had worked in an American hospital.

In both Greece and the United States, birth is treated as a pathological process fraught with potentially disastrous risks for woman and baby alike (for the United States, see Jordan 1993; Davis-Floyd 1992). In neither place does an institutionalized mechanism exist to distinguish a normal, uncomplicated birth from one that is in fact high risk. Unlike other European nations, such as Holland, Sweden, and increasingly, the United Kingdom, in which low-risk women, attended by midwives, give birth with a modicum of technological assistance, *all* births in Greece (as in the United States) are subject to much the same array of interventions (Jordan 1993, 61; DeVries et al. 2001). Thus, over the course of a typical pregnancy, a Greek woman visits her doctor a dozen or more times. As part of her routine prenatal care, she undergoes a battery of tests that usually include at least three or four—and increasingly in recent years, monthly—ultrasound scans. Almost without exception, she gives birth in a hospital setting, where upon admission she immediately receives an enema and a pubic shave. She is hooked up to an IV through which a cocktail of drugs is administered, including most prominently the hormone oxytocin (pitocin) to augment her uterine contractions. Today, she most likely receives prostaglandins (misoprostol, called cytotec in the United States) to soften her cervix. If a woman's water hasn't broken by the time she arrives at the hospital, her membrane is artificially ruptured. Her abdomen is encircled with an electronic fetal monitor that she will wear throughout her labor. Her vaginal opening is enlarged by an episiotomy, although she receives no pain medication beyond perhaps a local anesthetic injected directly into her perineum right before her incision is repaired. Throughout her labor, she is not permitted to eat or drink. When the time comes to give birth, she does so exclusively in the lithotomy position, flat on her back, on the surgical table called— unreassuringly for this native English speaker—the *boom*. Once she is positioned on the *boom*, her arms and legs are splayed out and sometimes strapped into place so that nearly all mobility on her part is impeded. In over a quarter of births, vacuum extraction, which involves attaching a suction device to the infant's skull, is used to deliver the baby.

When I began my hospital study in 1990, family members were not allowed in the delivery room. By 2000, hospital policy had changed, and husbands routinely stayed with their wives throughout the birth. This reversal in policy, the only major change in maternity care over this period, came about largely as a result of the demands of women and their families. (Coincidentally perhaps, this was the one reform *Birth Is Love* forcefully promoted.) By 2000, everyone expected a husband to stay with his wife throughout the birth—with or without a video camera. A senior midwife, for example, told me that in the few cases that a woman preferred to have her mother instead of her husband stay with her, she always talked the woman out of it. Telling women, as she put it, that "it was time to cut the umbilical cord," she managed to convince them that their husband was the more appropriate choice.

By the early 2000s, Greece's rate of caesarean sections—far and away "the most invasive and risk-bearing" of all birth technologies, according to Carol Sakala (1993, 1177)—had reached unprecedented levels.[20] In 1983, it stood at a modest 12 percent, well within the WHO global target rate of 10–15 percent of births (Tzoumaka-Bakoula 1990, 87). By 2005, over 40 percent of women gave birth via caesarean section. Because immigrants, who now comprise about one-tenth of the national population, tend to receive fewer caesareans, the rate for ethnic Greek women is actually higher still. A 2002 study in Athens, for instance, found that the caesarean rate for ethnic Greek women who delivered in public hospitals was 52.5 percent. For insured women who gave birth in private hospitals, it reached an astonishing 65 percent (Mossialos et al. 2005). I should point out that Greece's caesarean rate, while very high, is today not that unusual cross-culturally. Rather, it is best considered a local manifestation of what one critic has called the global "pandemic of medically unnecessary cesarean births" (Sakala 1993, 1189). In the end, when births by caesarean section are added to those by vacuum extraction, the total rate of what are known in obstetrics as "instrumental births" now approaches 100 percent (Skalkidis et al. 1996).

That a woman birthing in Greece will experience most or all of the procedures just mentioned is virtually guaranteed by the highly democratic access to the National Health System. Even if a patient is uninsured or cannot afford to pay for a procedure (for instance, an undocumented immigrant), it is unlikely that she will be denied prenatal or obstetrical care. For Dr. F., the obstetrician who had practiced both in the United States and Greece, this ability to treat patients free of charge if necessary was one of the most appealing aspects of the Greek health care system. In contrast to his experience in the United States, in Greece he felt freer to fulfill what he called the "romantic ideal" of medicine. He explained why:

> Everybody is basically covered here. If something happens to you in the States and you end up in the hospital, you might end up losing half your home. This doesn't really happen here. Patients without any insurance will come in and have their baby and probably won't even pay anything—because the system here is not organized completely. And so you can do things here to patients, be nice to patients and do procedures to help them out, easier than in the States. I can have a patient that's not well off and I can do an ultrasound for her, I can do her monitoring for free, I can do a minor procedure for free. It's easier to do in a Greek hospital—versus the States: as soon as you step in the door there, everything gets charged.

Because of this leeway, almost every birthing woman in Greece, from the posh private clinic patient in Athens to the itinerant Roma (Gypsy) farm worker, ultimately becomes enmeshed in a technologically intense and highly interventionist model of obstetrical care.[21]

Although all or most of the foregoing interventions are found wherever birth has become medicalized, it is essential to scrutinize each local example for "what is *not* shared in the emerging global order of reproduction," as well as for what is (Rapp 1994, 34). The global circulation of obstetrical technologies does not necessarily erase cultural difference or produce a jumbled "postmodern collage" (Lock 1997, 40). Cross-cultural comparison of technological configurations can be particularly valuable in deciphering the local inflections of biomedicine and the roles they play in fashioning particular kinds of knowledge and identities.

When examined from such a comparative perspective, Greek obstetrical practice stands out for the *intensity* with which technical interventions are deployed. A study of obstetrics in twelve countries (Stephenson et al. 1993) nearly two decades ago underscored this point.[22] Of the countries for which there was information, Greece had by far the highest rate of use of oxytocin to augment labor. Eighty percent of Greek women giving birth received oxytocin, compared to 20 percent in the United Kingdom and 12 percent in the United States. In the public hospital I observed in the early 1990s, the only women not receiving oxytocin were typically those who had arrived at the hospital relatively late in their labor and were already well dilated. The twelve-country study also found that Greece had the sharpest increase over the five-year study period in rates of instrumental vaginal delivery (mostly by vacuum extraction) and of caesarean sections. Today, Greece's caesarean rate is the highest in the European Union and one of the highest in the world (Mossialos et al. 2005). By all indications, the rate will continue to rise, if only because vaginal births after a caesarean delivery are still rarely attempted. The Rhodes hospital closely followed these national trends: in 1990, its caesarean section rate was already at 35 percent, up from 18 percent in 1985 (Georges 1996, 166).[23]

A notable aspect of obstetrical practice in Rhodes is the absence of anesthesia in childbirth.[24] In the past, Rhodian women would be put under general anesthesia toward the end of their labor, while their episiotomies were being repaired, and awakened some twenty minutes to a half hour after having given birth, but this practice has been abandoned. In public hospitals, mild painkilling drugs may be given from time to time during labor, but anesthesia is used only for caesarean sections. Epidurals are increasingly available in private clinics in Athens and other major cities. However, in Rhodes, neither the public hospital nor the private clinic offered them. The reason I was given by all of the obstetricians I asked was the acute shortage of anesthesiologists. In 2002, only four anesthesiologists were on staff to handle the needs of all the departments in the Rhodes hospital. This was a woefully inadequate number, not least because Rhodes's popularity with tourists has meant that the hospital had to handle an exceptionally high rate of trauma surgery from traffic accidents during the island's long tourist season. Additionally, very few anesthesiologists had the specialized training and skills needed to administer epidurals. In the face of the thousand or so births that took place in the hospital each year, epidurals for childbirth simply were not an option.

Some of the medical interventions that were now routine, such as the use of drugs to augment labor and the artificial breaking of membranes, can increase considerably the pain of childbirth. Rhodian women who had already had a child and knew what to expect, and others who had heard stories from friends and family, were often very afraid of giving birth. Not infrequently, this fear led women to ask—and in one prenatal visit I witnessed, desperately beg—their obstetrician to perform a caesarean.

The absence of anesthesia in public hospitals has created a market for alternative means for coping with the pain of childbirth that many women had come to dread. Professional midwives filled this niche by offering private lessons in what is known in Greece as "painfree childbirth" (*anodhinos toketos*). In addition to providing instructions on Lamaze-like breathing and guided imaging, these lessons tutored a woman in what to expect once she entered the hospital. If the midwife giving the classes also worked in the hospital in which the woman was to give birth, she also acted as her labor coach or doula. The special care and attention these midwives gave their clients during labor and delivery was always greatly appreciated by the women I interviewed. I hasten to note here that the term "doula," from the ancient Greek word for "slave," is an unfortunate coining of North American childbirth reformers. In Greece, birth activists roundly reject the term for its demeaning associations and are sincerely puzzled by its adoption and use in the United States and elsewhere.

The comparatively intensive use of technology also characterizes the management of pregnancy and prenatal care. Recent studies of prenatal care in the countries of the European Union have found that on the whole, Greek doctors and midwives held the most favorable attitudes toward interventions over the course of a woman's prenatal care. For instance, a recent EU-sponsored survey compared attitudes toward genetic testing in Greece, the Netherlands, England, and Finland. Greek physicians were found to be the most supportive and least critical of prenatal screening (Ettore 1999; see also Marangos and Adam 1999). Similarly, Greek midwives were several times more likely to support the use of technological interventions in prenatal care than were midwives in the other countries surveyed (Pechlivani and Adam 1999). The vast majority of Greek midwives were in favor of routine prenatal testing to detect fetal anomalies and genetic disorders. Overwhelmingly, they held the view that fetal ultrasound imaging, which can detect gross fetal anomalies; the thalassemia test, which can detect the serious hemoglobin disorder for which a high percentage of Greeks are carriers; and the MsAfp test, which screens for spina bifida and Down syndrome should be available to all pregnant women (95, 91, and 88 percent respectively). Nearly all (95 percent) believed that it was the state's obligation to ensure universal access to these tests. The great majority (78 percent) of the midwives surveyed also felt that prenatal screening did not raise ethical or social problems (Pechlivani and Adam 1999, 11–12). When asked specifically whether prenatal ultrasound promoted the medicalization of pregnancy, Greek midwives were much more likely to disagree than were English or Dutch midwives (Kooij et al. 1999, 11). At least in part, midwives' strong support for prenatal tests reflects the widespread awareness of the high burden of genetic disease in Greece. At the same time, survey findings such as these confirm Dr. F.'s impression, noted earlier, that Greek midwives tend to be, in his words, "aggressive." That is, they tend to hold highly favorable attitudes toward technological interventions of all kinds.

The Greek media also tend to portray the technologies of prenatal surveillance in a more favorable light than do the media elsewhere in Europe. The first nationally representative study of Greek women's awareness and use of prenatal testing recently found that the popular media served women as vitally important translators and purveyors of medical knowledge. This survey revealed that besides their doctors, the media were the most influential source of information on pregnancy and prenatal care (Mavrou, Metaxotou, and Trichopoulos 1998, 351). Against this finding, it is important to note that the Greek popular media overwhelmingly represent technological interventions in a positive and enthusiastic manner. Another recent study, which looked at print media coverage of a broad range of prenatal technologies, including ultrasound, amniocentesis, CVS, MSAfp, genetic screening, and genetic tests, found critical debate on their adoption and use to be virtually nonexistent. By and large, the Greek media tended to ignore the social and psychological entailments of these technologies and to focus almost exclusively on pragmatic issues. The authors conclude of their review of the Greek media:

> In general, the aim of the articles is to provide information for pregnant women, so that they can take advantage of all the potentials of modern biomedical technology available in Greece. The articles are characterized by a rather paternalistic or directive style and no particular debate is developed through them. The articles are based on the assumption that *more tests mean better health*. No particular dilemmas or options for prenatal screening are discussed. The articles seem to serve as promotion of any test available and a demand to take advantage of those not available. . . . There was no reference to ethical dilemmas concerning tests already available to Greek women and no questioning of the usefulness of any available diagnostic test could be found. (Lauren et al. 1999, 9–10, my emphasis)

In short, both the medical experts (doctors and midwives) and those who produce the mass-mediated popular translations of expert knowledge (journalists and authors of advice literature) converge in their optimistic narratives and positive representations of a broad array of technological interventions in obstetrical care.

Finally, though certainly not least, women themselves have played a complex role in the medicalization of pregnancy and birth in Greece. Rhodian women's narratives reveal the extent to which they share in the optimistic discourse of the experts and their popular translators. As consumers, women are of course "embedded in a network of social relations that limits and controls the technological choices that [they are] capable of making" (R. Cowan 1987, 262). Within the framework of these constraints, their demands have also had an important hand in shaping the specific profile of technological interventions. However, as discussed in the next section, the meanings women assign to these interventions also exceed the familiar modernist narrative of optimism and progress. In addition, women's perceptions are closely related to, and shaped by, long-standing assumptions of medical benevolence and by reconfigured cultural meanings that link these technologies to the personal project of becoming modern pregnant subjects and mothers.

Blurring the Boundaries of Consent and Constraint: Women and their Doctors

The quality of beneficence is a sine qua non that women expect from the doctor they have carefully chosen from what is, given the serious oversupply of doctors in Greece, a highly competitive field of candidates. Among other things, both the doctor's benevolence and his competence are expressed through, and judged by, the alacrity with which he intervenes, in women's own words "to help her" deal with the common issues and problems of pregnancy and birth—above all, anxiety, uncertainty, and pain.[25] Francesca, a twenty-five-year-old hairdresser, who had just given birth to her first child, described the importance of the confidence and trust she placed in her doctor to "help her" in terms similar to those I heard from many other women:

> My doctor helped me a lot. I could ask him about anything. He gave me support. That's why women say, "You've got to be bonded, *dhemeni*, with your doctor. . . ." Me, I go to my doctor with my eyes closed, *me ta matia klista*, with complete confidence. He's very good; he helped me a lot.

EG: How did he help you?

Francesca: When I got to the hospital, I was only dilated about two to three centimeters, although the pains had started several hours earlier. When I arrived, they gave me *oro* [oxytocin] right away. The doctor told me it was so that the contractions would come faster, so I could finish sooner, and not have to go through so much trouble and hardship, *na min taleporitho*. And after a few minutes I felt it, the pains got stronger, they came every minute and then every half-minute, and they got even stronger. The midwife helped me to breathe, because I wanted to yell. But I didn't yell, that is, I didn't until the doctor broke my water.

EG: Would you have preferred that they didn't do this?

Francesca: No, no—they gave me the IV and broke my water and I hurt badly for a few times [contractions] and that was it. *Kalitera etsi*, it's better that way, I think, instead of taking all day, they helped me to finish faster.

Ino, twenty-three, a secretary, who had just had her first child, told me she had gone straight to the bookstore as soon as she got the results of her pregnancy test. She bought several books, including *Birth Is Love*, and read them all. As she observed with a hint of pride, she arrived at the hospital an informed consumer:

> So, I knew what to expect when the time came to give birth. I knew all about the procedures and why they are done. I knew about everything that would happen. When I got to the hospital, they shaved me, gave me an enema and put in an IV, and gave me *oro*.
> EG: Why did they give you *oro*?
> Ino: Because it helps you to dilate, *na kanis dhiastoli*. They gave me oro and my stomach immediately became hard like a stone, *petrose*. The pains immediately got stronger—*a lot*, not a little! And then they got faster. First every fifteen minutes, then every few seconds. Dr. Z. was so good, he was trying hard to help me, to help me finish more quickly.

Toward the end of the interview, I asked Ino to describe the ideal birth. Her answer was typical, if more to the point than most women's: "Fast! The faster the better!"

The pain of childbirth has long figured as an important cultural resource in the fashioning and performance of maternal identities in Greece. As Dubisch (1995a, 215) first pointed out, women's expressions of pain and suffering "call attention to what they must endure in order to carry out their roles," especially their roles as mothers. And, as Paxson (2004, 97) further elaborates, "childbirth is the dramatic, painful moment that marks the beginning of the *social*, maternal relationship." For this reason, many women associated the pain of labor with the power to "complete" a woman's transformation as a mother. Zambeta, nineteen, who had dropped out of high school to marry her boyfriend when she became pregnant in her senior year, expressed this sentiment most eloquently:

> I didn't want to have a caesarean, because when you give birth naturally, *fisiologhika* [that is, vaginally], you are completed as a woman. If you don't feel the pains of birth, you can't call yourself a woman. You hurt, and you feel that with your troubles and efforts and your sweat, you bring your

baby, a new life, into the world. I didn't feel this thing, but I think that it is something important. But with a caesarean, it's a dead thing, *ena nekro praghma*, you go to sleep and you wake up.

However valued pain might be for effecting a woman's completion as a mother, allowing it to run a protracted course, when there were medical means available to curtail it, was decidedly *not* valued. For Ino, Francesca, and many others, appreciation of a speedy delivery reflected their desire to avoid prolonging pain that was often considerably augmented by interventions such as pitocin and amniotomy. As importantly, prolonged labor had come to be regarded as a physical strain that could pose a danger to the health of woman and infant alike. All births were treated as potentially fraught with risk, or *risko*. More colloquially, doctors, along with women and their families, often used the word "*taleporia*," which means hardship or suffering, to describe the process of labor. Labor was a *taleporia* for women, to be sure. But it posed the greatest hazards for the baby, who had to navigate the birth canal, and it was commonly felt that the risk of damage or other harm to the baby's health only increased as labor dragged on. Allowing a labor to run its course when the technical means were at hand to intervene would be regarded as a failure on the doctor's part to protect both mother and infant from potential harm. Thus, although pain retained its symbolic importance for many women, a little, it seemed, went a long way: "the faster the better!"[26]

Doctors are well aware of the woman's expectations that they "help" her to "finish quickly" and may feel compelled to oblige them. Dr. P., an obstetrician in his early forties who was moderately critical of the intensity with which interventions were applied in birth, described how these cultural expectations led to feelings of pressure from women and their families to "do something":

> The woman herself will say to you, "Doctor, help me to finish quickly." And if a woman passes her due date, the whole family panics. Mothers, grandmothers, everybody. "Something's going to happen to the baby. The baby's going to dry out. The baby's going to die, the baby's going to do this, the baby's going to do that." So there's a lot of pressure to do something.

Consistent with this logic, there was little tolerance on the part of doctors or women and their families for exceeding the due date. In fact, induction of labor for a postdate pregnancy typically occurs earlier in Greece than elsewhere in Europe (Alran et al. 2002).

If the due date is exceeded by more than a few days, the pressure to perform a caesarean section begins to mount. As caesareans have become common, many women's perceptions of the procedure have begun to change. The majority of women I spoke with, like Zambeta, said that they preferred vaginal birth. Some women, however, asked their doctors to perform a caesarean specifically so they could receive anesthesia. Still others held an ambivalent view of the operation. I interviewed Ritsa, a twenty-seven-year-old accountant, a few days after she gave birth to her second daughter by caesarean section. Remarkably relaxed, bubbly, and voluble, Ritsa had this to say about the procedure:

> Sometimes I think that I'm lucky I had a caesarean. I had wanted to deliver naturally after my first caesarean, but Dr. L. wouldn't consider it. I thought that feeling the pains of labor would make you more of a mother, that you would feel that the child is more yours. But now, I think it's better that I had a caesarean. I have friends [who delivered vaginally] who still can't make love with their husbands because of [complications from] the episiotomy, and another friend who, after all these years, still remembers the doctor sewing her up; she can't forget it. I think the time will come when all women will want a caesarean. [Why?] Because it doesn't interfere with your sex life. Nothing changes in that respect. Women today have another mentality, *ali nootropia*. They are more concerned about their sexuality than their mothers were. . . . A caesarean is just like any other intervention, *mia epemvasi opos oles i ales*.

As this quote reveals, Ritsa's opinion of the caesarean section clearly shifted over time, from a procedure she initially wanted to avoid to one she endowed with desirable qualities. At least in part, her narrative suggests, this shift occurred because the procedure had come to be associated with a new "mentality" that highlights sexuality as a central feature of Greek understandings of modern femininity. Free from the "taboos" of the past (which Ritsa tellingly refers to as the views held by her mother's generation), the expression of this sexuality is also a central ingredient in contemporary understandings of the modern companionate couple and of a successful conjugal life. Thus for Ritsa, the caesarean section accrued value for its ability to safeguard the quality of a woman's sexual expression within her marriage. Ironically, Ritsa did not value the caesarean section primarily because it prevented the vaginal damage sometimes attributed to "natural" childbirth, but because it protected her from the iatrogenic damage (both physical and psychological) that could result from the (inevitable) episiotomy. Toward the end of our conversation, Ritsa's mother came into her room to visit her, and as we began to talk about the birth once more, she offered her own reasons for preferring a caesarean birth. Ritsa's mother was glad that her daughter had had the procedure, she told me, so that she did not have to endure the hardship of childbirth. "It's better this way," she explained. "I didn't want to see my daughter suffer."

Although Rhodian women occasionally criticized the hospital staff or some feature of the hospital facilities they found inadequate, few expressed dissatisfaction over the array of procedures and interventions they experienced. Only one of the women I interviewed, Stavroula, told me that she had made an attempt to evade the standard hospital procedures. A striking twenty-five-year-old former secretary who had married her boss, Stavroula was a thoroughgoing contrarian with a mordant manner that left unscathed neither her doctor, nor her husband, nor herself. She was the only woman who told me that she would have preferred to give birth at home, as she put it, "so I could avoid having to use the hospital bathrooms," but that it was simply impossible to do so in Rhodes. She was also the only woman who refused to let me use a tape recorder during our interview, although she clearly enjoyed answering my questions at length and did not mind repeating an especially memorable turn of phrase until I wrote it down verbatim (as a result, our conversation lasted well over three hours).

Stavroula was unusual from the beginning to the end of her pregnancy. She went to see her doctor only twice after she learned she was pregnant, because "I don't get along well with doctors. They break my nerves very easily. And I don't want to wait hours to see them. As long as everything was okay, I didn't go." She rode her motorcycle and smoked throughout her pregnancy, pointing out with some satisfaction that her baby was nevertheless born healthy and "huge, over four kilos." Unlike so many of the other women I spoke with, she made no special preparations for the birth. Although a high school graduate, she differed from most other women with a similar level of education in that she had not read any books or magazines about pregnancy, nor had she attended childbirth classes. She felt sure that she knew what to do, "from instinct, *apo enstikto*." And anyway, she went on, "whatever you do, you're going to hurt." When her contractions began, she deliberately stayed away from the hospital as long as she could. "At home I could eat and drink whatever I wanted, especially eat. Because in the hospital they don't give you anything and you could die of hunger." Besides, "at home I would hurt, and in the hospital I would hurt." So she delayed going to the hospital—that is, until she saw some blood. Frightened, she called her doctor, who told her to come immediately. "What happened then?" I asked, curious to learn how far her contrariness would get her. "They gave me an enema, which I didn't want, and they shaved me, which I hated." "Did you ask them not to?" "Eh, who's going to listen to me? Whether I want it or don't want it, I was going to get it." Then they gave her oxytocin and the doctor stripped her membrane. "I asked them why, and they said so the pains will get stronger and you can finish more quickly." After about fifteen minutes, the contractions did get strong and very painful. "Would you have preferred not to have the oxytocin or your waters artificially broken?" I asked. She thought for a moment and then told me that she couldn't answer that question. You simply had to have it done. And, she said after some hesitation, you do get out faster, but then she ruefully added, "in theory, *sti theoria*."

I cannot explain why Stavroula differed from the other women I interviewed. As far as I could tell, her education and upbringing were entirely unremarkable. Her responses to the questions about contraception and abortion I routinely asked were also in line with those I heard from most of the other women. Intriguingly, Stavroula's story evokes some of the distinctive features of the current of Greek modernity that James Faubion has described in his ethnographic study of Athenian elites. Like them, she expresses "a sage suspicion of the security of any order, human or superhuman" (1993, 155). I had heard women express variants of this attitude with respect to other aspects of their lives, but Stavroula was unique in her outright suspicion and rejection of medical expertise over her pregnancy. Puzzling though it is, Stavroula's story is important because it demonstrates that, even in an overdetermined context such as Rhodes, a few women are able to tap into an alternative discourse of modernity that demotes the authority of experts and valorizes their own "instincts," that is, their own intuition and embodied knowledge as guides for navigating their pregnancies (see Davis-Floyd and Arvidson 1997). Of course, in the absence of alternatives to hospital birth, when all was said and done, even Stavroula experienced the full range of interventions, from enema to episiotomy.

"Putting the Baby on Television": Fetal Ultrasound Imaging and Rhodian Women's Experiences of Pregnancy

Technology, popularly referred to as "machines" (*mikhanes* or *mikhanimata*), plays a major role in Rhodian women's decisions as to where to give birth. In general, Greek families who can afford them prefer private clinics to the public maternity hospitals, which often have low prestige and mainly serve poor women, immigrants, and Greece's Roma population (Arnold 1985; Lefkarites 1992; Tzoumaka-Bakoula 1990). For Rhodian women, the ultimate sign of distinction is to go to Athens and give birth in a private clinic, where the

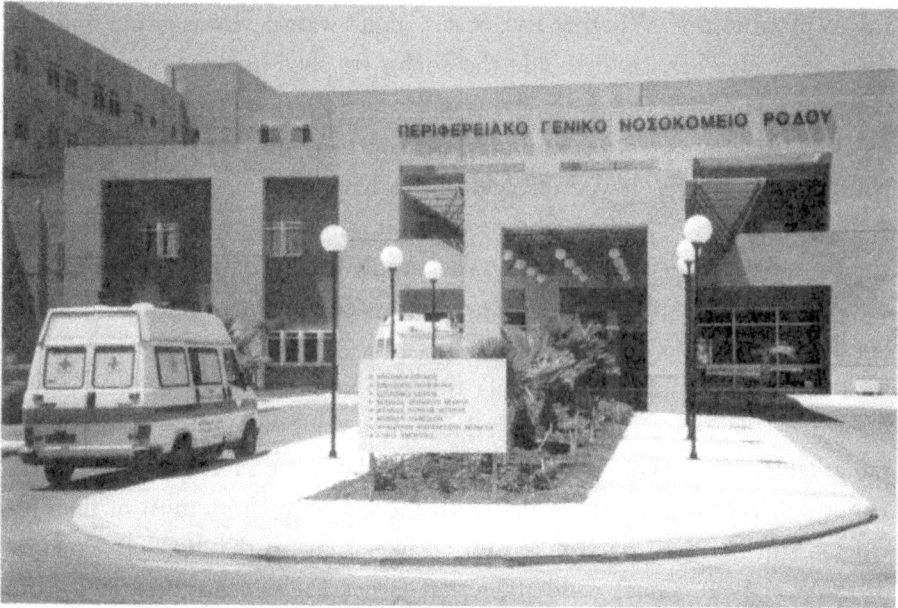

9. Rhodes General Hospital, completed in 2000.

most up-to-date "machines" and best doctors can be found. Rhodes is unusual, however, in that most women who give birth locally (as the majority do for practical reasons) choose the public hospital over the private clinic, even if they could easily afford to pay out of pocket for private care. Throughout Greece, doctors in the public and private sectors compete intensely for patients (Bartsocas 1997). In Rhodes, the public sector has won out as much for its superior stock of "machines" as for its reputation for employing the best doctors on the island. And so, each year about a thousand births take place in the Rhodes public hospital, out of a national total of about a hundred thousand (Fig. 9).

Without doubt, among the "machines" seen as vital to the successful management of pregnancy and birth, the most prominent is the fetal ultrasonograpic scanner (Fig. 10). Fetal ultrasound imaging was introduced in Greece in the 1970s, and by the early 1990s, it is safe to say, no pregnancy went unscanned. Rhodian women typically had three to five scans over the course of a normal pregnancy. In the early 1990s, the modal number for my sample of women was four, but a few women had seven or more. By 2000, regular monthly scans had become common, with an additional level II scan now recommended in the fifth month. I always asked pregnant women I happened to meet if they'd had an ultrasound. "*Ame!* For sure! And how! Every month," is an answer I got with increasing frequency in recent years. Such in-

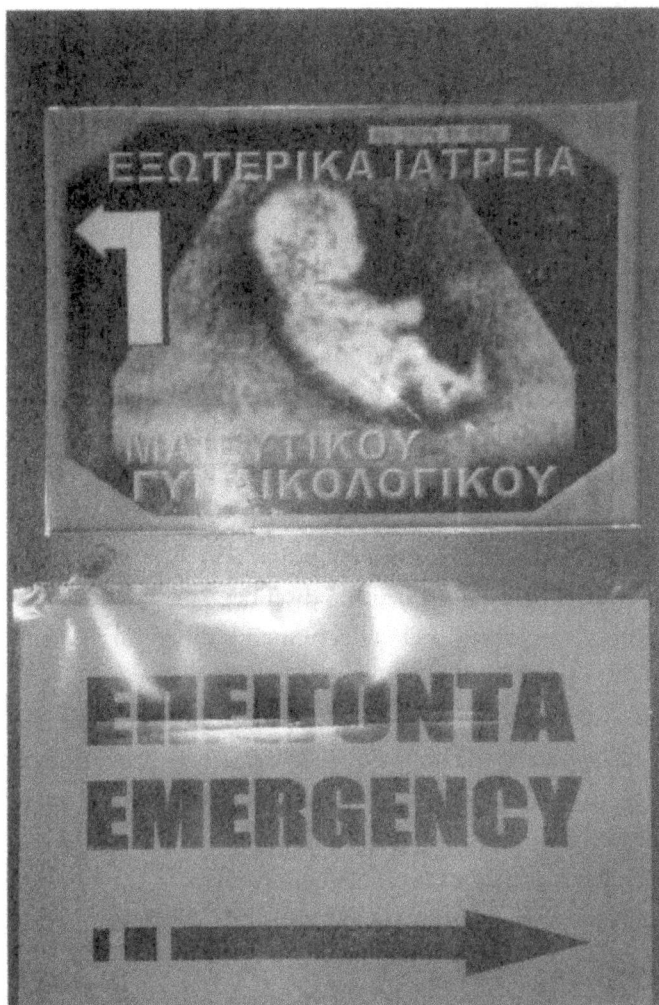

10. Sign for Obstetrics and Gynecology Clinic, Rhodes General Hospital.

tensive monitoring is not a regional aberration but reflects Greek obstetrical practice generally. Medical students in Athens are taught to do three scans per normal pregnancy, one in each trimester. A survey conducted in the early 1990s of more than five hundred normal pregnancies in Athens found that, in fact, nearly all women (93 percent) had had at least one fetal ultrasound scan, while about one-quarter experienced two or more in the third trimester alone (Breart et al. 1992). Normal pregnancies are scanned with ultrasound for a large variety of reasons, including to confirm a suspected pregnancy, chart fetal growth, establish due dates, ascertain presentation of the fetus, detect gross anomalies, and, surprisingly often, as I discuss later, respond to a woman's request to "see the baby."

In this section, I focus exclusively on ultrasound as a way of gaining a deeper sense of the processes that shape the specific configuration of intensive technological intervention in Greek obstetrical practice. Of course, because of the visual images it generates, ultrasound is not a typical intervention. The primacy attributed to vision is a widely remarked feature of modernity, and its historical ascendence in biomedicine has been well documented. Ultrasound, like many visualizing medical technologies, is the product in part of the modern "scopic drive" to render bodies visible.[27] Ultrasound also stands apart for its strong link to popular visual technologies. This association is explicitly recognized in Greek everyday usage, where ultrasound is commonly referred to as "television" (*tileorasi*), and doing an ultrasound is known as "putting the baby on television." Television is an apt metaphor for fetal ultrasound imaging in Greece. It is ubiquitous and provides a major vehicle for the dissemination of images of modernity and information about modern behavior throughout the country (Handman 1983; McNeill 1978). The women I interviewed were nearly all born around or after the time television was first introduced in Greece, 1966, and have thus grown up with its discursive conventions, not least of which is its "ability to carry a socially convincing sense of the real" (Fiske 1987, 21).

The ultrasound scan as performed in the hospital is a formulaic procedure that resonates with ritual overtones (Davis-Floyd 1992). Only level I ultrasounds are performed in the public hospital; higher-resolution level II scans had to be done in private clinics. The following description is of a typical session, which usually lasts about five minutes. For most women, it is replicated several times over the course of their pregnancies, with little variation and in near silence.

Toward the conclusion of a routine prenatal examination, the doctor (or the woman) may suggest "putting the baby on television." The woman then follows the doctor down the hospital corridor to a small room, lit dimly only by the shadowy gray light emanating from the ultrasound monitor. No other medical personnel are present during the session, but the woman may be accompanied by family members, usually her husband, and possibly a small child. The woman lies on the examining bed next to the apparatus and, generally without being instructed to do so (since she has usually done this before), wordlessly pulls her skirt or slacks and underwear down below her abdomen. The doctor squirts her exposed abdomen with a coupling gel and begins to probe its surface with the transducer.

The screen is generally turned toward the doctor. The woman can view it by craning her neck, but her eyes are often directed toward the doctor's face. Quickly and silently, the doctor scans the entire fetal image, then focuses on the genital area for a while. At this point, he may break his silence to announce, "Girl" or "Boy"—unless the woman has already jumped in to tell him she doesn't want to know the sex. Or he may tell the woman that the position or age of the fetus doesn't permit him to see the sex this time, and that he will look again next month. Finally, the doctor scans to the skull and freezes the image in order to measure the biparietal diameter (skull width). He checks a chart over the bed upon which the woman is lying and announces the age of the fetus, in weeks and days. If the doctor himself does not tell the woman at this point that "the baby is all right" (no anomaly was detected in the more than eighty sessions I observed), she will ask him. Most often, this is the only time she speaks. After wiping the gel from the woman's abdomen with a paper towel, the doctor leaves. If the woman's husband is with her, as was the case with about one-third of the women, they may exchange a few quick comments in the corridor, usually about the fetus's announced sex.

The Rhodian women I spoke with almost uniformly regarded ultrasound in a positive light. Their appreciation of the technology and of the various kinds of information and sensations it produced did not mean that they submitted themselves to the procedure automatically or unreflectively, however. During our interviews, I routinely prompted women to discuss the advantages (*pleonektimata*) and disadvantages (*mionektimata*) of the procedure. It was evident from their responses that most had considered the possibility of health risks to the fetus or to themselves. They usually thought of ultrasound's potential risk—or *risko*, the loan word many women used when discussing their deliberations—in terms of some form of radiation. Women routinely attempted to sort out the risk of delivering a "sick baby" from the risk of causing harm to the fetus by submitting to the ultrasound scan. Thus, for many women, enthusiasm for the scan was mixed with lingering doubt. Even if their concerns were dispelled, the questions that remained about the safety of the procedure revealed how their sense of maternal responsibility for the health of their offspring had now expanded and deepened to encompass the prenatal period.

As the following excerpts reveal, women often raised their concerns with their doctors and sought out additional information on their own in conversations with other women and by reading a variety of texts. Typically, the information they gathered reassured them. Stamatia, thirty, an officer in the army who had just had her second child, explained that she learned most about what she knew about ultrasound from her sister and her many friends who had had scans, but also had asked her doctor's opinion:

> I don't think it has any disadvantages or any effects on the baby. It doesn't work with X-rays [*aktines*]. I asked my doctor if there was any risk to the baby, but he told me there wasn't any, that it had no effect.

Khara, thirty-one, an engineer by training who was no longer working and who had just given birth to her first child, told me: "It doesn't do anything to the embryo, from what the doctor told me. It's not an X-ray."

Others, though reassured about its safety, still harbored some lingering doubts about the technology or about what experts might uncover in the future. Paraskevi, a twenty-four-year-old shopkeeper, who had just given birth to her second child, described how she learned about the procedure:

> I had heard about ultrasound before my first pregnancy. I'd read about it, and all the women have done it. I've read that some people have doubts about its safety [Paraskevi glanced at the pregnancy guide on the night table next to her bed.] I don't know, I don't think it has any risk. But maybe later they will find out [that it does].

Ritsa, the accountant whom I quoted earlier, explained how she dealt with her questions about the potential risks of the procedure:

> With my first child, I was afraid that the ultrasound would harm it. But the doctor explained that it worked with waves, not with radiation. With my second child, I wasn't afraid at all. I know that some scientists think that it's dangerous, that you shouldn't do it, but it helped me a lot.

As these excerpts indicate, women did not embrace prenatal ultrasound scans uncritically. Their generally favorable—and as will become apparent, often enthusiastic—responses to the scan took shape in dialogue with the opinions of influential others about the potential risks of the procedure. Whether through their exchanges with medical experts, their conversations with other women (many of whom themselves also had consulted experts), or popular guidebooks or other media, this dialogue almost always reassured them, even if, as some of the excerpts reveal, they still had some lingering doubts and concerns.

As informed consumers, women exerted a strong demand for fetal imaging that was in part a product of the machine's status as a metonym for the structural and symbolic superiority of modern medical science and technology. In the words of many women and their family members, technologies like ultrasound were important indices of "*tin iatriki ekseliksi pou ekhoume tora*, the medical development we have today" As noted earlier, this view was reflected in many women's expressed preference for the hospital because of its "machines." By 2000, pregnant women had come to expect, and not infrequently to request, ultrasound imaging at each prenatal visit. This expectation prompted Dr. P., the moderately critical obstetrician I quoted earlier, to complain of what he called the "overuse" (*katakhrisi*) of the procedure:

> When I tell them on a visit that they don't have to do an ultrasound, they look at me strangely. They say [he imagines], "This guy isn't doing his job." Every visit, they expect to get an ultrasound, but you [the doctor] aren't getting any more information.

Dr. P.'s experience was confirmed by Artemis, a twenty-five-year-old housewife, who had just given birth to her second child in the summer of 2001:

> I liked going to the doctor each month. In fact, I would have liked to have gone every fifteen days!
> EG: Why so frequently?
> Artemis: Because I liked to go to the doctor to see the embryo! [Laughs.]

Artemis's attachment to the ultrasound procedure may have been more extreme than most, but nearly all the women I spoke with regarded the procedure in a positive light.

Visualizing the Fetus/Seeing the Baby: Stories of Risk, Relationship, and Pleasure

Several themes recurred when women narrated their subjective experiences with fetal ultrasound imaging. First, there was the theme of women's dependence on the technology to assuage feelings of uncertainty and anxiety associated with the unpredictability of pregnancy and, more specifically, with the risk of giving birth to a sick or disabled infant, *ena arosto pedhi*. Although awareness of certain kinds of risks to fetal health has been heightened by women's exposure to biomedical discourse, and to the late modern discourse of risk more generally, physical and mental disabilities have historically been the object of considerable stigma in Greek culture (Arnold 1985, 257; Blue 1993; Blum and Blum 1965, 63; Velogiannis-Moutsopoulos and Bartsocas 1989, 230).[28] Disabilities of all kinds are dreaded not just for their direct consequences for the affected individual. Since many disabilities are believed to be hereditary (*soiako, klironomiko*), the birth of a sick child can stigmatize an entire family and negatively impact the marriage chances of its other members. An exemplar in this regard is the genetic disorder thalassemia, the blood disease that until recently doomed affected infants, like Kiria Eleftheria's son (see Chapter 3), to an early and painful death. Still today, those who have this disorder or who carry the trait are commonly referred to as having "*to stigma*," the stigma. So entrenched in everyday usage is this term that even doctors are compelled to use it. For example, a genetics counselor in Athens told me that she never uses this term because of its negative connotations, preferring to tell a patient that she is a carrier (*foreas*) or heterozygous (*eterozighos*). However, she went on to add, patients will then ask her, "What's that? In other words, do I have the stigma?"[29]

Today, as in the past, giving birth to a sick child is a danger recognized as inherent to any pregnancy. In the past, prophylactic steps—concealing the pregnancy, wearing amulets, and other apotropaic measures—were taken to keep the forces of harm at bay. Today, the pervasive contemporary discourse of risk, and the "biological prudence" (Rose 2007) to which it obligates women, have added another layer of complexity to this older sense of danger (many pregnant women still conspicuously sport blue beads as protection against the evil eye). Pregnant women, their partners, and other family members are all enmeshed in this discourse, disseminated most spectacularly through the media. As the following quote suggests, the heightened awareness of a proliferating number of risks has altered the structure of feeling of pregnancy from one generation to the next. During my interview with Adriana, her mother, Ksenia, a hotel manager in her late forties, dropped by and joined in our conversation. She had this to say about how her experience of pregnancy differed from her daughter's:

> Now, our children know what's going on, *kseroune ti tous ghinete*. We weren't like that. . . . I was completely in my own world when I was pregnant. I wasn't anxious, *dhen anisikhousa*. I ate whatever I wanted, I did chores without thinking, I did everything. But now, it's completely different. I see our children, who are well read, *dhiavasmena*, and they know. . . . As indifferent as I was toward myself, that's how much I've become concerned now about my daughter. I've become anxious, very anxious now, although that wasn't the case when I had my own children.

Ksenia's anxious commentary on her daughter's pregnancy resonates with that heightened awareness of risk that Beck (1992a) considers a hallmark of the "risk society." The particular salience Rhodian women gave to some risks, however, underscores the need to refine Beck's generalized typology, and in particular to consider how the specificities of place, culture, and history combine to distinctively shape local perceptions. On the one hand, some behaviors considered very risky in the United States, such as consuming even small amounts of alcohol when pregnant, were not of particular concern in Rhodes. The way the subject is treated in *Birth Is Love* suggests that this is the more general attitude as well. Alcohol is not even mentioned until the eighth edition; an expanded discussion in the ninth edition warns against excessive drinking but begins: "A beer, a glass of rosé wine, a little ouzo, in moments of high sprits, bring relaxation, well-being, *kefi*, and they stimulate the appetite" (Sikaki-Douka n.d., 127). On the other hand, some women regarded bathing in the sea (because of either the cold currents or microbes in the water) as a potential risk best avoided during pregnancy. Anxiety over radiation, however, was a theme that recurred in many narratives, not only over the ultrasound procedure, but also with respect to the pregnancy in general.

In part, this anxiety may reflect continuing uneasiness over the disastrous 1986 Chernobyl nuclear accident. Chernobyl had an immediate impact on the national birth rate at the time, causing it to plummet by about 10 percent, and concerns over its health consequences continue to circulate in Greece today (Emke-Poulopoulou 1994, 20–23). Evangelia, whom I mention in the introduction, is a poignant example of this lingering anxiety. She attributed the kidney problem found by her ultrasound scan to the contaminated rains that had drenched her more than a decade before she became pregnant (happily, when I saw her again the following year, I learned that her baby was born healthy after all). In 1999, the war in Kosovo prompted renewed anxiety over radiation. Doing fieldwork in Rhodes that summer, I was often caught up in discussions about the use by U.S. forces of bombs containing "depleted" but still radioactive uranium. This allegation, which I was able to confirm only with difficulty when I returned to the United States (Parsons 2001), had once again generated considerable anxiety over pregnancy outcomes, as well as cancer rates, the environment, and many other domains of daily life.[30] The pregnant women I spoke with that year were very worried about the possible effects of this radiation as they pictured it drifting its way across the Balkans and down to Greece.

However differently particular risks may be perceived, Rhodians, like most of us who live in late modern risk societies, must navigate a large amount of (probabilistic) information about hazards that are often "incalculable, unaccountable, uncompensatable and unlimited" (Lash and Urry 1994, 36). Furthermore, because so many modern hazards are invisible or hidden and thus imperceptible to the unaided human senses, ordinary people must rely on experts of various stripes to reveal and manage them. It is within this diffuse late or postmodern cultural logic of risk that some of the meanings of fetal ultrasound imaging must be examined.

Ultrasound imaging represents one significant, if not conclusive, technology for dealing with the "manufactured uncertainty" (Giddens 1991) that ensues from the pervasive discourse of risk. Although embedded in this discourse, ultrasound also reinforces long-standing fears surrounding pregnancy. Still, for the oldest generation, it was not pregnancy but the postpartum period that was fraught with the greatest sense of physical and spiritual danger. For the youngest generation, in contrast, it was pregnancy and birth that provoked the greatest anxiety and demanded the most attention. Pervasive and repetitive scanning seems to have increased this sense of anxiety among many of these women. Of course, in the overwhelming number of cases, the ultrasound scan also provides relief by allaying these anxieties. As Diane Beeson has cogently observed of prenatal diagnosis generally, just embarking on the process raises questions about the outcome of the pregnancy, despite there being "a 98–99 percent chance that no problem will be found in any given pregnancy" (1984, 164). As noted earlier, in the more than eighty ultrasound sessions I observed, no anomalies were in fact detected.[31]

Rhodian women commonly described feelings of "anxiety" (*ankhos*), "anguish" (*aghonia*), and "nervousness" (*trak*) just before the scan, in particular before their first scan, feelings that were usually put to rest once the doctor announced that "the baby is all right." This statement by Margharita, a twenty-five-year-old hairdresser, was typical:

> I had a lot of anxiety before my first ultrasound, because you can't know what's inside you. Until then, you only see your stomach. After, I felt more sure. You see that all is well.

All the women I spoke to took the doctor's assurance that "the baby is all right" to mean that the fetus was physically integral, or to use the women's words, that the "baby had its hands and feet," "all its organs," and was "whole" and "able-bodied" (*artimeles*). What it could not reveal, women generally agreed, was how these organs, including the brain, functioned. Despite this widely acknowledged limitation, the ultrasound scan nonetheless provided considerable relief and reassurance of fetal "health" to the great majority of women.

A second theme that recurred in women's narratives was their dependence on doctor and machine to mediate their contact with the fetus and to establish its reality. Only a small minority of the women I formally interviewed (three out of twenty-six) said that the ultrasound exam had not affected they way they experienced or thought of their pregnancy. For instance, Morfia, at thirty-six one of the oldest mothers I spoke with, tersely explained that the image on the screen had left her unmoved: "Just some shadows, *kati skies*, that's it, that's all I saw." Koula described the disorientation she experienced with her first ultrasound when she was pregnant at twenty with her first child:

> I felt strange, maybe because I was so young. I started laughing. You know, you don't feel anything yet and the doctor says, "This is what you have inside you." It was strange and I started laughing.

For most women, though, fetal ultrasound imaging played a critical role in reconfiguring what can be called "the structure of feeling of pregnancy," that is, the tangible ways that women lived and experienced their pregnancies (Probyn 1991; R. Williams 1961). Many described their reactions to the procedure in positive and often vivid terms. Of special note is the primacy of visualization over other forms of bodily experience in making the fetus "real," as heard in many women's statements. For instance, Popi, twenty-four years old and married to a taxi driver, said:

> I didn't believe I had a baby inside me. When you don't feel it or see it, it's hard to believe, it's something that you can't imagine—how the baby is, how it's growing, how it's moving. . . . After I saw it on the screen, I did believe it. I felt it was more alive in me. . . . I had also seen it [a fetus] on television but it's different to see your own.

And Stavroula, the contrarian former secretary who attempted to evade many of the hospital procedures when the time came for her to give birth, had this to say about the procedure:

> [With ultrasound] you have an idea of what you have inside you. I became conscious that it was a person. I hadn't felt it as much before, I had to see it first. At that moment, you feel that it's yours, the only thing that's yours.

For these women, quite different in terms of their education and class, as for many others, the murky ultrasonographic image furnishes readily recognizable "evidence" of fetal reality. Because the resolution of the image produced by the hospital's scanner is rather poor, women appear to actively read and interpret the fetal images according to the codes of objectivity and realism that underwrite modern visual technologies in general (television, videos, and photography) (Duden 1993; Fiske 1987; Petchesky 1987; Sontag 1989). Exposure to television from an early age may have also socialized this generation of Greek women (like Western European and North American women) to become "relatively flexible readers of images" (Condit 1990, 85). In this way, even though the fetal image is blurry and sometimes difficult to decipher, women were already primed and prepared to metaphorize the shadows that appear on the screen into "my baby." It is possible, too, that a common early experience with television and its realist representational codes may also account for the absence of class differences I observed in women's narratives (and for their striking similarities to North American women's responses to fetal ultrasound images; see Mitchell 2001). The "truthfulness" and authority of the image are further reinforced through the dramatic ability of the cameralike apparatus to compensate for the deficiencies of the human eye—both the doctor's and the woman's (see Crary 1990). In this regard, women's use of metaphors of other visualizing machines (television, camera, microscope) to refer to the ultrasound apparatus is especially revealing. In any case, with ultrasound a new commonsense mode of apprehending the "reality" of the fetus is established and positively valued early in the pregnancy.

Historical change in the sensory experience of this reality was reflected in an exchange that occurred between Stavroula and her mother, who came into her daughter's room toward the end of our interview. Stavroula's mother, a stylish woman in her fifties, interjected that she had felt what her daughter was describing when she first sensed the baby move inside her. To which Stavroula replied, "You feel it more intensely when you see it." For most women, due to the intensive use of fetal imaging, seeing (or rather, being shown) the fetus now usually precedes feeling it inside them. Besides this temporal precedence, these women's comments suggest that doctor- and machine-mediated seeing demotes the tactile sensations of the body to a secondary order of significance (an argument put forward in Duden 1993 regarding the obsolescence of the experience of quickening).

Yet women's comments often revealed greater complexity and hint at how ultrasonography might work to reconfigure women's sensory experiences by giving a tactile quality to the pregnancy through the visualization of what is, without the technology, impossible to see. As in Stavroula's case, many women explained that the fetus is *felt* as more alive, more present, when it's *seen*. Sometimes, seeing the image even seems to precipitate the tactile sensation of proprioception, as suggested in the following excerpt from my interview with Olga, twenty-three, a shop owner with a middle school education who was expecting her first child:

> It's good that you can see the baby and that the doctor explains things to you. Before I went in [for her first ultrasound] I was full of worry and anxiety, *aghonia.* I'd heard the heartbeat before [with the doppler] but I

still felt worried. The doctor pointed out the head, feet, spine—it looked like a zipper—the heart, everything, almost, and all were well. The baby was growing normally, *kanonika*, according to its age. I relaxed after that, I calmed down, and a few days later, I felt the baby move.

The ability of modern visualizing technologies to impart a material and tactile quality to what is seen was brilliantly explored early in this century by Walter Benjamin, whose work remains a source of insights into the operations of what he called "the optical unconscious" of mass culture (Taussig 1992, 144). Writing of medical photography in particular, Benjamin observed how new modalities of perception were made possible when bodily dimensions previously unseen or hidden were now rendered visible (Berlant 1997, 106). Several of the women I interviewed seemed to be making a similar point. By adding a tactile modality to the visual, the authority of the ultrasound to represent fetal reality is further enhanced, particularly early in the pregnancy, when women's sensual apprehensions of the fetus are to a large extent a product of their interactions with the machine and the information it creates.

A final theme to emerge from women's narratives of ultrasonography that merits mention is the strong pleasure that many of them derived from seeing the fetal image. For instance, Penelope, twenty, a comfortably middle-class woman who did not work, explained:

> The first time I saw the baby, I was crazy with happiness. It was a contact with the child. Every time I went to the doctor, I wanted to see the child again.

Evi, a twenty-eight-year-old former shopkeeper, described her delight on seeing the image:

> After my first ultrasound I felt like I did when I saw it after giving birth—that much happiness.

Tina, eighteen, a clerk in a bakery, exclaimed:

> I had four ultrasounds and that wasn't enough! When the doctor first suggested it, I couldn't wait to see it. I was so impatient, the minutes-long wait seemed eons . . . I thought it would be like on television, that I would see the little hands, like under a microscope. But I wasn't disappointed: I saw it move, I saw that it was healthy.

Ria, thirty, an economist who worked in the civil service and had just given birth to her first children, twin girls, after several years of unsuccessful attempts to conceive, had this to say:

> How did I feel when the doctor showed me the ultrasound? Happiness, tremendous happiness. Because I wanted it. That minute I felt love for everyone; I've never felt like that before.

Some women derived a pleasurable bonus from the possibility of sharing the ultrasound scan with others. Artemis, whom I quoted earlier, described how after every ultrasound, she got together to compare notes with a close friend who was also pregnant. "I liked going to see the embryo each month," she told me with a laugh. "Why, were you worried?" I asked her. "No, not after the first one. I liked going because I wanted to see its development. I had a friend who was one month ahead of me in her pregnancy, and each month we would get together for coffee and compare. 'Mine has grown so much, its foot, its hand, is so big.'" Fani, a nineteen-year-old middle school graduate who owns and runs a tourist shop with her husband, was similarly enthusiastic about ultrasound. Describing herself and her husband as a "modern couple" (*moderno zevghari*), she told me that one of the reasons she enjoyed her ultrasounds was that her husband went with her. As she explained, "When you have your husband with you, it's better, because you share everything together." This desire to share in Fani's experience also led her husband to convince her doctor, who was an old school chum, to give him permission to stay in the delivery room when she gave birth—one of the very few husbands in 1990 who were allowed to do so.[32]

The pleasure that many women enthusiastically express can be traced to multiple aspects of the scan. There is, first of all, pleasure in the assurance of fetal health, as Tina mentions ("I saw that it was healthy"). Pleasure also derives from the perception of realism it shares with television (see Fiske 1987). Thus, the ecstatic sensation of contact that Penelope describes is enabled, or at least enhanced, by ultrasonography's ability to reveal fetal movements in real time. Real-time ultrasonography, like live television, imparts a feeling of nowness that is symmetrical with the lived time of the pregnant woman and in the process promotes a sense of immediate contact with the fetus ("I saw it move," as Tina said). Akin to the sense of "spectatorial privilege" that John Fiske (1987, 25) identifies as a hallmark of "television culture," there is also the scopic pleasure of being all seeing and all knowing about the fetus ("You see how it is"). Knowledge of the sex of the fetus reinforces this ability and appears to be especially valued because the ideal gender composition of contemporary Greek families is often quite specific: one boy and one girl. Although women share this spectatorial privilege with the doctors, they move beyond the doctors' terse declarations of fetal age, sex, and health to actively appropriate the fetal image for themselves, endowing their fetuses with qualities and attributes that are meaningful to them alone ("You feel that it's yours, the only thing that's yours"; "I felt it was more alive"). Finally, for some women, there was also pleasure of a social nature to be derived from sharing this knowledge and sentiment with significant others in their lives.

Nonetheless, as Foucault (e.g., 1982) famously cautioned, the connections between pleasure and power, what he called the "positive" forms of power, must not be overlooked. To mediate between this desired visual contact with the fetus, women had to depend on doctor and machine. Without losing sight of the ways in which women creatively invest the technology and images it produces with personal meaning, it must be recognized that fetal imaging possesses many of the features of a classically Foucauldian biopolitical technology: by exciting and channeling desires and pleasures, it produces new subjects and objects of normalizing knowledge (Sawicki 1991, 83).

The determination of due dates is one notable example of this process. Each routine scan, in addtion to producing information that women desired, generated a precise dating of the pregnancy in weeks and days. By repeatedly comparing fetal anthropometric measurements taken from ultrasound images with antenatal growth charts compiled from survey data, the doctor is able to sustain a "constant web of observation around the normal individual" (Armstrong 1983, 101). With the aid of this observational web, individual pregnancies became synchronized with what might be called "doctor's time," and a "temporal symmetry" was established in which the rhythms of the pregnancy and the doctor's expectations came to coincide (Zerubavel 1981, cited in Barley 1988, 126–27). This artifactual synchronicity had important practical implications: if a woman's pregnancy failed to conform to expectations, the result was usually an attempt to induce labor via amniotomy, pitocin, and/or a caesarean section (for a fuller discussion, see Georges 1996).

Ultrasound and the Doctors

By the early 1990s most Greek obstetricians had an ultrasound scanner in their offices. As Dr. M., a clinical professor of obstetrics in Athens, commented to me, "Every obstetrician-gynecologist who gets a degree inevitably buys an ultrasound machine, or sends [his patients] to someone who has one. It's like a stethoscope—that is what ultrasound has become for every obstetrician."

As is the case in the United States, ultrasonography is not recognized as a separate specialty in Greece. The scanning technique appears deceptively simple, although in fact, of all the medical imaging technologies, ultrasound is the most dependent on the skill of the operator. Greek obstetricians learn to use ultrasound on rotation as part of their basic medical education, but few receive any additional training. As Dr. M. went on to lament, "Many do ultrasound, but they don't know what they're seeing." I should emphasize that the situation in the United States is not substantially different, prompting a leading ultrasonographer to a similar lament: "One would think that the number of incompetent or poorly trained practitioners would decline [with time]. This has not been the case" (Craig 1990, 561).

Whereas women almost uniformly regarded ultrasound in a positive light, a clear generational divide marked the views of the obstetricians in the public hospital. Doctors under forty saw the machine as indispensable, enabling them to practice modern obstetrics. To quote Dr. A., in his midthirties: "Obstetrics has made great progress in recent years because of fetal ultrasound. It provides information that just could not be gotten by other means. . . . Ultrasound is the single most important diagnostic tool we have." Nearly all the younger obstetricians held similar perceptions, despite the fact that hospital records revealed little or no change in outcome statistics since the introduction of routine imaging. The sole exception was the cesarean section rate, which had nearly doubled in four years: from 18 percent in 1985 (the year before the scanner was acquired) to 35 percent by the end of the decade.[33]

In contrast to the younger generation of obstetricians, the oldest obstetricians in the hospital were often critical of the ways in which the machine was routinely used. Arguing against what he considered to be a false sense of precision generated by ultrasonography, a senior obstetrician in his late fifties flatly asserted that "obstetrics is an art, not a science." Dr. P. criticized what he called the "overuse" (*katakhrisi*) of ultrasound and complained that it can "distance the doctor from the patient." Dr. L., another senior obstetrician, expressed annoyance and regret at the loss of value of his physical senses that had occurred as older hands-on methods, such as dating the pregnancy by measuring the height of the uterine fundus, have been completely eclipsed by ultrasound:

There are few things my hands can't find that the ultrasound machine can. My hands are my eyes . . . but patients think it's more modern to use a machine. They themselves would not trust just a manual exam. The doctor needs to show that he's modern too. That is, some will do an exam with a machine just because a woman will trust him more if he does. . . . Now machines are used as a way for doctors to advertise themselves.

Dr. L.'s statement suggests something of how obstetricians perceive the role of ultrasound, and in particular its association with narratives of progress and modernity, in buttressing their authority.

Dr. L.'s last sentence is also significant and hints at another factor at work in the proliferation of obstetrical interventions of all sorts. Throughout Greece, the relatively low salaries earned by doctors working for the National Health Service are often supplemented by gifts given in cash and kind by patients as expressions of gratitude for the care they have received. This practice is an integral aspect of the informal culture of the public health care system. Gift giving, which includes flower arrangements and assortments of pastries and chocolates, as well as cash, must be understood within the wider paternalistic and clientelistic ethos that characterizes doctor-patient relationships in Greece (Velogiannis-Moustopoulos and Bartsocas 1989). It is also necessary to distinguish this practice from the institution of the *fakelaki*, or "little envelope," which is an extra fee that doctors may occasionally demand in advance to expedite hospital care (Colombotos and Fakiolas 1993). Gift giving, in contrast, is a gesture—often insistent—made post facto by patients and their families to demonstrate appreciation and gratitude to the doctor (and other hospital staff) for their "help." "*Thelis ke to dhinis*, you give it because you want to," people insisted when I asked about this common practice. To illustrate this point, one friend told me about her uncle, a prominent doctor in Athens, who adamantly refused to accept gifts of any kind. His principled stand only forced his patients to resort to subterfuge, compelling them to cleverly hide expensive pens, bottles of whiskey, and other gifts when they visited his office. Similarly, a Rhodian woman told me that when she learned that her Athenian specialist absolutely refused to accept gifts, she inquired about his favorite charity (Doctors without Borders) and promptly made a donation. In the end, although individual sums given to doctors may be fairly modest, cumulatively they do offer some incentive to be responsive to patient demands, and thus they play a role in determining the contours of the Greek health care delivery system (Colombotos and Fakiolas 1993; Mossialos et al. 2005). For instance, the probability of receiving cash gratuities after a birth encourages doctors to provide continuity in prenatal and obstetrical care, something that women highly desire and appreciate. So, even though they are often overworked, salaried public sector doctors still want "to advertise themselves," as Dr. L. put it, that is, to attract and keep women, whom they treat as their individual, quasi-private patients, for the extra income they represent.

Informal expressions of gratitude also may have played a role in promoting the intensification of fetal scanning, and possibly of some other obstetrical procedures as well.[34] One doctor explained how this dynamic works:

> I can't survive on what the government pays me. I can't make it. I'm not a person who does unnecessary things. But if I don't do procedures, I don't get paid [informally]. If I send a patient home with a five-centimeter cyst, chances are it'll go away by itself. Two months later, 90 percent of them will be gone. But I won't get a gift. They'll say, "Thank you very much," and that's it. I do the procedure, and I'll get paid. And I need to get paid. I can't live on my salary. Now we have monthly ultrasounds. It's one way of doctors justifying their payment. You don't get paid [extra salary] to do an ultrasound. But you do an ultrasound for a patient, and it seems like you're doing something for them, you justify getting paid.

In this manner, fetal ultrasound scanning has been fitted into the preexisting informal political economy of health care, which it helps reinforce.

Many critics have publicly denounced the common practice of giving gratuities, and especially the *fakelaki*, to National Health Service doctors, as yet another example of the corruption and clientism endemic to Greek bureaucracies. Be this as it may, it is also possible to view gift giving from the clients' perspective as a form of resistance to the "externally imposed depersonalization of relations" (Tsoukalas 1991, 14) represented by huge public institutions like the National Health Service, and more generally as a form of resistance to the state and its labyrinthine regulations. By cultivating personal, clientelistic relationships with doctors and other hospital staff through such informal means, Greek women and their families are able to finesse and personalize an ostensibly rigid public bureaucratic structure.

Belated Modernity, Obstetrical Ritual, and Technological Rituals of Negation

The specific contours of maternity care in Greece are shaped, overdetermined even, by a multitude of metamedical forces that cut across many domains of Greek culture and society. Obstetricians, midwives, women, and their families alike have all embraced the routine, intensive, often repetitive use of a wide array of technological interventions in pregnancy and birth. This enthusiastic technological embrace is not, of course, peculiar to Greek maternity care. Rather, exceptionally high rates of obstetrical interventions can be found mainly in the United States and in many nations that have experienced rapid improvements in their standard of living in recent decades, such as Brazil, Chile, Taiwan, and the urban centers of India. Carol Sakala, an articulate critic of the globally skyrocketing rates of medically unnecessary caesarean sections, provides a blunt diagnosis of why this is the case:

> The U.S. seems to have had a perverse leadership role in international
> trends for high-technology obstetrics through the training of physicians
> who go on to practice in other nations, the exportation of medical
> technologies, the exportation of textbooks and professional journals,
> local production of medical technologies by subsidiaries of U.S. multi-
> national corporations, requirements for purchase of specific U.S. products
> in exchange for purchase of products of other nations or for foreign aid,
> and the general aura of prestige and efficacy attached to high-technology
> medicine. (1993, 1178)

Sakala's diagnosis highlights some of the critically significant political economic dimensions of the technological escalation in maternity care globally, but it is perhaps especially pertinent to Greece, where U.S. influence and the American variant of biomedicine came to dominate soon after World War II.

Within each nation, the particular structure of domestic health care and the organization of the medical professions also play important mediating roles in shaping the content of maternity care. As we have seen in this chapter, the majority of obstetricians in Greece work in the low-paid public sector. They have come to depend economically on the informal payments offered by patients who creatively use the power of this incentive to make the health care bureaucracy more responsive to their needs and preferences. Technological interventions of all kinds serve to justify patient largesse and help fuel their ever-escalating adoption and use. This economic incentive to doctors dovetails neatly with strong consumer demand from women and their families, stoked in part by uncritical media representations of any and every new medical development as a desirable advance.

Still another important factor influencing the technologically intense signature of maternity care in Greece is the absence of collective opposition to the current model of obstetrics, akin to the natural childbirth movements that have precipitated some measure of rethinking and reform elsewhere. It is worth reiterating the vital role that such oppositional discourses can play, at the very least, in enabling people to imagine alternatives to present practices (Davis-Floyd 1992). Such critical discourses historically have not comprised part of the reformative agenda of Greek feminism or consumer activism; they remain largely unsaid. Without such collectively imagined alternatives, whatever their sources, it is often difficult to identify problems and articulate solutions, and even the sporadic attempt to resist particular interventions, like the contrarian Stavroula's, comes to little. Organizations such as Evtokia are beginning to raise awareness of alternatives to the technocratic model of pregnancy and birth, but as yet, this voice is only a faint whisper.

Beyond the array of factors just reprised, a more complete understanding of Greek maternity care requires closer scrutiny of the symbolic dimensions of biomedical technology. Biomedical technology is widely perceived as both an index and a vehicle of modern medical progress (*i iatriki ekseliksi pou ekhoume tora*, as I was often told). Not just in Greece but throughout the world, this implicit valence has propelled the adoption of many obstetrical technologies in the absence of evidence that they do in fact work as they are imagined, or, as we have seen in this chapter, even in the face of massive evidence that they do not work at all. Furthermore, once a technology is adopted, there is a powerful drive to use it simply because it exists. The allure of this "technological imperative," yoked as it is to a modernist discourse of progress and optimism, often proves irresistible (Fuchs 1968; Koenig 1988; Tymstra 1989).

These well-documented processes apply across all societies in which biomedicine is hegemonic. Accounting for the particular signature of Greek maternity care requires that we also examine the locally specific inflections of these symbolic meanings in the process of their pragmatic negotiation and deployment. If technology is often a sign of the modern, in the Greek context, the meanings of the modern have their local and historical inflections, a theme I develop throughout this book. The "belated" nature of Greek modernity (Jusdanis 1992, 2001) has meant that the meanings of the modern have evolved in continual reference to definitions always already devised by more powerful outsiders. Assessing one's "progress" using the yardstick of these others is part of the larger experience of symbolic domination (Argyrou 1996, 2).

In ways that reflect and reinforce the political economic dimensions just discussed, the intensive and repetitive use of obstetrical technology may be interpreted as a kind of ritual of negation, an implicit "counterstatement" (Pfaffenberger 1992, 502) to the dividing practices of those influential others who would consign Greece to the category of the margins of Europe. From this perspective, the highly technological signature of Greek of maternity care can be described as "redressive" insofar as it enacts a symbolic response to technological domination that is intended to mitigate or subvert that domi-

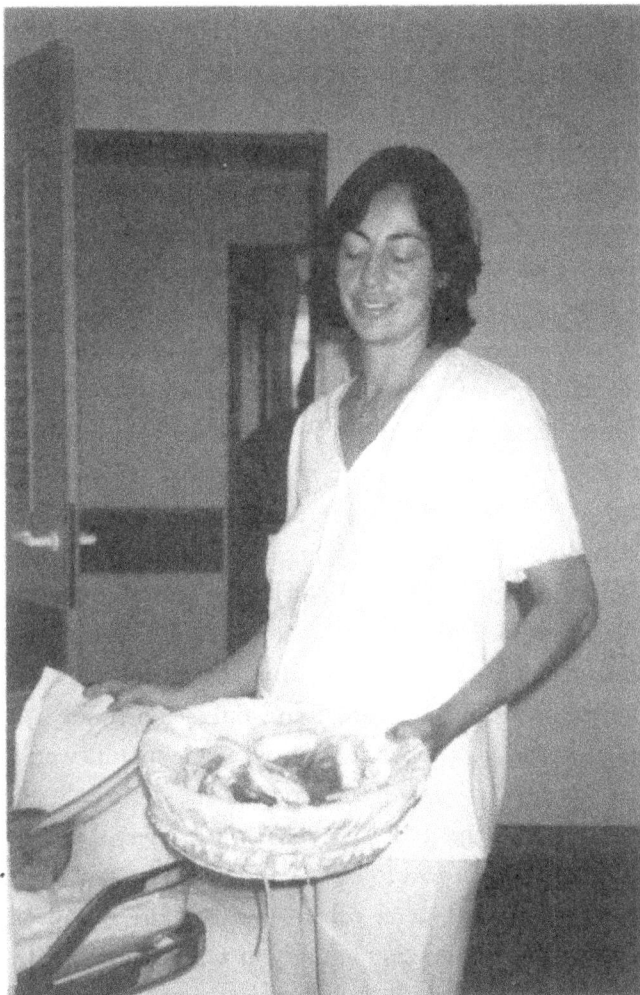

11. New mother with infant in hospital room, offering sweets to visitors.

nation (505). Thus, instead of a simple linear model of diffusion of obstetrical technologies from the more to the less industrially advanced nations, where they may be "inappropriately" adopted and used, it is perhaps more instructive to examine the relevant groups of social actors, each embedded in a specific social context of power relations, that shapes and reinforces their choices. As we have seen in this chapter, doctors and women both desire obstetrical technologies for a variety of symbolic and pragmatic reasons that may have little or nothing to do with technical efficacy. For the women who have been my main focus in this chapter, obstetrical technologies in general, and fetal ultrasound in particular, play an important part in fashioning their identities as (late) modern pregnant subjects.

However, at the same time that obstetrical technologies have been embraced and used with ever increasing intensity in Greece, many of these same technologies are being closely scrutinized in the world's centers of biomedical research. Ironically, given a growing awareness of these outcome studies and the increasing clamor emanating largely from the United States and the United Kingdom for the adoption of a more rational "evidence-based medicine," some cross-national comparisons now implicitly code high rates of obstetrical intervention as backward, Third World, or Mediterranean (e.g., Alran et al. 2002; Stephenson et al. 1993). A pattern intrinsic to the process of symbolic domination is thus repeated: modernity, ever elusive, "remains the terminus toward which non-Western peoples constantly edge—without actually arriving" (Comaroff and Comaroff 1993, xi). By this process, "redressive ritual" is transmogrified into "lagging emulation" (Friedl 1964).[35]

The example of the design and redesign of the obstetrical wing of the Rhodes General Hospital illustrates this point more concretely. When I first began my research there in 1990, the obstetrical wing, built during the Italian regime and reflecting the practice of its day, did not have a separate nursery. Newborns were kept in bassinets in their mothers' rooms (Fig. 11). Taking me for a tour of the wing early in my research, the then director of the Maternity Department assured me that this regrettable situation would soon end. Plans underway for a new wing provided for a separate nursery, where infants would be kept apart from their mothers, as was the practice in the United States when he had done his residency in the 1960s. A short while later, the head midwife of the department was sent abroad to attend an EU-sponsored seminar on childbirth. There, she learned that the other nations of the European Union now strongly recommended that mother and infant *not* be separated after birth. When she returned to Rhodes, she convinced the director to have the architectural plans altered to accommodate this more up-to-date view and the new hospital, completed in 2000, does not have a separate nursery. Ironically, of course, this had been the practice, *faute de mieux*, all along. But although the referent—mothers sharing a room with their infants—remained the same, its coding had now undergone a complete about-face: from backward to modern and up-to-date.

Chapter 6

Living with Contradictions: Contraception and Abortion and the Contemporary Greek Family

At the end of the Second World War, the birth rate in Greece began to tumble until, by the late 1990s, it approached a world-historical low.[1] Today, the one-to two-child family is the norm, if still not exactly the professed ideal. And so, in just a generation or two, the high-fertility regime described in Chapter 3 was replaced by one that is now below the level required to maintain the population. Baby-bust demographics similar to Greece's are common throughout Europe and declining birth rates are a global trend. What is intriguing about the Greek context is that this shift has been achieved largely through the seemingly anomalous combination of traditional birth control methods, mainly coitus interruptus and condoms, and intensive recourse to medical abortions. Only a small fraction of Greek women rely on medical means of contraception such as the pill and the IUD, and their numbers have barely changed over the last twenty years. Thus, whereas pregnancy and birth were swiftly and thoroughly medicalized, often with the active, even enthusiastic, collaboration of women themselves, the medicalization of contraception appears to have been roundly refused. At the same time, medical abortion is a commonplace, a procedure experienced, sometimes repeatedly, by up to half of Greek women over the course of their reproductive lives.

In this chapter, I explore some of the ostensibly puzzling contradictions that beset Greek birth control practices, contradictions that hamstring any attempt to tell a straightforward story of inevitable medicalization yoked to a relentlessly homogenizing process of modernization. As described in Chapter 5, Rhodian women hardly act like docile bodies in clinical encounters with their obstetricians; rather, they typically expect, demand, and appreciate the intensive use of prenatal and birth technologies. Outside and beyond the clinical encounter, they pursue additional biomedical knowledge through pregnancy guides and other media, endeavoring to tutor and transform themselves into scientifically literate, modern pregnant subjects. How, then, to reconcile their often eager embrace of biomedical knowledge and technological interventions in pregnancy and birth with their overwhelming rejection of biomedical technologies to control fertility? And, if biomedical technologies often serve as readily recognizable, even sublime, signifiers of a desired modernity, as I have suggested in previous chapters, why are some staunchly refused and others just as fervently embraced? I explore each of these apparent contradictions in turn, beginning with the broader context of the demographic problem that is widely lamented as bedeviling the Greek nation today.

The Demographic Problem, (Failed) Maternity, and the (Orthodox) National Body Politic

At the most general level, the demographic problem refers to the concern that the Greek population is somehow inadequate and must be increased for the sake of national welfare and security. Similar concerns date back almost to Greek independence, when undernatality was first recognized as a serious threat to the nascent nation building project. At that time, however, Greece's birth rate was high and showed no indication of decreasing. Instead, nineteenth-century discourse on undernatality focused on the high rates of infant and child mortality that were perceived to be sapping the nation's vigor and military strength, and ultimately thwarting its irredentist aspirations (known as the "Great Idea") to annex Greek-speaking populations still living under Ottoman rule. Medical and educational experts of the day concurred in identifying women's "wrong-headed," "superstitious," "irrational," and ultimately lethal child-care practices (feeding and swaddling in particular) as the root causes of high rates of infant and child death (Korasidou 2002). By the latter half of the twentieth century, concern over the state of the national population had surfaced once again to become the subject of public interest and debate. Today, the demographic problem refers almost exclusively to the nation's exceptionally low birth rate, although in the 1960s and 1970s, the effects of the large-scale migration of Greeks seeking employment as guest workers in Western Europe were also recognized as contributing factors. By the 1980s, blame for the stagnant and aging condition of the national population was increasingly attributed to the "undernatality" (*ipoghenitikotita*) of Greek women and, in particular, to their widespread resort to abortion (Athanasiou 2001; Halkias 2004; Paxson 2004; Skilogianis 2001).

In Greece today, there is broad consensus that women's undernatality poses a real danger to the vitality and very continuity of the nation. An especially clear sense of the scope of public endorsement of the idea that a serious problem exists emerges from a study that analyzed the content of articles and letters to the editor appearing in Greek newspapers in the 1990s (Halkias 1998). Across the political spectrum of the press—right-wing, centrist, and left-wing alike—the declining birth rate was consistently framed as one of the most critical threats to the nation. More to the point, an equally broad agreement existed on the etiology of the problem: "Greek women—'and couples' as the left importantly attempts to add—[are] those responsible." Abortion, in particular, "is clearly primarily identified as women's 'fault' and deployed as an explanation for the nation's difficulties" (Halkias 1998, 132). Repeatedly, the right-wing and centrist press, and to a surprising extent left-wing publications as well, assign blame for the high rate of abortion perceived to be bleeding the nation of its future citizens to women's "ignorance," "immaturity," "irrational preferences," lack of up-to-date scientific knowledge, and general "backwardness" (Halkias 2004, 315 and passim), terms that resoundingly echo the nineteenth-century discourse of blame for high rates of infant mortality. Besides the popular press, well-publicized books with titles such as *The Birthless Nation* and *The Demographic Problem* have appeared in recent years that further broadcast and reinforce the alarmist register that typifies much of contemporary demographic discourse.

Greece is by no means alone in representing declining birth rates as a grave problem and threat to the national body politic. Since at least the nineteenth century, demographic discourse has been part of the biopolitical projects of European elites (see, e.g., Cole 2000; Ipsen 1996). Despite the similarities, however, the discourse of demographic alarm inevitably reflects the contingencies of each nation's history and cultural politics. In Italy, for example, which ties with Japan in having the world's lowest birth rate (though Greece, Spain, and Portugal are not far behind), expert discourses circulating in the media also tend to blame women for "irrationally" refusing to have more than one child (Krause 2001, 586). There, nothing less is at stake than the survival of the "Italian 'race' and the disappearance of *European* culture" in the face of an alleged onslaught of racialized, largely immigrant, Others (595, my emphasis).

In Greece, too, the continuity of the Greek "race" and of Greek Orthodox civilization is represented as under siege. But here, demographic anxiety is also closely tied to the issue of Greece's military strength vis-à-vis potentially hostile neighboring states, among which the "Turkish threat" has historically loomed largest. Greece's shrinking birth rate is often unfavorably contrasted to Turkey's large and growing population—although in fact, Turkey's birth rate has also declined rapidly over the last couple of decades. In the aforementioned *Birthless Nation*, Fani Palli-Petralia, former member of Parliament and minister of human welfare under Mitsotakis's conservative New Democracy government (1992–1993), offers a particularly strident example of this rhetoric. In Palli-Petralia's view, a long line of military defeats (to the unnamed but implicit Turks), from the fall of Constantinople in 1453 to the Asia Minor Catastrophe of 1922, can be blamed on an insufficiency of Greeks ("*olighanthropian ton Ellinon*"). This dearth, she goes on to opine, has reached such a low point that Greece is now poised on the edge of definitive ethnic/national disappearance ("*ethnikis eksafanisis*") (1997, 12–13).

It would be irresponsible, however, to wave away such rhetoric as *merely* alarmist and exaggerated; to do so would be to ignore the particulars of Greece's history and its unusual geopolitical position within the European Union. As Richard Clogg (2002, 6) has acutely observed, critics often "fail to take account of the historical roots of present-day antagonisms and of the extreme sensitivity to perceived threats to national sovereignty that can arise in countries whose frontiers have only relatively recently been established." (Indeed, Rhodes and the Dodecanese joined the Greek nation only in 1947, and claims over some of the region's islands are still disputed.) The point, though, is not the reality of external threats, but rather how they have been framed and responsibility and blame assigned. Beginning in the nineteenth century and resurfacing at critical political moments in the twentieth, the discourse of demographic doom has consistently targeted women's failed maternity, in other words, their refusal to conform to appropriate gender expectations that privilege the reproductive dimensions of their identity. In the early 1990s, this venerable discourse got a second wind, as long-standing fears of being overrun and overcome by hostile, non-Christian Others were compounded by the unprecedented influx of new immigrants, particularly Albanians, who are also widely regarded as more fecund than Greeks.

The Greek state has fanned such widespread apprehensions with a stream of pronatalist rhetoric and policies aimed largely at women. In official speeches and other political discourse, women are repeatedly exhorted to bear more children as their patriotic duty, a duty sometimes explicitly compared to the compulsory military service of men (Kotsamanis 1988). Policies intended to promote larger families include employment protection for pregnant women, extended maternity leaves (very generous by U.S. standards), and the provision of free public nurseries and kindergartens, as well as such direct incentives as lump-sum birth payments and monthly subsidies to families with more than three children (the juridical category known as *politekni*, "many-children"), special pensions for *politekni* mothers, reduced military service for their sons, and tax exemptions, among a host of other special privileges (Symeonidou

2002, 17). By and large, however, public opinion views these inducements, or rather, their implementation on the ground, as seriously inadequate and inadequately serious (see also Paxson 2004, 200; Skilogianis 2001, 163). Typically, the men and women I spoke with endorsed the pronatalist position that large families are good for Greece. Just as typically, however, they scoffed at state policies for falling laughably short of the level of support needed by today's families. As Rhodians widely lamented, the economic demands of parenthood are greater and harder than ever to meet. On one memorable occasion, for instance, I overheard the husband of a Rhodian friend talking back to a politician on TV who was urging people to have more children: "Give me a hundred thousand drachmas a month," he retorted scornfully in those pre-euro days, "and I'll have another kid!" If the state expected its citizens to reproduce as their patriotic duty, then they in turn, it appeared, expected the state to act like a good father and meet its financial obligations. Because the state has manifestly failed to do so, its pronatalist rhetoric appears to have little purchase on a couple's actual reproductive decisions. Thus, despite a pervasive discourse that seeks to provoke a sense of the usefulness of women's bodies to a broader nationalist agenda, the overall trend has been, and continues to be, one of unremitting decline in the number of children Greek couples are having.

The Greek Orthodox Church has also endorsed and reinforced attempts by the state to encourage larger families. Although often flexible and forgiving in practice, officially the Church condemns all forms of birth control with the exceptions of rhythm and abstinence. Abortion is held to be a major sin and is equated with murder. The Church has long enjoyed a close, if not always harmonious, relationship with the Greek state and appears to have played a role in keeping medical methods of contraception illegal until the early 1980s (Naziri 1988). In an unprecedentedly activist move, the Church recently announced that it would offer income subsidies to *politekni* Greek Orthodox families living close to the Turkish border in order to offset the more fecund Muslim Greek minority populations concentrated in those areas.

The Macropolitics of Abortion and Contraception: Consistencies, Contradictions, and Entanglements

Consistent with the pronatalism of both state and Church, female methods of birth control remained illegal until 1980 (Paxson 2004, 113). Abortion was legalized in 1986. Prior to legalization, however, safe medical abortions were nonetheless readily available in Greece's cities, including Rhodes Town, whereas medical means of contraception, in contrast, were rarely prescribed by doctors. In the decades following the war, abortion in Greece was in effect an open secret best described as a "legalized illegality" (Naziri 1988). Never backstreet affairs, abortions were typically performed under general anesthetic by gynecologists in their private offices. In a relatively small society such as Rhodes, the names of doctors willing to perform abortions were widely known; in larger cities of Greece, abortions could be readily obtained in private hospitals and clinics. This availability of safe, only nominally illegal medical abortions was a direct consequence of doctors' success in evading the law. As members of a prestigious profession with access to influential networks, doctors were in an advantageous position to play the game of legal evasion, in any event, a widespread and entrenched feature of Greek political culture (Tsoukalas 1991). Thus, despite the large scale on which illegal abortions were performed, prosecutions of either the doctors or the women involved were almost nonexistent (Agrafiotis and Mandi 1997; Arnold 1985; Naziri 1988). In fact, legalization appears to have altered the abortion experience very little. For example, Iota, a forty-nine-year-old college teacher, had a total of four abortions, two before legalization and two after. The same gynecologist performed them all, in the same clinic, using similar procedures. Most importantly for understanding the role abortion came to play in Greek contraceptive culture, doctors' success in medicalizing abortion decades before it was officially legalized helped promote its routinization. Thus, in contrast to many other areas of the world in which abortion was illegal, Greek women did not have to face risks to their lives and the prospect of leaving children motherless every time they made their abortion decisions. In short, abortion became an entrenched method for limiting family size well before medical means of contraception were widely available. This historical pattern of "abortion before birth control" (as Norgren 2001 has shown for Japan) is an important element of the distinctive Greek contraceptive context that took shape in the postwar period.

In 1986, a new law effectively permitting abortion on demand for any reason up to the twelfth week of pregnancy placed Greece (together with Sweden, Norway, Denmark, and Austria) at the most liberal end of the spectrum of abortion law in Europe (Tribe 1990). Further, abortions were to be covered by the National Health Insurance system, making the procedure virtually free of cost for the majority of women (Stamiris 1986), although in practice most women preferred to pay for abortion out of pocket to ensure their privacy. Legalization had been part of the electoral platform of the socialist party (PASoK), which achieved power in 1981. However, despite the absence of an organized antiabortion movement in Greece, opposition from the conservative political parties that had ruled Greece for most of the postwar period and from the Greek Orthodox Church managed to produce a delay of some five years. The socialists' position on abortion was part of a package of progressive social and cultural reforms, as well as a response to pressure from the numerous Greek women's organizations that had begun to flourish after the fall of the military junta in 1974 (Stamiris 1986; Papagaroufali 1990). Nonetheless, legalizing abortion was not the burning issue for Greek women's organizations—which, as noted in Chapter 5, had focused their energies instead on the more pressing task of abolishing Greece's repressively patriarchal family laws—that it was for their U.S. counterparts. Ultimately, the large and glaring gap between relatively untrammeled abortion practice and abortion law became one of the most compelling arguments in favor of legalization. That Greece's high abortion rate was common knowledge discussed openly in the mass media signified to many a breakdown in the moral authority and political legitimacy of the state. Legalization thus became emblematic of the larger need to end the widespread practice of legal evasion and reestablish civic order (Naziri 1988).

Policies toward family planning also changed after the socialists' ascent to power. Prior to that time, only a handful of small private family-planning organizations operated in the urban centers. Family planning was largely the affair of individuals and the range of options was limited (Margharitidhou 1991; Paxson 2004). The pill had been imported into Greece since 1963 but legally could be prescribed only to correct menstrual irregularities (Siampos 1975, 343). Women who were determined to use oral contraceptives could purchase them without a prescription from a pharmacy, but few apparently did. Both male and female sterilization remained illegal until quite recently. In Rhodes, intrauterine devices were not widely available before the mid-1980s (like the pill, they were illegal until 1980). Except for condoms, which could be purchased in pharmacies and corner kiosks, birth control methods were not readily accessible and only rarely used.

When the socialist government established the National Health Service in 1983, it included a legal mandate to correct this situation by providing reliable information on medical techniques of contraception. Information was to be disseminated through the new health centers that were being built in every part of the country. After an initial rush of enthusiasm, however, government support for these centers waned. By the late 1980s, understaffed and undersupported, they were being used mainly for routine gynecological exams such as the Pap test. Similarly, the socialists' initial support for the mass dissemination of information on family planning quickly eroded. Also beginning in 1983, well-known actors had regularly appeared on informative short television programs, called *spots* in Greek, to offer detailed information on birth control (among a number of other health-related issues) on the state-controlled channels. As discussed in the preceding chapter, the media are an important source of information on health and medicine for Greek women. While birth control spots were fairly frequently aired in the socialists' early years, by the late 1980s broadcasts had stopped altogether. Greek family planners attribute the elimination of these spots, which reached a wide national audience, and the more general erosion of support for family planning services, to the intensification of nationalism during the 1980s. Heightened nationalist sentiment was inextricably linked in official discourse to the demographic problem and more specifically to the undernatality of women (Margharitidhou 1991; Katsoudas 1987).

The Medical Profession: Gatekeepers to Contraception

There is a perception among some sectors of Greek society that doctors were responsible, at least in some measure, for the low levels of medical contraceptive use and the high rates of abortion. Reflecting a more abstract and generalized mistrust of the medical profession (that usually does not extend to one's *own* doctor, however), and indeed of all professionals, doctors are said to profit from abortion and may be accused of having consistently blocked efforts to disseminate medical methods of birth control in order to sustain a more lucrative trade in abortion (Arnold 1985; Naziri 1988; Margharitidhou 1991). Even some doctors I spoke with shared this opinion. For example, an Athenian gynecologist who had once held a prominent position in the family-planning section of the National Health Service not only agreed, but also claimed that doctors were partially responsible for spreading negative reports about the pill in order to promote abortions. Such perceptions, it could be argued, reflect a more widespread cultural mistrust of the motives of others, and especially of those in positions of authority (Herzfeld 1997). *Simferon* (self-interest) is not infrequently suspected of underlying other people's intentions and the justifications they give for their actions. Attributions of self-interest to the medical profession are certainly not unique to Greek culture and have frequently been adduced to explain the obstruction of access to birth control elsewhere as well. Although such beliefs may circulate widely in a given society, their veracity is notoriously difficult to document and the evidence almost always remains circumstantial (Norgren 2001, 111). Still, the occasional candid comment from a medical professional did offer some support for this perception. One midwife, for instance, told me it was the unofficial policy at the large Athenian hospital where she'd trained in the early 1980s not to advise women on birth control after an abortion. And a doctor interviewed by anthropologist Marlene Arnold (1985, 124) as part of her study of reproduction in Crete, also conducted in the early 1980s, told her: "Of course I don't freely offer birth control information. Do you think I could keep a clinic like this open, if I only had fees from births?" In a more recent study of abortion among Athenian women, Joanna Skilogianis concluded from her interviews and observations at conferences devoted to sexual education and family planning that "'modern contraception' continues to be infrequently used largely because of the lack of firm and unified support from the medical profession in favor of such options" (2001, 221).

Whatever role self-interest may have played in doctors' resistance to the birth control pill, it is undoubtedly the case that many held genuine reservations about the long-term health consequences of ingesting hormones on a daily basis. Because of such reservations, many gynecologists continue to be reluctant to prescribe hormone replacement therapy (HRT) for menopausal women, a treatment that for the physicians posed no economic disincentive and even some possibility of economic gain. A middle-aged Athenian friend told me, for example, that she had asked her highly regarded (and U.S.-trained) doctor for HRT to treat her hot flashes, but that he refused because of its association with cancer. It is also important to keep in mind that the legalization of oral contraceptives in Greece came on the heels of a decadelong "flight from the pill" and barrage of negative news reports about its health risks, as well as those of the IUD, in the United States, Japan, and Europe (Henshaw 1990, 80). Over the next decade or so, doctors remained cautious about the pill's links with cancer, and as Heather Paxson (2004, 108) has observed, they "passed on to their patients a wariness that approached mortal fear."

One final factor that must also be considered in understanding the medical profession's attitudes toward birth control is that, until fairly recently, doctors themselves were not taught about contraception as part of their medical education. All Greek medical schools, like nearly all universities in the country, are public and state financed; only after medical contraception was fully legalized in 1980 did the subject become part of the medical school curriculum (Comninos 1988). Not surprisingly, one overview of family planning conducted in the mid-1970s concluded that because of this lack of exposure, "knowledge of contraception among practicing doctors is very limited" (Siampos 1975, 343).

In the last decade or so, this situation has begun to change. New attitudes were particularly evident in the younger generation of doctors I interviewed and observed in the public hospital in Rhodes. For example, one young resident was appalled when he overheard the midwife just mentioned tell me about the absence of routine contraceptive counseling after abortion in her Athens hospital. In his opinion, such conduct was "absolutely unethical." He himself, like some of the other young doctors I interviewed, regards abortion with some distaste: "I became a doctor to give life, not to take it," he explained. Doctor A., who told me he closely follows the antiabortion movement in the United States via CNN, not only tries to talk women into medical contraception—including, unsuccessfully, his own wife—but also tries to talk them out of abortions. In the numerous clinical encounters I observed, when women asked these doctors about birth control, they were usually provided with detailed information.[2]

Since the establishment of the National Health Service and its mandated family-planning services in the 1980s, doctors and professional midwives continue to play an important role as gatekeepers to contraceptive choice, now channeling women toward certain birth control methods while blocking others. Today, Greek women have basically two medical methods readily available to them, the pill and the IUD. Other options, such as contraceptive sponges and injectables, are not readily available. Because the IUD is associated with a risk of infection that can ultimately result in infertility, doctors routinely advise women against using this method until they have completed their families (Skilogianis 2001, 216). As a consequence, almost no Rhodian woman under thirty or so used the IUD. Female barrier methods, such as the diaphragm, were held in very low esteem by all the gynecologists with whom I spoke. In any case, spermicides, which must be imported, were only intermittently available in Rhodes. In the most recent national survey of contraceptive use, conducted in 1999, 0 percent of Greek women reported using a diaphragm (Symeonidou 2002, 87). Vivi, a thirty-nine-year-old shopkeeper who had lived in Australia for more than ten years, described her frustration in trying to obtain a new diaphragm once she resettled in Rhodes. The gynecologist she consulted was unfamiliar with the device, suggesting that she use the IUD instead. She had in fact tried it some years before, but had it removed because of the severe and continuous bleeding it caused. Ultimately, Vivi overrode her embarrassment and wrote to her son who was still living in Australia, instructing him to go to the National Health Service, have her diaphragm prescription renewed, and send it to her.

Sterilization was also illegal until recently. Today, tubal ligations are usually performed only on older women, women with numerous children, or women undergoing a second caesarean section. Vasectomies are almost unthinkable, and only a negligible 0.2 percent of Greek men have been sterilized (Symeonidou et al. 2000, 65). Negative attitudes on the part of providers may have influenced access to sterilization—as has been the case in France, Spain, and Japan (Jones et al. 1989). For example, a professor of obstetrics and gynecology in Athens suggests sterilization only to women who have already had numerous children, and never to men, because, as he explained:

> Somehow [the husband] will feel he is less a man, that he is diminished somehow as a man. Also women have that impression—if you do tubal ligation, something will be missing. Women ask, "What will happen to me afterward?" So imagine what a man will say!

Rhodian women who told me that they wanted to be sterilized sometimes had to convince their doctors to perform the operation. They did not always succeed. After Fotoula gave birth to her second child at the age of thirty-two, she asked her obstetrician to perform a tubal ligation. He refused, telling her that he would do it for her after she turned thirty-five but not now, as "there was no turning back" and she might change her mind and want a third child.[3]

The history and politics of contraception and abortion in Greece sketched in this section provide an important context for grasping how official discourses and expert practices narrowed the range of possibilities and interpretive frameworks available to women for thinking about and making sense of medical contraception. In the next section, I look more closely at how women pragmatically made do within the context of these constraints as they struggled with rapidly changing cultural understandings of the family and of themselves as mothers and wives.

Greek Contraceptive Culture: Abortion before Birth Control

Cross-national comparisons reveal that most societies possess their own idiosyncratic contraceptive culture. That is, each nation tends to exhibit an enduring pattern in which, over time, just a few birth control methods, often only one or two from the palette of available options, come to predominate (J. Potter 1999). Despite the fact that demographers conventionally index medical means of contraception as "modern" and all others as "traditional," contraceptive cultures exhibit startlingly wide variation from country to country that manifestly invalidates such simple dichotomies. Globally, the medicalization of contraception has in fact been wildly uneven, and the mix of methods dominating any given national context often bears little or no relationship to overall socioeconomic development or modernity. For instance, Vietnam and France, by any conventional measure at opposite ends of the development spectrum, are characterized by some of the highest rates of IUD use in the world, while in the United States this method was all but abandoned in the 1970s (because of deaths associated with the Dalkon Shield). Women in Belguim and Thailand rely heavily on the pill, in contrast to less than 1 percent of Japanese women, who, like Greeks, depend mostly on condoms and coitus interruptus. The Dominican Republic and the United States have some of the world's highest levels of female sterilization. The highest rates of male sterilization are found in the United States, Korea, and Nepal, while the procedure is virtually absent in France, Kenya, and Romania (J. Potter 1999, 706, table 1). And, defying some stereotypical representations of rampant Turkish fecundity, some 40 percent of Turkish women use the IUD or the pill, as compared to about 10 percent of Greek women (Alpu and Fidan 2006). Such marked global variation strongly suggests that in each locale, the particularities of national policies, the dynamics of competing interest groups, and the contingencies of history play significant roles in shaping patterns of contraceptive preferences (J. Potter 1999; Norgren 2001). Furthermore, any attempt to understand a specific contraceptive culture must also consider the fact that everywhere, contraception and abortion are "necessarily linked" in complex ways, as Rosalind Petchesky (1990) has importantly observed. In short, to be properly understood, the specific contraceptive culture of a given society must be situated within the local politics and practice of abortion as well (Greenhalgh 1995).

In Greek contraceptive culture, a conceptual distinction is made between medical methods of birth control, called "contraception" (*antisilipsi*), and the use of nonmedical techniques, expressed as "being careful" (*prosekho*)—as in "We are careful" (*Prosekhoume*), or more typically, "My husband is careful" (*O andras mou prosekhi*). Although "contraception" has been massively rejected, married couples throughout Greece do have high, and ever increasing, rates of "being careful," largely through the use of coitus interruptus or withdrawal (called *travighma*, "pulling out") and condoms (Comninos 1988; Symeonidou 2000). The rhythm method, the only method besides abstinence condoned by the Greek Orthodox Church, was used exclusively by only a handful of Rhodian women. Generally speaking, older women tended to be either uncertain or mistaken about where in their cycle their fertile days fell. A commonly expressed belief was that a woman is fertile some four to seven days before or after her period, or both, a Hippocratic belief linked to the "openness" of the womb during menstruation and therefore its greater receptivity to conception at that time. However, it was highly unlikely for these women to have used traditional understandings of rhythm to regulate their fertility. In fact, many of the oldest women who had relied on coitus interruptus and condoms expected their husbands to "be careful" each and every time the couple had intercourse, the implication being that there was no reliable safe period. Younger women who had learned their biomedical lessons regarding the female reproductive cycle—typically, from a popular health manual or friends or perhaps from their doctor—sometimes used the rhythm method, almost always in conjunction with coitus interruptus, condoms, or both (see also Halkias 2004). Reliance on *antisilipsi*, which in the Greek understanding essentially refers to the pill and the IUD, characterized roughly the same low proportion of Rhodian women I interviewed (11 percent) as it did women nationally (between 7 percent and 12 percent; Symeonidou 2000, 2002).

As this brief overview of Greek contraceptive culture reveals, birth control practices remain largely outside the purview of the medical profession. For the women and men who came of age during and immediately following the devastation and hardship of World War II, and who were the first to sharply curtail the size of their families, the *only* means of fertility control readily available were those that demographers typically classify as "male-dominated" or "traditional" methods, condoms and coitus interruptus, and for many women, abortions so numerous they sometimes lost count. In the immediate postwar years, medical abortions and ethnomedical abortifacients coexisted as alternatives that women could use interchangeably, according to their circumstances. Recall the examples of Kiria Khariklia, who went to a doctor only after unsuccessfully trying to abort, first, by drinking rue and later, brewed onion-skins, and Kiria Evanthia, who used rue as a last resort because she was unable to pay for a medical abortion without her husband's knowledge. These examples point to an important continuity in the cultural logic of abortion in the prewar and postwar periods. While medical abortion entailed a departure from more ambiguous ethnogynecological understandings and practices that had offered women some insulation from the moral burden of abortion, it also followed a well-established cultural pattern of actively tinkering with and attempting to influence pregnancy outcomes. Medical abortion was new for most of these women, but the logic and experience of abortion were not.

Under the new demographic regime taking shape after the war, many women simultaneously experienced the intensification of abortion and its medicalization. As importantly, at the same time that the birth rate was plummeting, a growing number of doctors willing to perform abortions appeared on the scene. At the obstetrician-run private clinics that sprouted up throughout Greece, women could obtain safe medical abortions that were only nominally illegal (Valaoras et al. 1965). In this manner, the pattern of "abortion before birth control" (Norgren 2001) became established and remained firmly in place when the next generation began to marry and form their families.

When the pill and the IUD later came on the scene, doctors could have ignored and circumvented their illegality, as they had with abortion. However, for the reasons discussed they generally did not, and over the next decade or two most remained ambivalent at best about these new methods. Other methods, such as douches and foams, could be found sporadically in pharmacies in Rhodes Town, but very few women used them on a regular basis. With options for *antisilipsi* thus severely curtailed, women who married and began establishing their families in the decades following the war had little choice but to rely on their husbands to "be careful, *na prosekhoun*," that is, to practice coitus interruptus or use a condom. But, as I was often told, husbands were not consistently careful. Initially, the dramatic social changes of the postwar period, especially the expanded educational goals for children and new ideologies of parenthood that I discuss later, no doubt affected mothers more than fathers, as they lost household help and had to sacrifice themselves to further their children's studies. Women of the transitional generation often told me that they wanted fewer children than their husbands did.[4] When they found themselves undesirably pregnant, this conjugal dissonance with respect to ideal family size sometimes led them to take matters into their own hands and arrange abortions without consulting their husbands (as they had previously done with ethnogynecological abortifacients). Although there are no official records of the number of abortions performed during this period, most scholars agree that they were considerably more numerous in the 1960s and 1970s than in the 1980s and 1990s (Symeonidou et al. 2000). The large number of abortions characterizing the postwar decades, estimated at up to three hundred thousand a year (a figure roughly three times the annual number of live births), coupled with women's sometimes unilateral decisions to abort, suggests, among other things, a certain dissonance between women's and men's reproductive projects at the time. At the very least, it illustrates the fierce determination on the part of some women, like Kiria Evanthia, to end pregnancies their husbands had not been conscientious enough to prevent or might have preferred to keep.

In contrast, the youngest generation of women and men, those who formed their families in the 1980s and 1990s, almost always made abortion decisions jointly.[5] If I am right in regarding the abortion rate (in part) as an index of conjugal dissonance, then this notable generational change suggests a growing convergence of men's and women's reproductive goals, as well as the ascendance of a more companionate ideal of marriage. Interestingly, some young women did, however, occasionally hide their abortions from their mothers, from whom they expected pressure to keep the pregnancy, especially if they had only had one or two children. Conflict over reproductive goals and notions of ideal family size was thus sometimes more evident between junior and

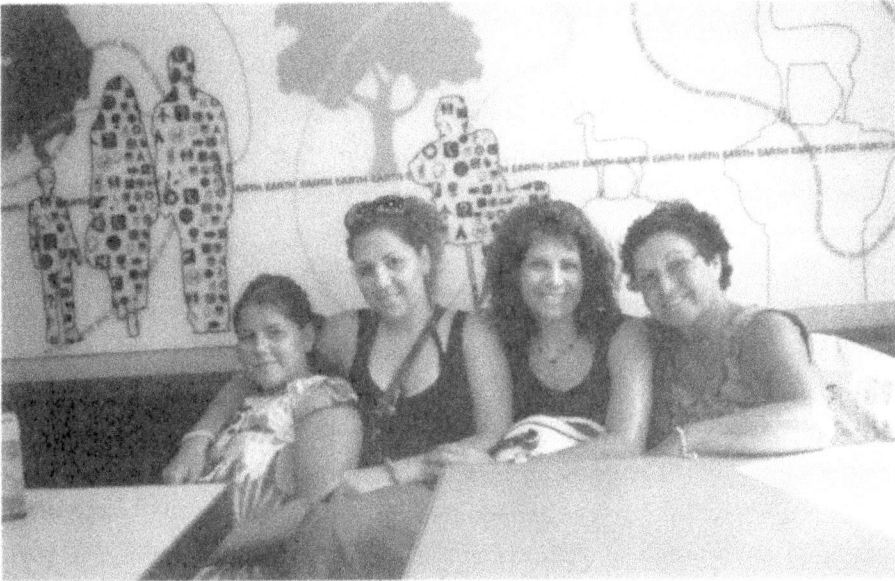

12. Three generations on a lunch break in downtown Rhodes.

senior *women* than between husbands and wives of the youngest generation. For example, when Toula and her husband agreed to stop (at least for the fore-seeable future) after one boy, Toula's mother and her mother-in-law both kept after her to have another child. More precisely, they urged her "to make a girl" in order to complete *to zevgharaki*, the "little couple" (a boy and a girl) that today generally represents the ideal family. Toula, a shopkeeper in her thir-ties, remembered her mother insisting: "I gave birth to four—you can have one more," which after some initial resistance, she eventually did. Khrisi, an architect also in her thirties, described the more discreet manner with which her mother-in-law, a kind and considerate women with whom she got along quite well, would broach the subject of another child. "You know, Khrisi, I had a dream last night," she would confide to her daughter-in-law from time to time, and then proceed to describe how she had seen Khrisi in her dreams radiantly pregnant, or just having given birth to a healthy baby. Because per-haps the majority of daughters still receive dowry houses or apartments when they marry, a tendency toward matrilocality persists even in Rhodes Town, where small multistoried apartment buildings are often inhabited by matrilin-eal kin, layered by generation. Social contact across the generations tends to be frequent and close (Fig. 12). Coupled with the dependence of many working women on their mothers for child care and household chores, these living ar-rangements create abundant opportunities for maternal surveillance. Although this closeness sometimes caused tensions, and the pronatalist pressure issuing from a woman's mother was occasionally unwelcome, it could also serve as an important resource. For instance, when Dora, who had one child, was unable to conceive a second because of fertility problems, her husband, Nikos, was content to leave it at that; it was Dora's mother who insisted on going back to work as a chambermaid to pay for her daughter's in vitro fertilization treatments.

In Rhodes, women who had only one child felt by far the strongest pressure. Having two children was widely regarded as desirable both for the company and close bond that siblings share and, most importantly, women told me, *mi kako*—knock on wood—for the prudent hedge it provides parents. High infant and child mortality is now well in the past, but traffic accidents in particular are frighteningly frequent in Greece today and can randomly strike the one-child family childless. As the mother of an only child, I too was often admonished by older women that "one is no better than none" (only the truncated version of the old saying is heard today). Or, as my friend Sophia's mother, a hard-working farmer, direly warned me—to her daughter's acute embarrassment—upon meeting me for the first time, "*Ena pedhi, ena mati!* One child [is the same as having only], one eye!" Sophia's negative reaction notwithstanding, I interpreted these warnings, and the practical advice that often accompanied them, as extensions of the old female ethos of care for other women's reproductive success and well-being that I described in Chapter 3. On another occasion, I experienced a simultaneously touching and amusing example of this ethos. My husband had come to visit us in the field and we had gone to the town of Lindos, a major tourist destination on the island, to show him its beautiful acropolis perched high above the improbably perfect circle of St. Paul's Bay. My husband had gone on ahead, and my five-year-old daughter and I trudged slowly up the hill behind him. During the day, the narrow footpath to the acropolis is lined with Lindian women selling lace-trimmed tablecloths, spread out on the surrounding boulders to entice the tourists. I stopped to rest and chat with two of these women, and soon found myself fielding the volley of questions I was by now quite used to answering: "No other children?" "Why not?" "Where's your husband?" Hearing that he was visiting us only for a short while, these women I had only just met offered to mind my daughter that night so my husband and I could spend the evening alone and, with a little luck, eventually provide her with a sibling.

By the mid 1980s, contraceptive options had increased considerably, and for the first time woman-controlled medical methods became accessible and readily available. As noted earlier, doctors' attitudes also began to change, especially with respect to the pill. Nonetheless, with a few notable exceptions, the basic features of Greek contraceptive culture remained essentially stable.

Table 1. Principal Methods of Contraception, 1983, 1997, 1999

Contraceptive Method	1983 (n=507) %	1997 (n=502) %	1999 (n=1,786)* %
Pill	1.2	4.2	2.5
IUD	2.0	7.4	4.2
Diaphragm	0.2	0.0	0.0
Spermicides	1.0	0.0	n/a
Douches	1.2	2.8	n/a
Condom	27.4	40.8	25.6
Coitus interruptus	35.1	30.7	29.5
Periodic abstinence	0.0	1.6	2.8
Tubal ligation	0.8	1.6	5.8
Vasectomy	0.0	0.2	0.2
No methods	22.8	8.7	28.8
All other methods	8.3	2.0	0.0

Sources: H. Symeonidou et al. 2000 (65, table 5.2); H. Symeonidou 2002 (87, table 19).
*Based on national sample of 2,062 women, 1,786 of whom were fecund, nonpregnant,
  and sexually active at the time of the survey.

Table 1 summarizes information from a series of national surveys of women's contraceptive choices conducted over the last two decades by the demographer Haris Symeonidou and colleagues. Symeonidou et al. (2000) surveyed some five hundred women about birth control in 1983, interviewing them again in 1997 to ask about the method they had most often relied on in the intervening years. Table 1 presents findings from Symeonidou's 1983 and 1997 surveys, as well as the results of a much larger national survey conducted in 1999. As this table clearly indicates, women's refusal of medical means of contraception has been both formidable and steadfast. In 1983, a negligible 1.2 percent of women of reproductive age were using the pill. Fourteen years later, this figure had increased by a mere 3 percentage points. Rates for the IUD were somewhat higher, but still comparatively very low. Only one man in Symeonidou's 1997 study, and none of the roughly one hundred men interviewed as part of the 1999 survey, reported a vasectomy. A total of 6 percent of women had had a tubal ligation. Throughout this period, more than half the women surveyed continued to rely on condoms and withdrawal.

The general impression that Greek women's use of medical methods of contraception is changing at a glacial pace is importantly qualified, however,

Table 2. Women's Use of Medical Birth Control in 1999 by Age Group

Age Year of birth	20–29 1970–1979	30–39 1960–1969	40–49 1950–1959
Pill	5.1	2.9	0.9
IUD	4.4	4.2	2.4
Sterilization	0.5	3.7	11.4

Source: H. Symeonidou 2002 (87, table 19).

when the rates for each age group in the 1999 national sample are examined separately. A glance at table 2 reveals that by far the biggest change in birth control use was the relatively large proportion (11.4 percent) of women between 40 and 49 who had been sterilized. Indeed, for the oldest women in the sample, those between the ages of 45 and 49, this figure reached 12.8 percent. By contrast, only 3.7 percent of women 30 to 39 years of age had undergone the procedure. Clearly, it was the oldest cohort of fertile women, those who in my Rhodian sample fell into what I have called the transitional generation, that had turned in greatest numbers to a modern medical birth control method—and to the most definitive one at that.[6] I will revisit this notable development further on.

Many scholars have attempted to explain the distinctive signature of Greek contraceptive culture, in particular, why the great majority of Greek women have refused to adopt modern medical means of contraception and have continued to rely on the presumably less reliable traditional methods such as coitus interruptus and condoms. Prominent demographers, doctors, and family planners may blame women's "ignorance" or, more charitably, their lack of scientific literacy and "lack of information" on up-to-date methods (e.g., Symeonidou et al. 2000, 67). Social scientists, in turn, have offered a dizzying array of cultural and psychological explanations. Some have suggested that women turn their back on medical methods because of the high value traditionally placed on female fertility and maternity in Greece. By choosing less dependable methods such as coitus interruptus, they argue, women unconsciously leave the door open to a pregnancy that periodically ratifies their fertility and displays their potential for motherhood. Given the profound changes in ideal family size, however, women following this imperative must inevitably resort to abortion, a cycle that some have referred to as Greek women's "abortion syndrome" (Naziri 1988; see also Arnold 1985; Loizos and Papataxiarchis

1991b).[7] Others have argued that women have rejected medical methods because, being woman controlled, they represent a challenge to a couple's gendered relations of power. Behaving in an appropriately feminine manner, according to this perspective, mandates that Greek women cede contraceptive control to their male partner (Paxson 2002, 2004). Still others have argued that when Greek women refuse medical contraception and rely instead on coitus interruptus, they are in essence proving the loyalty and trust they have for their partner. On a grander scale, they are performing their allegiance to a Greek national spirit whose understanding of love resists the calculating rationality and individualism of the West as symbolized by regimes of medical contraception. By this logic, reliance on withdrawal, and the abortions that often result from this reliance, become transgressive acts against a broader system of symbolic domination (Halkias 2004). In the following section, I draw on the narratives of Rhodian women to offer my own interpretation of the distinctive signature that characterizes Greek contraceptive culture today.

Risk, Reflexivity, and Late Modern Contraceptive Culture in Rhodes

The Rhodian women I spoke with were decidedly not ignorant of the most commonly available methods of contraception and almost always had something to say about their advantages and disadvantages. The majority readily acknowledged that medical methods were highly reliable. They rejected them nonetheless largely because of fears and misgivings over their long-term consequences for their health and fertility. Pervading women's narratives of refusal was a discourse of risk, rendered today in Greek, as noted earlier, by the loan word *risko*. The ways women talked about risk as they assessed their contraceptive options and justified their decisions revealed a complex braiding of at least four elements: the scientific knowledge they had gleaned and often actively sought out from medical experts, the media, and popular guides and pamphlets; their own embodied experiences with medical methods; the embodied experiences and views of other women in their social networks; and the web of local perceptions and meanings associated with an ever-expanding array of manufactured risks issuing from medicine, science, and technology. Women drew on this repertoire of elements, as I describe in this section, in variable and often creative ways as they attempted to interpret and evaluate the implications of each method for their everyday lives and to justify their choices. Yet, because each of these elements tended to reinforce the other, they usually worked together to support and cement women's overwhelmingly negative views of medical contraception. By doing so, they have ultimately helped sustain the distinctive Greek contraceptive culture that began to take shape at the end of World War II.

Risko

Like Greek women surveyed nationally (Tountas et al. 2004), Rhodian women explain their reluctance to use medical contraception largely in terms of the potentially harmful consequences for their health. The most frequently mentioned reason for rejecting the pill was the risk of cancer, often specified by site (breast, uterus), a concern that features in the narratives of women from Athens and Thessaloniki as well (Halkias 2004; Naziri 1988; Paxson 2004; Skilogianis 2001). Cancer (*karkino*) is a disease so greatly feared in Greece that until recently, people avoided even uttering the word. Women of the oldest generation, for example, might refer to cancer euphemistically as "the bad disease, *i kaki arostia, to kako*." Although younger Rhodian women rarely resorted to such locutions, cancer did not appear to have lost any of its negative charge. Indeed, nondisclosure of a cancer diagnosis continues to be standard practice in Greek oncology.[8]

Women had been hearing about the relationship between hormones and cancer in the Greek media since negative reports began to circulate in the 1970s. That is, a decade before the pill was legalized for contraceptive purposes, its potential hazards to women's bodily health and well‑being had already been widely publicized. To further put this moment in historical perspective, just as the pill became legal in Greece, Dutch women were abandoning it in large numbers (Henshaw 1990). As many did during their pregnancies, Rhodian women often consulted their health encyclopedias, pamphlets, and other popular medical guides to educate themselves in greater detail about the pill. As a rule, these materials tended to highlight risks, contraindications, and side effects. For example, one guide a Rhodian woman shared with me entitled *The Doctor Advises* summarized the advantages of the pill in a couple of sentences; the author then went on for the next page and a half to describe the many and various health risks associated with the ingestion of hormones on a long-term basis. The more recent appearance of low-dose pills has had to contend with this deeply entrenched association, as illustrated in an exchange I had with Dr. A., the antiabortion obstetrician who was unable to convince his own wife to take the pill. In the following excerpt, he describes his experiences counseling patients about birth control:

I manage to convince some of the women, especially the younger ones, to take the pill, to convince them that the new pills protect against cancer generally, especially breast cancer. But most of the time I don't succeed.

EG: Why not?

Dr. A.: Because of the mentality, *nootropia*. They prefer withdrawal, *ekso* [literally, "outside"].

EG: Why?

Dr. A.: Because they are afraid of getting sick, of getting cancer; . . . one woman learns from the other that the pill causes cancer and they are afraid.

At this point in our interview, I asked his opinion of the theory that, ultimately, withdrawal is preferred because it allows men to retain control over contraception and fertility in general:

No, no, I don't agree. Not now, not this generation anyway. It's more the mentality—one man learns it from another, just as women learn from each other about the pill. They are afraid that their wives will get sick in general, and that they will get cancer.

Rhodian women also drew heavily on their own embodied experiences as deterrents to pill use—about twice as many of the women I interviewed had tried the pill at some point as were currently using it—as well as those of their relatives and friends. Among the reasons most frequently cited were such undesirable "side effects" (*parenerghies*) as weight gain, nausea, dizziness, phlebitis, "nerves," and difficulty in becoming pregnant after quitting, as well as the fear of forgetting to take the pills.[9] After listing several reasons for rejecting the pill, Tina, the bakery worker, concisely summed up a common attitude: "If I knew they wouldn't do me harm, I would use them." Some of the younger doctors, like Dr. A., complained that by giving up too soon, women were depriving their bodies of the opportunity to become habituated to the pill. However, given the almost uniformly negative interpretive frameworks available to women for making sense of their unpleasant, and occasionally even alarming, bodily experiences—whether derived from the media, medical professionals, or other women in their social networks—it is not difficult to understand why many stopped taking the pill after a few months or so.

When women did decide to take the pill, it was often in spite of their own uneasiness and the pressure from friends, mothers, boyfriends, or husbands, and in some cases their mothers-in-law, to stop lest they ruin their health and future ability to bear children. Ghiorghia, a graduate student in her twenties, had been on the pill for several years without any adverse effects. Although she was very satisfied, she complained that she was tired of dealing with the negative reactions of her women friends and classmates at the university when they learned she was taking the pill: "*Dhen tha khapakonome egho*, I'm not going to stuff *myself* with pills," Ghiorghia told me they might typically respond—to her steadily growing annoyance. And no wonder: "*khapakonome*" is a slang term derived from *khapi* (pill), and carries negative connotations of wanton pill popping and even drug abuse. Nelly, a twenty-seven-year-old mother of two who had quit her job to raise her children, had been on the pill for several years and, like Ghiorghia, was quite satisfied. After our interview, Nelly kindly offered to arrange an appointment for me to talk with her mother as well. Before calling, though, she specifically requested that I not mention that she was using the pill, to avoid potential arguments with her mother down the line.

The IUD was considered somewhat less risky than the pill and was therefore a more acceptable method, at least for women who had completed their families and no longer had to worry about protecting their fertility. But, here too, personal experience and other women's accounts of side effects deterred many from using the device. Even women who experienced no adverse effects would periodically stop taking the pill for a while or have the IUD removed, to "give the body a rest" (as Skilogianis [2001, 200] also found among Athenian women).[10] Implicit in this practice was a sense that both methods somehow imposed a burden on a woman's body (*fortoni to soma*), which therefore needed periods of respite and removal to recover. In some cases, women ultimately, and sometimes reluctantly, turned to the pill or the IUD only after experiencing numerous abortions.[11]

By the mid-1980s, when medical means of contraception were becoming increasingly accessible and accepted by critically situated gatekeepers, such as doctors, midwives, and family planners, the essential features of Greek contraceptive culture had been in place for roughly three decades. Despite the appearance of a new generation of low-dose pills, and with the intriguing exception of tubal ligation, contraceptive preferences had barely changed (although the rate of condom use has nearly doubled, a development that some Greek researchers attribute to the "AIDS information epidemic" in the Greek media [Agrafiotis and Mandi 1997, 564]). Taking a cross-national perspective once again, it becomes apparent that what the demographer Joseph Potter has identified as a pattern of "inertia" in contraceptive cultures over time is more the norm than the exception. This widespread phenomenon of stasis or inertia has led him to conclude that "contraceptive regimes that evolved in one set of circumstances can persist long after they no longer make sense" and further, to advise that explanations not be sought "solely in terms of deep-seated cultural preferences or the present-day incentive structure" (1999, 704).

Potter's point that the history and politics of reproduction play major roles in shaping contraceptive cultures and accounting for their persistence offers a valuable correction to explanations that lean perhaps too heavily on psycho-cultural factors. However, I would also insist that to endure, contraceptive regimes *do* have to "make sense" to those who live and operate within them. Rhodian women and men frequently turned to a culturally meaningful network of binary oppositions to think about and evaluate the various methods of contraception available to them, and to justify their choices. By attending to the terms of this cultural logic and, as importantly, to the strategic ways these terms are deployed as women attempt to justify their choices, we may begin to unravel the ostensible puzzle of avidly modern mothers and fathers relying stubbornly on traditional methods of birth control. As I discuss in the next section, Rhodians expressed their preference for what demographers typically code as "traditional" methods in terms that reflected distinctively (late) modern concerns and anxieties over the manufactured risks and iatrogenic side effects of medical contraception. Attending to the ways women and men talk about and make sense of the various options available to them ultimately suggests that "imposing a traditional/modern taxonomy on these methods distracts us from the possibility that those who use them may classify these methods in other ways" (Hirsch and Nathanson 2001, 414).

Appeals to Nature and the Cultural Logic of Medical Refusal

Coitus interruptus is often coded as a traditional birth control method, not only because it is not medicalized, but also because it presumably disempowers women by ensuring that control over contraception remains in the hands of men. However, as Schneider and Schneider have shown in their historical study of the Sicilian town of Villamura, coitus interruptus has meanings and uses that vary over time and across social context. From a practice associated with hedonism and self-indulgence in eighteenth-century Europe, coitus interruptus was later reconfigured into the emblem of a new conjugal sensibility, one in which men "sacrificed" a degree of sexual pleasure in exchange the social improvement and respectability entailed by having smaller families. The practice eventually came to be regarded as a sign of self-control, a technique for taming or "civilizing" animal instincts—in contrast to couples that continued to have large families who were said to behave like "rabbits" or "mice." Because it relied on communication and cooperation between spouses, coitus interruptus also reflected a spreading ideal of companionate marriage predicated upon sentiments of conjugal mutuality (if not necessarily equality) and a new emotional focus on children and their well-being (1991, 887). More recently, Hirsch and Nathanson have found the practice to reflect ideals of emotional intimacy and joint decision making among contemporary Mexican couples as well. Mexican women, like Rhodian women, refer to their husbands as "taking care" of them (*él me cuida*) when they practice withdrawal. Like Rhodian women too, they regarded medical contraception as "extremely dangerous" to their bodies and appreciated the "sacrifice" their husbands made to protect their health by practicing withdrawal. As the authors conclude of Mexican men's role in birth control: "The physical restraint of desire becomes a private performance of the shared goal of having a more modern family" (2001, 421).

Suspending the conventional typologies that classify coitus interruptus and other presumably male-controlled methods such as condoms as traditional and medical methods as modern thus allows us to attend more closely to the meanings and valences that Rhodians themselves attach to these methods and in doing so, I would argue, helps clarify the processes that have led to the seemingly paradoxical unevenness of the medicalization of reproduction in contemporary Greece. As I show in this section, narratives of contraceptive refusal often drew on familiar cultural idioms that offered women (as well as the smaller number men I spoke with) a flexible logic with which to think about and evaluate the potential risks to health and fertility posed by medical contraception. Among the most salient of these were the opposed pairs natural/unnatural and inside/outside.

Appeals to "nature" and the "natural" are often intimately bound up with attempts to make moral sense of new reproductive technologies of all sorts (Traina et al., 2008). Although from the perspective of science, nature belongs to an order distinct from the moral, in popular usage "nature" often serves as a "moral touchstone, the effects of which are especially evident at the culturally constructed margins between 'nature' and 'culture'" (Lock and Kaufert 1998, 20). These insights are particularly helpful when attempting to understand the ways in which Rhodian women appealed to nature as they talked about their contraceptive choices. Their largely negative perceptions of the pill and the IUD were typically voiced in terms of a concern over the risks involved in introducing "unnatural" substances and "foreign" objects into the interior of the body on a long-term basis. When women spoke of "nature" and "the natural" in their attempts to explain and justify their contraceptive choices, however, they were not invoking an inviolable sacralized order of things or making religious appeals, at least not in the conventional Greek Orthodox sense. In fact, many young women were unaware that the Church prohibited medical contraceptive methods—as good an indication as any of the relatively low key of the Church's opposition. Rather, their appeals to "nature" and "the natural" were linked to a broader network of concerns about the risks and potentially adverse consequences of particular medico-technological interventions for their bodily health and fertility. In the Rhodian context, then, "nature" and "the natural" stood in opposition to the "artificial" and "the manufactured," that is, to the potentially risky and injurious products of modern medicine and science. Implicit in this opposition was a moral obligation to avoid risks to one's health and fertility by keeping these potentially harmful products from entering the "inside" of the body.[12] When assessing contraceptive options, women spoke in particular of the fear and anxiety provoked by the idea of introducing "chemicals" (*khimika*), "medicines" (*farmaka*, which in Greek means both "medicine" and "poison"), "hormones" (*ormones*) and other "manufactured substances" and objects (*tekhnikous tropous*) into the body's interior on a long-term basis. It is important to point out that apprehension and ambivalence over these manufactured risks was by no means restricted to the domain of medical contraception. Anxiety over the health effects of chemicals, medicines, hormones, and radiation (as discussed in Chapter 5) was grounded in a broader concern over the potential risks, hazards, and unintended consequences of modern science and technology that extends across many domains of contemporary Greek society. The cultural salience of these terms is suggested by their traffic across these diverse domains. To give one pertinent example: organic produce may be described as being produced "*khoris ormones*, without hormones," or "without *farmaka*" (unlike the United States, where the reference is usually to the absence of pesticides or chemical fertilizers).

Such reflexive concern over manufactured risks and hazards, while globally diffused today, is arguably more intense in some locations than in others. Compared to the United States, public opinion across Europe (and Japan) demonstrates considerably higher levels of anxiety over all kinds of biotechnological interventions into nature and lower levels of trust in the protective intent of governmental regulatory institutions (Hoban 1997). For instance, unlike Americans, but like other consumers across the European Union, Greeks are very wary of genetically modified foods. Confirming this widespread apprehension, Theodoros Koliopanos, a former deputy minister of the environment, wryly observed in a recent interview that "all political parties are opposed [to GMOs], which is odd because we disagree on everything else" (Rosenthal 2006). Without discounting the seriousness or sincerity of Rhodian women's fears regarding the bodily risks of medical contraception, it is also possible to interpret their talk of "nature" and "the natural" when justifying refusal as a way of expressing or performing their sensibility as reflexive, late modern subjects who are alert to the dilemmatic aspects of contemporary medicine—with its tangled mix of desirable benefits and potentially iatrogenic risks to health and body. Unwittingly, then, the late modern valence that attaches to women's justifications for refusing medical contraception may also help reinforce the inertia or stasis so apparent in Greek contraceptive culture over the last several decades.

When I asked Melina, a primary school teacher in her midthirties, to explain her reasons for rejecting the pill, she simply said: "I've never taken the pill. I consider it an unnatural intervention, *mia afisiki paremvasi*." When this otherwise thoughtful and articulate woman stopped there, as many women did, assuming perhaps that the implicit meanings packed into her appeal to nature would be transparent to me, I asked her to elaborate:

> Why? Because it interferes with the natural functioning of the body. Since there are other methods available that you can use without interfering with nature, in the functioning of the body, why not use them? The pill intervenes hormonally. Me, I don't want the hormones, because they are a drug, *ena farmako*, and what's more, a drug that has so many effects on the body. Now, I don't know the biology exactly. But I believe it intervenes in the body in an unnatural way, isn't that right, *etsi dhen ine*? You intervene with manufactured means, *me tekhnikous tropous*, with other substances, *me ala mesa*. It's an irritation to the woman's body.

In making their evaluative claims and justifying their choices among contraceptive options, women often linked the natural/unnatural contrast with the paired idioms of inside/outside. As many anthropologists have observed, inside/outside is an opposition that is among the most salient and productive tropes in Greek culture, used in various and flexible ways to construct and comment upon the social order (Dubisch 1986). For example, in the domain of social relations, "inside" is associated with those who are classified as "our own" (*dhiki mas*), an elastically shifting category of inclusion whose membership varies depending on the context; that which is "outside" connotes the "foreign" or the "other" (*kseno*). The inside/outside distinction is pertinent to the discourse of health maintenance as well. For both the social and the physical body, the "foreign," with its disruptive potential, is usually suspect, potentially polluting and injurious to well-being (Arnold 1985; Dubisch 1986). In the classic anthropological formulation, the "foreign" is thus matter dangerously out of place (Douglas 1966). However, as the ethnogynecological use of pessaries and the internal manipulations of the mammi (or the popularity of tampons today) suggest, it is not necessarily the violation of bodily boundaries per se to which women objected. Rather, women used the inside/outside contrast to express their anxieties and fears over the perceived *nature* or attributes of the matter being introduced into the body. In the case of contraception, it is the intrusion of manufactured objects (*tekhnikous tropous*) and substances into the body's interior and their potential iatrogenic risks that tend to be coded as "unnatural" and thus potentially injurious. By this logic, taking the pill was often framed as "unnatural" because it entailed ingesting "foreign" (*kseno*) substances such as "hormones," "medicines," "chemicals," and "drugs" on a long-term basis. As Keti, a thirty-two-year-old store clerk and mother of two explained: "I didn't want to take birth control pills, because they are a foreign . . . a foreign organism [*sic*] inside your organism. . . . I don't like to take any medicines—even an aspirin you take, it's a foreign organism, *ksenos orghanismos.*"

The inside/outside binary also implicitly informed many Rhodian women's reluctance to use the IUD. The most commonly heard objection was the formulaic: "The IUD is a foreign body, *kseno soma,* inside my body." When pressed, women elaborated on the variety of dangers and anomalous consequences attendant upon violating the integrity of body boundaries. Thus, "the IUD can become one with your flesh; it will be impossible to remove it." "I'm doing something not entirely natural. I've introduced something inside me. I do damage to nature, to my organism." Occasionally, women asked me what contraceptive method I used. When I described the diaphragm, they sometimes objected that this method too was problematic or "unnatural" because I was introducing foreign substances and objects inside my body. Initially, I was puzzled by these objections. Coming of age as I did in the era of the Dalkon Shield and under the influence of Barbara Seaman's germinal *The Doctor's Case against the Pill,* published in 1969, I confess that I had no difficulty understanding women's reasons for rejecting the medical contraceptives available to them. For me, the diaphragm had always represented an indispensable (if still at times resented) alternative to what I also perceived to be the unacceptable health risks associated with the pill and the IUD. Eventually, though, the arguments women used to make sense of an essentially unknown method such as the diaphragm helped to clarify the often implicit cultural logic that guided their evaluations of medical contraception in general.

Although pills and the IUD were usually coded as "unnatural" and coitus interruptus and, to a lesser extent, condoms as "natural," these idioms were also used in flexible and creative ways. In a particularly revealing rhetorical move, women who had adopted a medical method of contraception might invert the conventional meanings associated with the natural/unnatural and inside/outside binaries when justifying their decisions. Given the often strongly negative reactions from friends and family, women's appropriation of these terms to defend their choices can be interpreted as a pragmatic bid to deflect the common criticism that they were carelessly toying with their health and fertility. Keti, who had rejected the pill, as we saw earlier, because it was "a foreign organism" "inside" her body, went on to explain that she ultimately turned to the IUD because unlike the pill, "it is *outside* of the organism, *outside* of the uterus" (my emphasis). More notable still were the several women who had been sterilized who described tubal ligation as "the most natural method." Kiki, a restaurant cook in her early forties with three children, and a self-described modern woman ("*moderna ghineka*"), told me she was very happy with her tubal ligation. When she learned that her last child was to be delivered by caesarean, she seized the opportunity to ask her doctor to perform the procedure, because, as she put it, "it is the most natural method." Sterilization was "natural," Kiki went on explain, because "you have sexual ease, *seksualiki anesi*; you're not afraid of getting pregnant. And all the rest is normal, you see a normal period, you feel normal, without drugs and without risks or side effects." Kiria Alexandra had also been sterilized along with her caesarean delivery. After years of relying on withdrawal, which had led to two abortions, she, like Kiki, expressed great satisfaction with her sterilization: "It's the best method, it's the most natural. It doesn't change anything inside." Given women's concerns with the potential risks and hazards of the pill and IUD, perhaps it shouldn't be surprising that tubal ligation is the fastest-growing birth control method in Greece, at least among older women who have completed their families. Of course, the high rate of caesarean deliveries (now over 40 percent) would also seem to facilitate women's decisions to undergo the procedure. For the present argument, what is most significant about these excerpts is the insight they offer into how women creatively appropriate an enduringly salient and morally charged network of cultural idioms to justify their contraceptive choices, in this case, by flexibly recoding as "natural" a surgical intervention that results in permanent sterilization.

Of all the birth control methods commonly used in Greece, coitus interruptus is the likeliest to be described as the most natural ("*to pio fisiologhiko, pio fisiko*"). Other scholars, also noting this distinction, have suggested that what makes coitus interruptus "natural" and thus preferable to the more reliable medical methods is the possibility of conception it leaves open. On this view, as previously mentioned, Greek women regard sex and conception as inseparable; without the possibility of pregnancy, it is further argued, women could not experience sex as pleasurable or desirable. When Rhodian women indexed medical methods as "unnatural," however, this was not because contraception itself was seen as an unnatural act. As already noted, not a single

Rhodian woman I spoke with referenced the Greek Orthodox Church's opposition to medical methods as a reason for rejection. Nor, as Paxson (2002, 314) also found for Athenian women, did Rhodian women object to contraception on the grounds that it prevented women from proving their fertility. Rather, as I have just suggested, use of the idiom of "naturalness" appeared to reflect women's expressed anxiety over the health and fertility risks of introducing "unnatural," "foreign," or "chemical" substances and objects such as the IUD and the pill into the body on a long-term basis. Because coitus interruptus and sometimes condoms (although women might object to them on other grounds) did not involve such risks, they were usually regarded as more "natural" methods.

The heavy reliance on withdrawal did not mean that this method was regarded as ideal, however. Even though women tended to label withdrawal as "more natural," reservations and complaints about the method were also fairly common. The major problem, I was told, was that even if a partner were very skilled and careful, "just a single drop" accidentally emitted could result in pregnancy. For this reason, withdrawal routinely left open the possibility of abortion. Although abortion is a commonplace experience, few women took the procedure lightly.[13] Aside from the religious and moral issues it raises, abortion is widely perceived to carry its own medical risks. These include the risks and side effects from the general anesthesia that is routinely used when performing abortions, as well as from the procedure itself, which women feared might damage or "wound" their reproductive organs and potentially cause sterility (see also Skilogianis 2001). Eva, a thirty-three-year-old shop clerk and mother of a six-year-old daughter, discussed with me her fears and concerns over the abortion procedure. Eva had been on the pill for some five years, and although quite satisfied, she had switched to withdrawal when she turned thirty because of her age and because she smoked. "I prefer it, I risk it, *to riskaro*," she said of withdrawal. "But every month, I have anxiety, a terrible anxiety, *ena fovero ankhos*." When I asked her why, since she had just told me that she did not believe abortion was a sin, and since abortion was legal and readily available, she responded, "Yes, that's true, but the anesthesia? What do you do with that? And the scraping they do inside, *to skalisma*, what are you going to do with that too? Look, it's an operation." The potential medical risks and health consequences of the abortion she would inevitably face if withdrawal failed caused Eva considerable anxiety but at the end of the day were outweighed by an even stronger fear of the long-term ingestion of chemicals and hormones, given her particular circumstances (age and smoking).

Some women also complained that by interrupting the course of the sex act, withdrawal interfered with their pleasure. For others, the nagging fear of an unwanted pregnancy also negatively affected their sexual experience. Some twenty years ago, Yewoubdar Beyene (1989, 114) observed in her study of a village on the island of Evia that "stress for Greek women was caused by constant worry about unwanted pregnancy." This impression is confirmed by Kiria Alexandra, who provided a vivid description of her embodied experience of withdrawal before her tubal ligation:

> When a woman isn't afraid of getting pregnant, she is more sexual, *pio seksualikia*, more OK, *pio sosti*. Just the thought that she might get pregnant totally stops everything, *ta stamata ola*. Even if her body wants it, her mind will turn things back, *ta ghirnai piso*, because of her fear of getting pregnant.

And Roula, a thirty-nine-year-old shopkeeper and mother of two, offered this tart commentary on her years of relying on withdrawal before turning to the IUD: "It's the worst! You're afraid all the time [of getting pregnant]. And when the two don't finish together, *as mou'lipe to visino!*" This last idiomatic expression, which literally translates as "I could have done without the cherry," refers to the sour cherry preserves hostesses traditionally offered their guests when they came to visit. In using this expression, Roula is saying that the implied exchange—a sweet treat for a (boring or unpleasant) visit, limited pleasure for lingering anxiety—was simply not worth it.

The Sexual Politics of Coitus Interruptus

Debates over the nature of gender relations in Greece, on the one hand, and over the sexual politics of coitus interruptus, on the other, converge on the vexed issue of the degree of power women exercise in conjugal relationships. As previously noted, coitus interruptus has often been coded as a "traditional" birth control method because it is believed to ensure that men retain control over contraception. Rhodian women's narratives also suggest that while it is true in one sense that reliance on coitus interruptus is a means of "pass[ing] the responsibility of birth control to men" (Loizos and Papataxiarchis 1991b, 225), it is equally true that, as others have proposed, women's assertions of their own needs are often necessary to ensure men's effective cooperation (Petchesky 1990; Flandrin 1979; McLaren 1990). Thus, Kiriaki, a twenty-nine-year-old middle-class housewife, told me she and her husband relied solely on coitus interruptus, but "if I don't remind him, he forgets to." I asked Irini, an eighteen-year-old working-class housewife, if the fact that they always used this method didn't bother her or her husband. She assured me it didn't, explaining that she found it no obstacle to her own sexual satisfaction (although obviously some women, like Kiria Alexandra, did). As for her husband, she said, "It's only a moment," and he was "used to it." Smaro, twenty-four years old, was blunt: "So let the man's pleasure be diminished." A hospital social worker who frequently counseled Rhodians on contraception summarized women's feelings toward the use of coitus interruptus as a major means of birth control by using a common Greek expression: "Why me and not him? *Ghiati egho ke okhi ekinos?*" In other words, she went on to explain, why should I be the one to take the health risks and bear the discomforts of contraception?

None of the women (or the fifteen men) I interviewed explicitly referred to coitus interruptus as a burden or sacrifice, as Schneider and Schneider (1991) describe for rural Sicily and Hirsch and Nathanson (2001) for Mexico. Still, a sense that it might represent something of a sacrifice of the man's pleasure was nonetheless sometimes implicit. This sense emerges from the following excerpt of a conversation I had with Khristos, an engineer in his midthirties. Through my friendship with his wife, Melina, I'd come to know Khristos fairly well and felt comfortable enough to talk to him on the topic of withdrawal:

> EG: Is withdrawal a sacrifice for you?
> Khristos: Not a very important one, *okhi simantiko.* Everything is relative;
>   . . . it's the easiest method. No preparation, no forgetting to take a
>   pill—
> Melina [interjecting]: I never seriously considered taking the pill.
> EG: Women often tell me that withdrawal is the most natural method. Is
>   it natural?
> Khristos: Anything in which you interrupt the natural course of the
>   process is not natural. It's the *best* method for women, because they're
>   not taking any chemicals, but it's not natural. You have less pleasure
>   . . . but if I eat one piece of chocolate instead of two, it's not a big
>   difference.

Khristos's chocolate-eating analogy good-naturedly hints at the sense of deprivation that may accompany some men's embodied experience of withdrawal. At the same time, it exemplifies the degree to which men share their wives' perception that the health risks of the birth control pill are unacceptable— even if they may simultaneously reject their wives' appeals to nature and the natural to justify reliance on withdrawal. Confirming Dr. A.'s opinion of men's attitudes toward medical contraception, eleven of the fifteen married men I was able to interview on the topic also phrased their objections in terms of the adverse health effects for their wives. Finally, Khristos's evaluation of with-drawal gestures toward a companionate ideal of conjugal relations in which the husband has a responsibility to take care of his wife's person and bodily well-being and protect her from harm. As Heather Paxson (2002, 320) con-cludes based on her research in Athens: "Women can view men's responsibility in contraceptive practices as a signal of their love (*aghapi*) and caring." In this section, I have argued that "caring" and "being careful" have multiple mean-ings. For my purposes, what is particularly noteworthy is that men and women *both* tended to justify their reliance on coitus interruptus as a way of avoiding the health risks associated with medicalized contraception. In deploying this shared discourse of risk (even as the meanings assigned to some key idioms, such as "natural," may differ radically) these men can also be seen as express-ing, among other things, their sensibilities as caring late modern husbands.

The Making of the (Late) Modern Greek Family

Today, husbands and wives generally agree that the two-child family is the ideal, although in practice many families have only one child.[14] While Rho-dians may sometimes express admiration for the large families of the past or nod to official pronatalist discourse by declaring that "large families are good for Greece," they, like the Sicilians studied by Schneider and Schneider (1991), may also disparage women who bear many children by calling them "rabbits" (*kouneles*). In this section, I argue that the recent shifts in both ideal and ac-tual family size can be adequately grasped only against the background of sig-nificant transformations in understandings of motherhood, fatherhood, and childhood in contemporary Greece. Given the overwhelming reliance on non-medical means of contraception described in the preceding section, for many couples, today's one- to two-child family can be attained only by resorting to abortion. (In the concluding section, I address how Rhodians face and attempt to resolve the moral contradictions and dilemmas inherent in this situation.)

Conceptions and practices of mothering and the appropriate care of chil-dren had undergone some notable transformations across the three generations of women I interviewed. As described in Chapter 3, rural women of the oldest generation were caught in a demanding and endless cycle of productive activi-ties, toiling in the wheat fields, tending the tree crops, and herding the goats and sheep. Essential to the survival of the household, these activities often kept them away from their homes for long hours each day, or even weeks at a time during the harvest season. Women also faced a heavy workload in the home, where they bore the primary responsibility for weaving cloth and making the family's clothing, preparing the meals, collecting firewood and water, washing clothes, looking after children, and performing the family religious rituals, among many other tasks. These multiple demands on their time and labor could be managed only with the help of a variety of "mother-centered" practices and technologies that freed at least some of their attention from child care (Ross 1993). Swaddling infants to keep them safely immobilized, carrying nursing infants along to the fields and hanging them from tree branches, enlisting daughters to act as their adjuncts, and elsewhere, feeding infants poppy seed tea to tranquilize them—all were important mother-centered practices that endured into the 1950s or early 1960s.[15] Even so, mothers often carefully curtailed their own consumption, sacrificing themselves to meet their families' basic needs and to fulfill the parental moral mandate "to augment and multiply what is passed on from one generation to the next" (Vlahoutsikou 1997, 295)

When Rhodian women of the transitional generation married and began to form their families, they did so under very different circumstances. Women who came of age in the 1960s and 1970s were the first to attend school for any extended period of time and the first for whom literacy was a given. Economic growth, urbanization, rising living standards, and the increase in leisure time relative to the amount their mothers had enjoyed made possible an unprecedentedly widespread embourgeoisement of Greek women. A far greater proportion of Rhodian women were now able to conform to the norms of respectable femininity as shaped by the ideal of the *nikokira*. The figure of the *nikokira* is familiar from the now classic ethnographies of Greece, which, not coincidentally, were based on fieldwork conducted mainly in the 1960s and 1970s (Bakalaki 1994).[16] In this model, husband and wife perform complementary roles that correspond to the public and private spheres, respectively. Married women generally did not work for pay (although, as discussed in Chapter 2, some Rhodian women quickly responded to the tourist boom by setting up businesses based in their homes). Those who did often quit after the birth of the first child to commit their full attention to its care and upbringing. Ideally, a married woman devoted herself exclusively to the domestic arts of mothercraft and housecraft: cooking, cleaning, raising her children, safeguarding the family's health and well-being, and creating needlepoint and crocheted handicrafts for household decoration. Still, as was true for the oldest generation, women were expected to judiciously exercise their management skills and economic restraint, and to sacrifice their own consumption for the advancement of the next generation. Ultimately, the *nikokira's* self-esteem and prestige derived from the successful management of her household and the promotion of its class mobility (Salamone and Stanton 1986; S. Sutton 1986).[17]

By the 1980s and 1990s, the nikokira ideal was being reshaped by new understandings of what it meant to be a mother, a wife, and—in a novel turn, as the theme of gender equality became part of everyday public discourse—"a person" (Papagaroufali 1990; J. Cowan 1996). This was a period anchored at the outset by Greece's accession to full membership the European Union in 1981 and punctuated throughout by a series of notable social and economic changes that have had a particularly significant impact on women. In 1983, the radically egalitarian Family Law was put into effect, in part as the result of unified pressure from Greek women's organizations, and in part from the European Community requirement that member nations comply with a liberal European discourse of rights (J. Cowan 1996, 71). After declining in the 1970s, women's formal participation in the labor force began to climb, officially reaching 39 percent by 1997 (Close 2002, 217). More impressive still was the growing number of women in institutions of higher learning, where, by the late 1990s, they formed the large majority of graduates (ibid.). Although "feminism" (*feminismos*) is today a somewhat tarnished term (for many Rhodians, it denoted an unacceptable dominance of women *over* men), the discourse of gender equality (*isotita*) is nonetheless part of mainstream understandings of contemporary young women. When, for instance, educational researchers in 1991 asked a sample of fifteen-year-old girls in Thessaloniki to describe how they saw themselves ten years hence, the futures they imagined inevitably embraced both "a successful career and a good husband" (Delighiani-Kwimsi 1993b).

Yet, the 1980s and 1990s were also fraught with a growing sense of economic insecurity and uncertainty about the future. Greece's engagement with globalization, which has been mediated largely through the European Union, has entailed a loss of local sovereignty over many domains. To take just one example, removal of the last of the barriers and tariffs that had historically protected the Greek economy has resulted in unsettling declines in both industry and agriculture (Close 2002, 172). At the same time, EU membership has led to increasing integration into the consumption patterns of the European core (Costa 1993, 83). The process of Europeanization underway in the European Union is inextricably linked with what has been called the "bourgeoiseification" of everyday life (Borneman and Fowler 1997, 494). These implicit dimensions of class and social distinction mean that, as Chouliaras (1993, 112) ironically observes, "'non-European' Europeans can be found [even] in the center of Western Europe." For Greeks and others on the southern rim of the European Union, consumption has represented perhaps the most important source of symbolic capital and route through which European affiliation is constituted and expressed and by which European and modern subjectivities may be created and displayed (Costa 1993; Moutsatsos 2001; Vlahoutsikou 1997). As Chrisy Moutsatsos (2001) has shown in her unique study of the beauty practices of Athenian women, Europeanization is a profoundly gendered (and racialized) process, not just inscribed on the surface of women's bodies but deeply etched into their embodied subjectivities as well. Today, alongside the newly intensified model of motherhood that I describe shortly, a widely diffused ideal of European bourgeois femininity that dictates greater investment in women's self-care and appearance makes additional demands on women's time, energy, and, of course, money. According to this ideal, women (at least through middle age) should strive to be *peripiimeni*, roughly, "soignée": stylishly dressed, well coifed, devoid of overly prominent "Mediterranean" hips and thighs, and, through the strenuous and regular efforts of their aesthetologists (a rapidly growing occupational niche in recent years), possessed of smooth-textured, light-colored, hairless skin. By 2000, a plastic surgeon had opened a practice in Rhodes Town to help women surgically approach this ideal.

In Rhodes, where the local economy was stronger than the national average thanks to tourism, the trend toward high levels of consumption and public display were perhaps even more apparent than elsewhere. A quick sense of consumption levels on the island can be gleaned from municipal surveys done in 2000 and 2004. These surveys found that nearly all households had a TV, 91 percent had a washing machine, 76 percent had cell phones, 58 percent had a VCR, 27 percent had a dishwasher, 36 percent had personal computers and 16 percent had air conditioning. In addition, 75 percent of those surveyed owned a car (Dhimos Rodhion 2002, 2007).

Yet wages in Greece, as in the other nations of Europe's South, remain low. As a result, Greeks must work almost twice as long to purchase the same basket of goods as those who live in the nations of the EU core (Bozaninou 1996). Not surprisingly, despite the dramatic recent increase in consumption levels, Greeks in general were more pessimistic than other EU citizens about their material prospects (Close 2002, 285, citing a survey in *To Vima*, December 17, 2000). Growing pessimism about the future was reflected in the term *neoftokhi*, "the newly poor," which circulated with increasing frequency alongside the older *neoplouti*, "nouveaux riches," long used to stereotype Rhodians, sometimes by Rhodians themselves.

The combination of high levels of consumption and relatively low wages makes enormous demands on a family's resources. For most, meeting these demands entailed long hours of work, second jobs, multiple wage earners—including mothers with small children, who previously might have quit working—and not least, considerable transfers of wealth and other resources between the generations. By far the most important intergenerational transfer of wealth is the dowry house. The 2000 Rhodian municipal survey referred to earlier found that an impressive three-quarters of Rhodians owned their own homes (67 percent) or lived rent-free (7 percent). About one-quarter owned a second house. Extrapolating from my research, I can venture with some confidence that many of these houses were acquired as dowry. Among those who lived rent-free, it was not uncommon to find a woman's brother living in her dowry house because she and her husband had built a newer and larger residence.[18]

Everyone knows, of course, that the dowry, *prika*, was legally abolished in the 1980s by the new Family Law. Some young women even laughed when I mentioned the word, which has acquired a distinctly negative cast. As David Sutton (1998a, 101) points out: "The association of dowry with 'rural backwardness' is clearly a widespread phenomenon in Greece" and is taken to represent the nation's most "un-modern" elements. Some Rhodian women also disparaged the term because it connoted a traditional understanding of marriage based on economic calculation (as evidenced in the pejorative term *prikothiras*, "dowry-monger") as opposed to a modern conjugality predicated on sexual attraction and romantic love. Yet, while the word "dowry" may have fallen into disfavor, endowing a daughter with a house or apartment when she married remained an ideal that families aspired to and often succeeded in realizing—surprisingly often, given the huge expense involved. Homeownership represented an important foundation of the enduring family project of social mobility; without it, the goal of improving status might be thwarted or even reversed. The minority of women I spoke with who did not have a residence when they married considered their situation to be unfortunate because of the ensuing necessity to divert so much of the family's income to rent. A few other women, like one of the midwives I interviewed, had worked and saved to buy an apartment on their own before marrying. But in Rhodes, perhaps more than in other parts of Greece, parents strived to provide their daughters with their own residence when they married.

The cost of dowering a daughter on Rhodes today encompasses a great deal more than constructing a dwelling. When they marry, daughters may receive residences that are literally fully furnished: kitchens are equipped with the latest-model appliances; cupboards are stocked with pots and pans, dishware, glasses, and silver; closets are crammed with sheets, towels, and blankets; and shelves and curio stands brim with name-brand figurines and other knickknacks. Grooms are expected to cover the cost of some of the furniture and appliances, if they can afford to do so. But the great bulk of the expense falls to the bride's parents. To accomplish this massive project of accumulation, mothers usually begin when their daughters are still very young. Kiria Loukia, who owned a tourist shop in the Old Town, described her purchasing strategies for me. When her daughters were three or four, she began collecting those items, such as silverware, that were least subject to fashion and thus unlikely to become outmoded. Items such as art and curios, for which tastes might change, she purchased last. The extent of parental largesse was often impressive. As Kiria Loukia went on to explain, "When I was buying dowry goods (*prikiaka*) for my daughters, I always asked, 'Which is the most expensive? Which is the best?' and I would start from there. Porcelain? That would be Lladro. Glass? That would be Murano. And so I would buy the most expensive piece I could afford." A poignant example of this long-term accumulation strategy gone awry was the story of one father who for years had been collecting wine with which to stock his daughter's dowry house. She married rather later than expected, however, and when she served the wine at her first dinner party, she discovered that bottle after bottle had turned to vinegar. Sometimes, as noted in Chapter 2, daughters may even receive two houses, one in town and a smaller one in a rustic style in their natal village for weekend and holiday use.

Because it enabled the younger generation to avoid the cost of rent and liberated income for other expenses, the dowry house was widely appreciated and valued as one of the most important forms of assistance (*voithia*) parents could offer their children in meeting modern standards of consumption and actively promoting their social mobility. Rather than a traditional obligation or duty, as it presumably was in the past, giving a house to one's children was now perceived as something every parent "naturally" desires to do if it is in their power.[19] "You give because you want to, *thelis ke dhinis*," I was often told. Or, as Ksenia responded when I asked about the new house she and her husband had just built for their daughter: "Whoever has something, won't they want to give it to their child? Won't they want to help them? Won't they want to make them a little house?" To Ksenia, the answer to these rhetorical questions is self-evident; it reflects, as Collier (1997, 15) observes of "modern" behaviors in rural Spain, "what any rational person would do." In the end, the ruefully traditional connotations of the dowry house were dealt with simply by replacing the term "*prika*" with "*voithia*."

In Rhodes today, parental transfers of wealth in the form of housing may even extend over two generations. Kiria Loukia's sister, Nena, a fifty-two-year-old mother of two and grandmother of three, owns and runs with her husband a small ceramics factory that produces the colorful souvenir plates that Rhodes is known for and that are quite popular with tourists. Well-off, although not inordinately so, she had built and fully furnished houses for both her daughters (for the youngest, she had hired an interior decorator from Athens, a growing trend on Rhodes among those who can afford it). Now, she had already begun the process of building a house for her four-year-old granddaughter. Nena explained why:

> I've married both my daughters, now I work for my grandchildren, because what my husband makes is more than enough for us. [I work] because it's harder to live now, harder for our children to make money than when we were young. I worry for my children, for my grandchildren. There are more taxes now, more expenses, many more expenses. . . . Whatever we made, my husband and I, we made it together as a couple. Now, you need more people to make what we made. Grandmothers, grandfathers, all have to help too. Otherwise, the children can't do it on their own.

As this narrative excerpt suggests, when Rhodian parents imagined the future, they were often anxious that their own standards of living would be difficult or impossible for their children and grandchildren to achieve, let alone exceed—at least not without considerable help.

Child care was another critical form of assistance that the older generation generously gave their children. Throughout Greece, the available public nurseries fall far short of demand and Rhodes was no exception. With more mothers than ever working for wages, the child-care gap has come to be filled largely by grandmothers. Such child-care arrangements were often facilitated by the matrivicinal residence patterns that resulted from local dowry practices. For example, Ghogho, a twenty-eight-year-old divorced mother of a seven-year-old, worked ten-hour shifts at a tourist shop six days a week during the saison. Ghogho lived in a three-story apartment building that her father, a taxi driver, had constructed piecemeal over the years as his savings allowed. Her apartment, which had been given to her when she married, was across the hall from her parents. Her brother lived in the top-floor apartment, which his parents had also built for him after he married a (dowryless) Scandinavian woman. Every school day, Ghogho's mother picked up Ghogho's daughter after classes, brought her home, and took care of her until Ghogho returned from work. She also had dinner ready when Ghogho came home each night and even ironed her clothes for her. On weekends, when Ghogho or her brother and his wife went out socially, they simply dropped their children off at their mother's flat. By performing the crucial service of child care, women like Ghogho's mother gave their daughters and daughters-in-law the opportunity to earn a salary for their households as well as the occasional leisure time that made it possible for them to maintain contemporary middle-class standards of consumption.

Working women who did not have a mother or mother-in-law available or able to help them increasingly turned to the pool of new immigrants, which had expanded dramatically in the 1990s. Previously, only well-to-do families employed household help, usually young women from the Philippines. Employing a *filipineza* is still a sign of distinction, but today Rhodians of far more modest means hire women from Eastern Europe and the Balkans.[20] And it is not only child care that has become commoditized. Although women are working outside the home in record numbers, the division of household labor by gender has not changed appreciably (Symeonidou 2000). By 2000, women I knew who in the early 1990s had done all their own housework were hiring immigrant women to clean for them. New immigrants could also be found in the countryside. Throughout Greece, the rural sector has been revitalized to some extent by the recent influx of cheap labor, especially from Albania. In Rhodes, where agriculture is in severe decline, Albanians living in the countryside were usually employed to care for infirm and elderly villagers, a responsibility that once fell to such villagers' daughters. Occasionally, the flood of immigrant women available for domestic labor even figured into a couple's reproductive decision making. For instance, when Soula found herself unexpectedly pregnant only a year after the birth of her second daughter, she seriously contemplated having an abortion. She knew that her husband, Mikhalis, wanted to try for a son, although he didn't come right out and say so. As Soula recalled their conversations over what course to take, Mikhalis told her that, since he already put in twelve-hour workdays, he was not in a position to provide additional help with the children; the decision, therefore, was ultimately hers. However, he went on to add, if she did decide to keep the pregnancy, he promised her that he would pay for "a woman, *mia ghineka*," by which he meant a full-time immigrant domestic worker, to help her raise the children. In the end, Soula kept the pregnancy, gave birth to a boy, and had already cycled through two child-care helpers, one from Romania and the other from Bulgaria, by the time I saw her again.

Even with help from their mothers or paid domestic workers, women of the youngest generation often perceived motherhood to be fraught with stress (*stres*) and anxiety (*ankhos*). For these women, conceptions of motherhood have been profoundly reshaped by new consumerist understandings that are intensely child centered, emotionally demanding, and financially taxing.[21] As Nena's quote suggested, in the contemporary context of global restructuring, which in Greece has been heavily mediated by EU membership, children's futures are imagined as increasingly uncertain. Beyond any doubt, globalization has punished the world's impoverished children most harshly, yet "the materially privileged are affected too, as the conditions for economic wellbeing appear ever more tenuous and the future well-being of children ever more uncertain" (Stephens 1995, 20). The discourse of stress is today so pervasive that the 2000 survey of Rhodian households mentioned earlier, an otherwise routine government-sponsored socioeconomic survey, included questions on how often respondents experienced *stres* and *ankhos* in their daily lives. An astonishing 42 percent of women (and 37 percent of men) reported feeling either or both "frequently" or "permanently" (Dhimos Rodhion 2002, table 8.4.1).

Much of parental stress and anxiety revolves around the theme of education. The Greek context stands out for the intensity with which children's higher education is culturally valued as a means for confronting what is widely perceived as an increasingly uncertain future (Tsoukalas 1976). In Greece, the intricately tiered higher education system is controlled and regulated by the state. Entry into the coveted upper echelons of this system is determined by how well a student performs on the highly competitive Panhellenic university entrance exams. Through its control of this critical filter, the Greek state plays a key role in mediating between children and national, regional, and global markets. As in other countries in which the state occupies a similar gatekeeping position (e.g., Japan, Korea, Indonesia, and India; see, e.g., Stephens 1995), passing the university entrance exam often becomes a concerted family project. Across social classes, there is a strong cultural expectation that parents will make every effort to ensure their children's success in achieving this goal. Almost obligatorily, given the widely lamented inadequacy of public education, this involved enrolling children in the "shadow education" system of costly private tutorial schools, the *frondisteria*.

Education in Greece today typically encompasses a mix of formal schooling and the parallel world of the *frondisteria*, as well as an array of additional extracurricular private lessons. While still in primary school, children may begin to attend private afternoon classes in computers and in the dominant languages of the European Union, English and German. Learning at least one foreign language increases their future job marketability, confers an aura of social distinction, and makes it possible for them to attend a university elsewhere in the European Union if they do not succeed in passing the Greek entrance exam. In fact, on a per capita basis, Greece is the largest exporter of students in the world today.[22] By the late 1990s, for instance, some thirty thousand Greek students were enrolled in British universities alone (Clogg 2002, 227). Preparation for the eventuality of going abroad to study has become part of the imagined future of many young Rhodians. Readers may recall the example of twelve-year-old Elena (mentioned in Chapter 2, note 7), who, when asked in her English class to make a drawing that illustrated her identity (she drew overlapping Greek and Irish flags), provided the following caption: "I'm pleased to know that when I grow up I'll be able to attend university in either Ireland or Greece. There will be a great choice for my future education." In middle school, many children begin attending academic tutorial schools in the afternoons and evenings. As children got older, the pressures to perform well in school increased exponentially. By high school, most students were severely taxed by their double day of classes and cram schools and by the long hours of studying into the night as they geared up for the imminent "exam hell" in their senior year.

The cost in parents' time, effort, and financial resources was also high. Helping younger children work through their mounds of daily homework was a task that usually fell to mothers, but fathers helped too. Mothers often forfeited help with household chores to give children more time to study or, to combat the effects of so much schoolwork on their health, to go out and relax with friends (see also Paxson 2004). The perception that childhood was under siege and in a state of unhealthy deterioration was not uncommon. On several occasions, for instance, the principal of my daughter's elementary school admonished parents who'd brought their children to school and lingered for the morning assembly to ease up on the extracurricular lessons and allow children more time for play. "Let your children be children!" he scolded us. "Children need time to play." Driving overscheduled children from lesson to lesson was a time-consuming chore that often fell to fathers. In addition to the time involved, the financial costs of these extracurricular classes could be staggering, especially as students started preparing for university entrance exams. As one woman wearily joked, once children enter high school, "the parent becomes just a wallet and a taxi driver, *portofoli kai taksidzis.*"

The "structure of feeling" of parenthood has changed in some other significant ways (R. Williams 1961). Women *and* men of the youngest generation typically endorsed an emotionally intensified and time-consuming model of parenting that placed high value on accessibility, good communication, and a less authoritarian approach than that which they typically attributed to their parents. As they had over the course of their pregnancies, many of these women had consulted guides for expert advice on childrearing techniques, among which the psychologist Penelope Leach's appeared to be the most popular. Ismini, a store clerk in her late twenties, explicitly defined her ideal of motherhood in opposition to her own mother's approach, which she considered to have been too remote and too strict:

A good mother needs to be patient; she needs lots of patience, not to be a dictator. She needs to devote a lot of time to listening and explaining things to her child, and not simply imposing her own view: "Don't do this, don't do that." She should be its friend. . . . Not like *ta palia miala*, the old minds.

Kostas, a thirty-nine-year-old father of two who owned a small restaurant that catered to tourists, enumerated the qualities of a good father in very similar terms:

> Open communication, spending time with the children, supporting them emotionally, being their friend. . . . You can't be old school, *palion arkhon* [literally, "of the old principles"]; you have to be of today's times, not to do what our mothers and fathers did.

Ideally, mothers (and fathers) required deep reserves of patience in order to provide the guidance and explanations that over time would nurture their child's own ability to make the right decisions and choices, and not simply impose their own rules in an authoritarian manner. Tellingly, both Kostas and Ismini deploy terms like "*palion arkhon*" and "*palia miala*" to distinguish their approaches to mothering and fathering from those of the previous generaton.

Given the enormous demands on their emotional and financial resources, it is perhaps not surprising that *both* mothers and fathers often described contemporary child rearing as more stressful than in the past (as M. Doumanis [1983] and Salamone and Stanton [1986] also report for other parts of Greece). Among the youngest generation of Rhodian women, the older idioms of maternal suffering and sacrifice, rooted in the gendered cosmology of the Greek Orthodox Church and implicitly endorsed and reinforced by the state, are today attenuated and increasingly supplanted by a medicalized discourse of stress and anxiety. Notably, these new medicalized idioms of distress were now as likely to be heard from fathers as from mothers. For instance, in response to my question about the number of children he would ideally have liked, Panos, thirty-three, a hotel employee and father of two, replied:

> I would have liked four, five, six children, if we're talking about what's good for Greece, but I can't cope. The needs have grown. A family with just one wage earner can't cope. A child needs a computer, the Internet, a cell phone, tutorial schools—the neighbor's kids can't have these things and yours not have them too. Me, I just finished primary school and I got

a job; now the anxiety, the stress, is greater. If I'd finished high school, I could have gotten a better job.[23]

In their unique study of Greek men and fatherhood, the psychologists Thalia Dragona and Despoina Naziri also found that "stress," "anxiety," and "responsibility" were among the outstanding themes in men's constructions of fatherhood. In an uncanny echo of Panos's sentiments, one of their respondents told them:

> When I first learned my wife was pregnant, *the only thing I felt was anxiety.* That's why the first thing I did was get a second job, to gather some money, so that I wouldn't deprive my child of whatever the other little children have. I went to the market to do some research to see what things cost and what I needed to buy. (1995, 100; my translation and emphasis)

In the context of these substantial changes, women, who bear the brunt of child caretaking, and men, who may still shoulder most of the responsibility for ensuring the family's material success and for maintaining or augmenting its levels of consumption, usually come to agree on the necessity of severely limiting family size in order to be good parents. Maria, a thirty-four-year-old chambermaid, expressed a view commonly heard from women from a range of social backgrounds (although most women usually specified higher educational goals than Maria's):

> Of course it's good to have only a few children, because we can help them advance in society better. When you have four or five children, you can't take care of them equally as well as you can two. It's not a question of saying [as in the past], "Children are happiness, *ine eftikhia ta pedhia*." The question is, how are you going to raise them, how are you going to help them to advance in their studies—to finish middle school, go to a technical school, learn a foreign language—help them with money, economically and socially, everywhere.[24]

With its cascade of obligations, Maria's narrative excerpt suggests the extent to which mothering has become intensified in contemporary Rhodes: to be a "good mother," still a primary social identity for most women, typically involves a far greater investment of time, attention, energy, money, responsibility, and, according to many women, stress and anxiety than in the past. On their part, fathers continue to be primarily responsible for, and derive prestige from, providing the economic means to maintain or improve the social position of the family (even when mothers work, as more than half now do). But, as is widely lamented, the demands of child rearing, both financial and emotional, are greater than ever. Under these circumstances, although the great majority of men and women endorsed the pronatalist position that "large families are good for Greece," they also saw them as incompatible with contemporary ideals of good parenthood.

Sin and Pity: Adapting Theology to Alternative Moralities of Abortion

Against the context of the preceding discussion, I conclude this chapter with a look at the dilemmas that arise when a contraceptive culture that relies heavily on abortion collides with a Greek Orthodox sensibility that condemns the practice as a major sin morally equivalent to murder. As described in Chapter 3, the ethnomedical regime that prevailed until World War II had cloaked early pregnancy in an interpretive ambiguity that enabled women of the oldest generation to bypass some of the moral onus associated with abortion. Once medicalization definitively erased this ambiguity, subsequent generations had to face head-on the challenge of making moral sense of themselves as Greek Orthodox women who aborted, often time and again. What is more, despite contemporary couples' overall agreement on the need to severely limit the number of children, by abortion if need be, it is still primarily women who must come to moral terms with the practice. As one woman put it, "The sin is on my back, not his [her husband's]," suggesting how profoundly the sense of transgression is gendered. The increasing secularization of Greek society notwithstanding, women's narratives revealed the extent to which they remain in active dialogue with the Church's position on abortion. As I describe shortly, Greek Orthodox theology continues to offer women a set of familiar and emotionally powerful terms with which to think about and come to grips with their abortion experiences. Few women rejected these terms outright. Rather, most engaged in an implicit dialogue with the Church, creatively and pragmatically adapting and redeploying its tenets and terms as they attempted to make moral sense of their everyday predicaments, in particular of the contradictions inherent in their position as women whose sense of personal and national identity is still intimately entwined with Greek Orthodoxy.

Rhodian women tended to interpret their abortions in one of three ways. A handful, typically young (in their twenties or early thirties) and usually well educated, flatly rejected the Church's position that abortion was a sin. Although these women sometimes found abortion problematic for psychological or health reasons, they refused—a few of them vehemently—to entertain theology as valid grounds for objection. Another minority, usually (though not always) in their late thirties or older, agreed unequivocally with the Church's absolutist doctrine that equates abortion with the murder of a "child" or a "person." These women held to a nonnegotiable ecclesiastical sense of sin, even when, as some did, they repeatedly violated it. As Niki, a twenty-nine-year-old housewife who had four abortions in a span of seven years, explained, "It's forbidden by religion. Every time, I regretted it, of course. But every time, I had to do it." When women like Niki aborted, their sense of sin might prevent them from taking part in the ritually purifying sacrament of Holy Communion, as dictated by the Church. Others might confess to a priest, who, more often than not, offered them forgiveness and comfort. Interestingly, their stories reveal that pastoral practice might often be flexible and pragmatic and, at times, touchingly compassionate. Niki, for instance, abstained from taking Communion over the seven years during which she underwent her multiple abortions because, as she explained, "knowing that it was forbidden, I did not want to mock God." After her last abortion, the feelings of remorse she had experienced to some extent from her first abortion became even more troubling, prompting her to go to confession. According to Niki, "I asked forgiveness and I confessed. He [the priest] blessed my belly with holy water and told me, 'Look, once God can forgive you. He can't forgive you over and over.' And I believe God forgave me. I want to believe that. Also the Church forgave me." Niki began taking Communion again and was seven months pregnant with her second child when I interviewed her. Similarly, Despina, an economically comfortable housewife in her late forties, had abstained from taking Communion for fifteen years because of her repeated abortions (a total of seven). When she finally confessed, the priest responded that fifteen years without Communion had been penance enough: she should resume taking it immediately. This disjuncture between Church doctrine and everyday practice may be related to the fact that Orthodox priests, obliged to marry and paid a low wage, face the same mundane parental obligations and dilemmas as most everyone else. Historically, as Sant Cassia with Bada (1992) has suggested, the sexual status of the priest and his often popular social origins may have helped keep the Church open to local practices and beliefs, especially regarding personal matters such as sexuality, and the related issues of contraception and abortion within marriage. In any case, the Orthodox Church has never been as staunch or vocal a public opponent of abortion as has the Catholic Church (Agrafiotis and Mandi 1997; Stamiris 1986).[25]

Very recently, women of the youngest generation have been exposed to new discourses that have sometimes led them to rethink their views of abortion. Evangelia, for example, told me that in the past she had no problem under-standing when some of her unmarried friends had abortions; however, her po-sition had begun to change after she saw the ultrasound images of the fetal heart beating during her pregnancy. She contrasted her view with that of her mother, who had suggested an abortion when Evangelia's fetus was diagnosed with a kidney problem:

> I think that younger women are more aware that it's a person from the start. We've seen the pamphlets from the Society for the Unborn Child. If you read those, you will get goose bumps. And if you've been pregnant and seen the little hands, heart, feet, you feel bad, you feel that you can't do it.

The Society for the Unborn Child, although tiny, managed in 2000 to project its antiabortion message onto a million telephone cards issued by the state-owned Greek Organization of Telecommunications (OTE), prompting pro-tests by Athenian feminist groups (Athanasiou 2001, 173). That same year, an Athenian genetics counselor who specializes in thalassemia told me that for the first time in her fifteen-year career, she had a young patient who refused to have an abortion after learning that her child had this serious disease. She attributed this refusal to the influence of Greek antiabortion organizations like the Society for the Unborn Child, which, although weak in comparison to their U.S. counterparts, have managed to influence the views of at least a few young women today.

The majority of women I spoke with, however, adapted and reinterpreted the Greek Orthodox Church's terms as they attempted to justify their abor-tions and exonerate themselves. Most women did not deny that abortion was a sin (*mia amartia*). Nor did they attempt to mute or challenge the status of personhood that the Church's teachings conferred on the fetus. In informal speech, in fact, women commonly referred to abortion as "*rikhno to pedhi*" or "*vghazo to pedhi*" (literally, to "cast" or "take out" the "child"). Unlike more passive and euphemized constructions such as "to have an abortion," the sense conveyed by these idiomatic Greek usages is one of agency on the part of the woman. Similarly, the use of the word "*pedhi*" confers a personhood to the fe-tus that is consistent with the tenets of the Church but offers no emotional insulation to the woman who aborts. On the surface, the ecclesiastical inter-pretation of the fetus as a person, and thus of abortion as a major sin, appears uncontested. Yet, even as they spoke of "sin" and of the "child" when narrat-ing their experiences, women went on to adapt the multiple meanings packed

into these culturally resonant terms to explain, justify, and ultimately exonerate their abortions. Thus, most women, after affirming the Orthodox theological position that abortion was a "sin," proceeded to draw upon and interweave
the many meanings of the word, which in addition to the religious include
the sense that something is a pity, or an unnecessary waste: "Yes, it's a sin,
mia amartia," women typically acknowledged, but it was also an amartia and,
many added, "a *bigger* amartia" (simultaneously a sin, a pity, and a waste) to
raise a child when you can't fulfill your considerable obligations "to help them
. . . everywhere," to use Maria's words once more.[26]

The majority of women thus explained their abortions through an idiom of
social morality, that is, a morality in which accountability to other humans—
in this case, almost always the unborn "child" conceptualized as a potential
family member—took first place. Moreover, this was a morality that was implicitly, and sometimes explicitly, critical of the ecclesiastical notion of sin.
Thus, Ghitsa, a twenty-seven-year-old medical resident, explained her abortion: "The Orthodox Church forbids it. And I revere it [the Church]. But beyond that, I believe there are other things too. If there are no prospects for
keeping another child, how can you do it?" Nadhia, forty years old and married to a bank manager, offered this explanation for her recent abortion: "It's
wrong to bring a child into the world to go hungry." Was the abortion a sin, I
asked? "It's a sin, *amartia*," she replied, "but it's also a pity, *amartia*, to keep it,
when you can't cope economically. . . . I think God will understand." Had she
had confessed her abortion to a priest? "No," Nadhia replied somewhat scornfully, "this is only between God and myself." In the following quote, Maria,
whom I cited earlier, reveals more elaborately the semantic slipperiness inherent in the way many women used the idiom of amartia:

> Maria: On the one side, it's an amartia [to abort], but on the other,
>   it s also an amartia to raise a child who won't live under good
>   circumstances, when you don't have the [economic] ease to raise them.
>   That's an amartia too.
> EG: In what sense of the word?
> Maria: Look, it's an amartia [emphatically] not to be able to give your
>   child enough to eat. Better to take it out [abort], so that the child
>   won't have to spend every day, not just with one amartia on its back,
>   but many.

Here, Maria, adhering to a social morality in which "sin" is tempered by, and
in her case, inextricably commingled with, "pity," refused to choose between
the two senses of amartia. Maria's and Nadhia's deployment of this multiva-

lent idiom can be interpreted as a strategic move toward self-exoneration that bypasses the formal institutions of the Church. Both imagined themselves vis-à-vis a compassionate and forgiving God, and neither felt she would be punished for her abortions: "I think God will understand."

Also noteworthy in these women's statements is the salience of "hunger" as a justification for abortions. In the relatively prosperous Rhodian context, however, hunger was almost never a serious threat—indeed, obesity has become a national health problem in recent years. As Nadhia, who was after all fairly well-off, clarified: "Well, figuratively speaking, *o loghos to lei*. Of course, it wouldn't go hungry. But it wouldn't have all that my other two children have, the luxuries—*politelies*, one pair of shoes, where my other children had three."[27] Still, the idiom of hunger, whose connotations, as Michael Herzfeld (1985) has pointed out, derive historical and emotional force from the Ottoman occupation and from the hardship and famine of recent wars, continues to circulate widely in Greece today.[28] For the rural Cretan shepherds that were the subject of Herzfeld's study, hunger represented a key rhetorical strategy for dealing with the moral tensions inherent in the animal theft in which they routinely engaged. More to the point, as Herzfeld goes on to explain, their strategic use of hunger as a motivation shifted the blame for animal theft onto the state and its indifferent bureaucracies. Although their circumstances differ greatly, Nadhia and other Rhodian women I interviewed also used the idiom of hunger to negotiate the moral tensions inherent in *their* identities as Orthodox mothers who nonetheless abort. Like rural Cretan men, they implicitly blame the state for its failure to provide for their future children's welfare. In sum, through the rhetoric of hunger, Rhodian women and Cretan shepherds alike "can always represent their own position as one of moral advantage" (Herzfeld 1985, 37–38).

The alternative socially embedded morality articulated by many Rhodian women is akin to what Rosalind Petchesky (1990), speaking of the abortion decisions of women in the United States, has described as the "morality of praxis." Arising from the accumulation of women's lived experiences—including, importantly, the social and practical aspects of their reproductive experiences—it is a morality that gives greater weight to responsibilities to others and that, in the process, justifies and exonerates abortion. Feminist ethicists have also underscored the contextualized, relational considerations that go into U.S. women's deliberations about abortion (Sherwin 1994). Similarly, when Rhodian women speak of aborting "the child," they are not referring to an abstract metaphysical notion of personhood but imagining a potential member of their family to whom considerable obligations accrue. Yet, the logic of their decisions is embedded in, and inflected by, characteristically Greek idioms of moral discourse. In the semantic gray areas that surround the usage of "*amartia*" and "*pedhi*," Rhodian women challenge the position of their Church with what might be called a "reverse discourse of sin" (Foucault 1978 [1990]). That is, they confront and resist the Church's hegemonic position on abortion by adopting the same terms and categories used by the Church to condemn the practice. Thus, most Rhodian women continue to regard abortion as a sin. In doing so, they acknowledge and affirm the continued significance of Greek Orthodoxy to their sense of personal and national identity.[29] At the same time, however, through their appropriation and redefinition of the Church's own categories, they confront and qualify its absolutism: not fulfilling the cascade of obligations associated with contemporary motherhood and consigning "the child" to relative deprivation (to "hunger") is a still greater amartia than abortion: both a "sin" and a "pity." Ultimately, it would appear, the imperatives of late modern motherhood carry greater moral weight than, and trump the tenets of, Church doctrine.

Chapter 7

Global and Local
Bodies of Knowledge

Rhodian women's ethnomedicine and the biomedicine that replaced it in the postwar decades are both best understood as local articulations of global medical traditions. Many of the ethnogynecological and ethno-obstetric principles and practices that I describe in the first chapters of this book will be recognizable to anyone familiar with ethnographic descriptions of fertility control and enhancement and pregnancy and birth in Latin America, South and Southeast Asia, and the Middle East, or with historical reconstructions of midwifery traditions and women's medicine that endured in Europe through the early modern period and, in some places, into the twentieth century. That these similarities have gone largely unnoticed to date is due at least in part to the fact that Greek ethnomedicine has not been studied as a comprehensive body of knowledge but rather as individual beliefs and practices or as essentially isomorphic with religious and ritual healing. In those chapters I hope to have shown that, when systematically reconstructed and carefully examined alongside the body of learned ancient medicine whose principles and practices informed so many health care systems around the globe prior to medicalization, the resonances are as clear as they are compelling.

As I also have argued, however, these resonances should not be read as evidence of an essentially timeless Greek countryside from which the shards of ancient medical traditions can be excavated from the "folk medicine" of contemporary villagers. Instead, my overview of the enduring influence of the medical theories and therapeutic modalities advanced by Galen, Soranus, and a host of others who followed in their footsteps over the longue durée of the Ancient, Byzantine, and Ottoman years suggests a fluid and complex, if still not well-understood, interplay of oral and literate routes of transmission over time. One such thread of transmission, I have proposed, can be found in the lowly genre of vernacular texts that appear to have played a significant role in preserving and broadcasting this body of medical knowledge in the Greek-speaking world. Some of these texts, like the *Geoponicon*, were published in multiple editions and circulated widely over a period of several centuries; others, like the handwritten school notebook composed by the practical healer Nikolaos Theodorakis of the Cretan village of Meronas, were intended for the private use of individual healers and their heirs. Official medicine during the Ottoman centuries also was heavily influenced by Galen and other Greek theorists. Combined with subsequent advances made by renowned physicians of the Islamicate world, this Ottoman version of Greco-Islamic medicine enjoyed privileged status and remained the official medicine of the empire until well into the nineteenth century. Much remains to be learned about the dynamic relationships that surely existed among ethnic Greek populations, their popular medical practitioners, and both official and popular Ottoman medicine before independence. No doubt future historical research on the vernacular iatrosophia genre will uncover creative innovations and local variations on the classical principles. Still, one of the most intriguing findings that emerges from the reconstruction of women's medicine on Rhodes is its remarkable continuity and consistency with the knowledge and practices espoused by Galen, Soranus, and those who were influenced by them and who popularized their work over the course of nearly two millennia and across large regions of the globe.

Beyond its ethnographic interest, Rhodian ethnomedicine also has implications for contemporary debates over the nature of globalization. The corpus of knowledge and practices described in the first chapters of the book supports a view of globalization as a historically deep process in which local bodies become intimately and actively implicated. In rural Rhodes, women's understandings of their bodily functioning and the therapeutic modalities at their disposal to manage their procreative concerns drew their persuasive force from a blend of secular and mechanistic humoral discourse on the one hand, and spiritually charged symbols and practices whose meanings were deeply rooted in the Greek Orthodox Christian tradition on the other. In many instances, the same object or substance (e.g., blood) or practice (e.g., salting the infant, secluding the lekhona) condensed diverse meanings derived from the two distinct traditions with no apparent conceptual dissonance. This blending was literally embodied in the person of the mammi, the village midwife, who was simultaneously a specialist in the knowledge and techniques needed to manage birth and the postpartum and in the informal rituals that initiated the gradual incorporation of the newborn into the human community.

Such blending or hybridization illustrates the creative process of "global localization" or "local globalization" (Nederveen Pierterse 2004) that took place time and again as ancient systems of medical knowledge were disseminated and took hold in many parts of the world. Observing this phenomenon across highly diverse Islamic societies, Good and DelVecchio Good (1992, 257) ponder the question of how principles rooted in classical Greek medical traditions became the paradigms for making sense of and managing illness and distress "from urban North Africa to small tribal societies, in Muslim India and Pakistan, and in many other Asian societies." A similar question might be asked of diverse Christian societies. As a growing number of historical studies of pregnancy and childbirth in early modern England (Cressy 1997; Hobby 1999), France, and Germany (Gelis 1991) demonstrate, there too ancient gynecological and obstetrical principles appear to have coexisted comfortably with both Protestant and Catholic religious traditions. One reason that has been repeatedly proposed to explain this seemingly paradoxical compatibility is that Galeno-Hippocratic anatomical and physiological principles (e.g., the one-sex model that theorized women as imperfect men) provided medical justification for dominant gender ideologies in Europe (Laqueur 1990; Martin 1987), as well as in Islamic societies (Good and DelVecchio Good 1992; Ze'evi 2006). The examples of Rhodian ethnogynecology and ethno-obstetrics suggest another reason as well: in its popular version, this body of knowledge offered women a valued set of meanings and practices *largely under their own control,* at hand when needed to pragmatically address the critical issues of health and illness, fertility and procreation, that inevitably arose over the course of their lives.

For anthropologists, hybridized medical traditions that simultaneously reflect and reconfigure global and local bodies of knowledge are significant for other reasons as well, not the least because of the challenges they pose to conventional understandings of boundaries and, by implication, of cultural difference. The many shared features found across Rhodian, Greco-Islamic, Ottoman, and early modern European medicine illustrate the point that Greek villages like Ermia and others I visited on Rhodes are best conceived as belonging to a "contingent countryside" (S. Sutton 2000) shaped and reshaped time and again by their interconnections with influential others. These hybridized medical traditions thus inevitably problematize any attempt to study local ethnomedicine without careful consideration of broader historical and transcultural flows of knowledge, people, texts, and practices. Finally, and in a related point, they also speak to recent critiques that have been leveled at ethnographic representations of rural life in Greece, as well as in the Mediterranean more generally (Argyrou 1996; Bakalaki 1994; Goddard, Llobera, and Shore 1994). The thrust of these critiques is that anthropology's obsession with finding difference, specificity, and otherness at the margins of Europe has served to obscure commmonalities that also exist across diverse societies and as a consequence has helped perpetuate the exoticization of the Mediterranean, and the reification of the West as its opposite. When ethnographers pay careful attention to cultural resonances as well as to difference, as Bakalaki (1994) and Argyrou (1996) do, for instance, in their research on dominant gender constructs in rural Greece and Cyprus, such ultimately ahistorical dichotomies become increasingly untenable.

In the second half of the book, I describe some of the ways in which the presumably global biomedical specialty of obstetrics and gynecology achieved hegemonic status in the postwar period at the same time it acquired its own distinctive signature. The example of Rhodes offers several insights into the process of medicalization that in recent decades has reconfigured the experience of reproduction in many parts of the world. In particular, it demonstrates that despite a more or less common package of discursive and technoscientific features that tend to travel together, medicalization is not a simple one-directional process or a juggernaut of inevitable uniformity and standardization. On the whole, Rhodian women and their doctors shared in the widespread modernist narrative that promotes medicalization by optimistically linking biomedical interventions and technologies to notions of progress, improvement in the standard of living, and increased control over the quality of life, including perhaps most importantly the quality of new life. But even as the medicalization of reproduction on Rhodes shares features with the process as it has unfolded elsewhere, it has evolved its own particular signature that bears the imprint of local configurations of power and the contingencies of Greek culture and history.

A notable feature of the medicalization process in Greece in the postwar period is its unevenness: the intensive medicalization of pregnancy and birth contrasted with the wholesale evasion of medicalized contraception. The factors responsible for this bifurcated pattern, as I have attempted to show in these later chapters, are complex and contingent on the intersecting influences of a variety of powerful institutions and discourses. Their effects have at times collided, and at others colluded, in shaping the ways women came to understand and respond to the new reproductive technologies that began to circulate in the postwar period. By the late twentieth century, the generally optimistic narrative of biomedical progress had been joined, and sometimes qualified by, other more anxious discourses of late modernity. A heightened awareness of a multitude of risks, fed by a stream of mass-mediated reports, intensified an older sense of responsibility on the part of women for the health of their children and family members. Increasingly, new meanings and discourses obligated a woman not only to seek expert advice to manage the growing array of risks associated with reproduction, but also to become a responsible "expert of herself" by means of self-education. These diverse discourses intersected one another in ways that were usually mutually reinforcing, as in the case of pre-natal care and childbirth, where technical interventions of all sorts were desired and demanded by women and their families to minimize risks and maximize the health and well-being of both mother and infant. In other contexts, however, these diverse discourses competed or clashed, as in the case of medical contraception. Despite their promise for rationalizing sex and increasing a woman's control over her fertility, medical technologies of contraception collided with the late modern discourse of risk and the expectation that a woman be responsibly informed and "biologically prudent" (Rose 2007) in the face of untold contemporary manufactured risks to her health and future fertility.

Rhodian women's enthusiastic embrace of and demand for some reproductive technologies and their simultaneous rejection of others thus represent neither a logical inconsistency nor an example of a postmodern consumerist mélange selected from the global supermarket of biomedical technologies. Instead, their distinctive pattern of responses to different technologies reflects the fragmentation of discourses that is another hallmark of the late modern experience. One consequence of this fragmentation, as Margaret Lock (1993b, xxi) has asserted in her study of menopause and aging, "has been the generation of knowledge within ever increasingly differentiated disciplines and sub-disciplines, so that there exist today, for example, several powerful competing discourses about the aging body, most of which regard their methods as scientific." This observation applies equally well to the domain of reproduction where contradictory discourses have helped foster a "dilemmatic disposition" toward contemporary biomedicine and its technologies.

Finally, it is important to point out that even when certain aspects of the medicalization of reproduction on Rhodes appear to closely resemble those found elsewhere, detailed ethnographic accounts often reveal an underlying diversity in women's responses. Cross-cultural comparison helps bring to light the variety of factors that may be masked behind common rates and figures and thus provides a more nuanced understanding of the processes that have helped shape these resemblances. What the World Health Organization has called the "global epidemic of medically unnecessary caesarean sections" is a case in point. Ethnographic studies of the comparably high caesarean rates in Taiwan and Brazil and for privileged women in Calcutta, for example, reveal important commonalities with Rhodes. Like Rhodian women, for instance, many Brazilian and Indian women have come to regard caesareans as desirable not only as a way to avoid pain but also, and as importantly, as a safer way to give birth (De Mello e Souza 1994; Donner 2004). But there are significant differences across each location as well. In Brazil, officials have responded to the high caesarean rate with national campaigns to demedicalize birth. As Dominque Behague (2002) has shown, these efforts have been met with distrust by poor women, however, who see them as yet another strategy for excluding them from the high-quality medical care usually reserved for the rich. Women with the social resources or political patronage to negotiate the medical system engage in a determined struggle to gain access to the highly technological regimes of maternity care, and in particular to birth by caesarean section. In doing so, they demonstrate their power to redress inequalities within the larger politics of Brazil's stratified system of reproductive health care (high-quality care featuring very high caesarean rates for wealthier women, vaginal births for the poor).

In the case of Calcutta, women's view of and demand for caesareans also is shaped by the local circumstances of their lives. In this patrilocal context, where women move into the house of their in-laws when they marry, caesareans have accrued value for the leverage they give young women in negotiating with affines over their domestic duties and responsibilities in the postpartum period. Before antenatal care and childbirth became medicalized in the 1960s, married women typically traveled to their natal homes to give birth; afterward, they stayed on to be taken care of by their mothers until the conclusion of their confinement. With medicalization, and the continuity of prenatal care it demanded, this customary right no longer applied. As a consequence, young women have come to appreciate birth by caesarean as a way to negotiate a more substantial period of rest and recovery from their mothers-in-law than they would have been given if they had delivered vaginally. Being able to use the cultural authority of modern medicine to achieve this goal was described as an empowering experience for these middle-class women. In contrast, poor, low-caste women who relied on their manual labor to survive preferred to avoid caesareans precisely because they disrupted their ability to keep working and thus imperiled their livelihood (Donner 2004). In the case of Taiwan, in contrast, demand for caesareans tends to be stronger among less-educated women. There, enhanced concerns for the quality of children have led to a marked tendency to schedule caesareans for the most auspicious day and hour as determined beforehand by the Pe-Ji or "Eight Characters of Nature" (Hsu, Liao, and Hwang 2008; Lo 2003). Without the benefit of such cross-cultural comparisons, the profoundly diverse factors that shape women's responses to caesareans in these different contexts would be masked behind their uniformly high rates.

When added to studies of the medicalization of reproduction such as these, the example of Rhodes expands our sense of the possible, and sometimes even the unexpected, ways in which global processes have come to be played out in particular contexts. As I hope to have shown in this book, within the constraints of powerful institutions and discourses and anchored in the specificities of their life circumstances, women actively evaluate and selectively respond to the range of reproductive technologies on offer. In the end, one of the most important contributions that the anthropology of reproduction can make to our understanding of the process of medicalization is through the empirical, theoretical, and practical challenges that its detailed accounts pose to abstract generalizations about the local effects of global phenomena.

Notes

Chapter 1

1. Two major incidents occurred over the course of my fieldwork that raised general alarm. First, the threat of mad cow disease spreading from Northern Europe raised troubling questions about the safety of the food supply. The second incident involved a scandal in which it was revealed that a Belgian company had been pumping animal feed contaminated with dioxins throughout the EU food chain. Many Rhodians I knew promptly dumped the contents of their cupboards and refrigerators; shopkeepers, hoping to reassure their customers, posted signs declaring the local origins of their foodstuffs; and mothers, trying to protect their children, snapped up the limited supply of (presumably) grass-fed Rhodian dairy products as soon as they appeared in the shops.

2. "Ermia" is a pseudonym, as are the names of all the people I interviewed for this book.

3. However intensified today, as Susan Sutton's extensive research has shown, such traffic is far from a recent phenomenon. See especially S. Sutton 1999, 2000.

4. Recent anthropological research has also addressed such diverse medical health-related topics as organ donation (Papagaroufali 1999, 2002), psychiatry (Blue 1993), and the evil-eye complex (Veikou 1998).

Chapter 2

1. As is the custom on Rhodes and elsewhere in Greece, I refer to women and men senior to me by the titles "Kiria" and "Kirios."

2. Hostility and conflict often characterize relations between the Greek archeological service and the inhabitants of sites that have been judged to be "historic." For a detailed case study, see Herzfeld 1991.

3. Tourists from the United States and Canada do not figure into this local taxonomy, either because they are greatly outnumbered by other tourists or because, at least in the case of Americans, the majority come on cruise ships and stay for only a day or less.

4. The true figure was probably much higher, because Rhodians, like Greeks generally,

tend to underreport personal income, a practice made possible by the robust parallel economy in which many people participate (see Koliopoulos and Veremis 2002, 177).

5. Perhaps the best-known film representation of such fantasies is *Shirley Valentine*, whose protagonist has since become a familiar feature of British popular culture (Ware 1997). After a single day on the island of Mykonos, which she describes as "the far side of paradise," Shirley claims to "hardly recognize" herself. This transformation has little to do with her fling with a local *kamaki*, she assures a disapproving friend: "The only holiday romance I've had is with myself." Lawrence Durrell uses almost identical language when he describes a sojourn on Corfu as ending with the "discovery of yourself" (cited in Roessel 2002, 272).

6. Cross-cultural marriage between foreign women and Greek men, largely ignored by anthropologists to date (but see Smith 2002), has been the subject of fictional and autobiographical accounts; see, e.g. Beverly Farmer's (1995) memoir, *The House in the Light*.

7. This objective is drilled into children from a young age. For an art exhibit in which students of the English Association's language classes were asked to illustrate their sense of identity, a student named Elena, age twelve, composed the following caption to her drawing of overlapping Irish and Greek flags: "I'm pleased to know that when I grow up I'll be able to attend university in either Ireland or Greece. There will be a great choice for my future education."

8. In an other example of the robot metaphor, Shirley Valentine, that familiar figure of British popular culture who epitomizes the subversive potential of a Greek holiday, refers to herself as "strutting around like R2 bleeding D2" in her daily round of household chores in London (cited in Placas 2001, 8).

9. At the same time, some forty-five thousand Greek immigrants in the United States returned to join the Greek army and fight in the Balkan Wars (Moskos 1989, cited in Jusdanis 2001, 170), an indication that dense social networks and return flows do not characterize only today's transnational migrants.

10. A recent study found that a quarter of all people randomly surveyed on Rhodes owned a second house (Dhimos Rodhion 2002.) Given that many non-native-born inhabitants were included in this survey, the proportion of native Rhodians who own a second house is probably higher still.

11. These opposed images of country and city are much in evidence in Eugenia Fakinou's 1991 novel, *Astradeni*, which tells the story of a young girl who migrates with her family to Athens from the Dodecanese island of Symi, located just a few kilometers from Rhodes. Narrated in the first person, the novel represents Symi through the eyes of Astradeni, and thus inextricably links the island with the idea of childhood innocence, a time "of delighted absorption in our own world, from which, eventually, in the course of growing up, we are distanced and separated, so that it and the world become things we observe" (R. Williams 1973, 297). In the novel, Athens is that world apart that Astradeni observes with distance and detachment. Fakinou portrays Athens as the dark foil of Symi— a place of confinement, as the family is forced to live in a dim and dank basement apartment; of disenchantment, where classmates, to Astradeni's shock, do not believe in God, whom she persists in addressing with the intimacy and affection made possible by the Greek diminutive as *"theoulli"* (my little/ dear God); and ultimately, of sexual assault and debasement.

12. A totally revised version of *I Ghlossa Mou* has recently replaced this earlier edition.

13. The demographer Haris Symeonidou (2002, 18) has referred to the widespread cultural expectation that mothers and grandmothers provide extensive household help to their grown children as "compulsory altruism."

Chapter 3

1. The Greek Orthodox Cathedral of St. Nicholas in Tarpon Springs, Florida, where I was baptized and went to church every Sunday through my adolescence, had only one common entrance. I remember, though, going to church when I had my period and attempting to conceal this fact, as my grandmother had carefully instructed me, by pretending to kiss the icons. Following her directions, I would feint a jab with my puckered lips that respectfully stopped just short of the icon's protective glass case, furtively hoping all the while that my performance was convincing enough that no bystanders would be able to guess my state.
2. Similar premedicalized terms occurred elsewhere Europe as well. In French and Spanish, for example, règles and regla, derived from the Latin regola, meaning "rule" or "order," were used to refer to menstruation.
3. In this chapter and the following, I use the term "procreation" rather than "reproduction." The latter, obviously rooted in the metaphor of production, connotes a "natural" process. The former, just as transparently derived from "creation," connotes a theological or ontological process. The term "reproduction" began to circulate in scientific and medical discourse in the nineteenth century and reflects the naturalistic worldview of medical science (see Duden 1991, 22; Martin 1987; Yanagisako and Delaney 1995, 9). "Procreation" is thus more apt for the premedicalized bodies of knowledge and practice that I describe in these chapters, even though the term tends to slight the fundamentally secular and mechanical principles that underpin the humoral model.
4. Technically, rural Greece was best characterized by what Ong calls "residual orality." See Tziovas 1989.
5. Echoes of this network of symbolic associations reverberate in early twentieth-century medicine. In Freud's interpretation of dreams, the rooms of a house represented "symbols of the genital orifice" to be opened by keys that are "decidedly male symbol[s]" (Freud 1963, quoted in Benthien 2002, 26).
6. See Dimitriou-Kotsoni (1993, 69) for other Aegean variants of this saying.
7. That the preference for boys continues to be strong was jokingly played with in an expression I heard from many younger Rhodians: "The gender of the baby doesn't matter, as long as it's healthy, and [pause for effect]—pees standing up."
8. "God forgive her" (Theos sinkhores' tin) is a formulaic expression used when speaking of the dead and does not imply any wrongdoing on the part of Kiria Rena's mother.
9. Representations of motherhood in rural Greece are largely based on fieldwork conducted in the 1960s and 1970s, and thus describe what I call in this book the "transitional generation." By this time, the agrarian sector was experiencing important (although unevenly distributed) transformations. For instance, in her classic comparison of rural and urban ideologies of motherhood in Greece, Mariella Doumanis (1983) notes in passing the tractors that lumbered through the village she studied. Salamone and Stanton (1986) produced their classic study of the *nikokira*

and women's roles on the island of Amouliani where agriculture was negligible and the tourist boom and fishing industry were offering a measure of prosperity; notably, they remark on the "relative leisure of Amouliani's women compared to their counterparts who lived in farming communities or worked in factory jobs" (1986, 112). Kenna (1992, 155) is one of the few to note women's embodied experience of the "unremitting and draining hard work" and the constant aches and pains associated with village life on the island she studied in the 1960s.

10. In the past, Rhodes was so heavily infested with snakes that it was nicknamed Rodhos Fidhousa (Snake-filled Rhodes).

11. All snakes are said to be strongly attracted to milk. Even in Rhodes Town before the war, milk was routinely put out for the (nonpoisonous) "house snake" (*fidhi tou spitiou*) that kept down the population of rats and mice. My own grandmother often commented when I was a child that I drank milk, of which I was very fond, "like a snake, *san to fidhi*."

12. This well-known practice was another salient symbol of Karpathian "backwardness" for many Rhodians.

13. Susan Buck Sutton (1999, 76), for example, cites evidence that, nationally, two-thirds of migrant remittances go to housing.

14. The influence of Soranus of Ephesus is also apparent in Paul's compendium, but it is Galen who ultimately dominates the gynecological portions of the text (Green 1985, 79ff).

15. Identical language can also be found in Jane Sharp's 1671 midwifery treatise to describe conception: "man . . . is the agent and tiller and sower of the ground, woman is the patient or ground to be tilled" (Hobby 1999, 32).

16. Compare this with the following advice from *Aristotle's Master-Piece*, the phenomenally successful English sex guide that was reprinted dozens of times in the eighteenth and nineteenth centuries: "It is also highly necessary, that in their mutual embraces, they [husband and wife] meet each other with equal ardor; for if the spirit flag on either part, they will fall short of what nature requires, and the woman must either miss of conception or else the children will prove weak in their bodies, or defective in their understanding. I do advise them, before they begin their conjugal embraces, to invigorate their mutual desires, and make their flames burn with a fierce ardor" (cited in Porter and Hall 1995, 44). In the same guide, the one-sex model also informs the following limerick:

    For those that have the strictest searchers been
    Find women are but men turn'd outside in . . .

    And that, tho' they of different sexes be,
    Yet in whole they are the same as we. (ibid., 52)

    The English midwife Jane Sharp, writing in 1671, also taught that conception occurred only when both partners experienced orgasm (Hobby 1999, xx; see also Eccles 1982, 35–36, for Tudor and Stuart England).

17. But see Chapter 4, where I discuss a possible underlying association between milk and blood in the context of practices aimed at increasing a nursing mother's milk production.

18. Note the parallel with women's use of the clean/dirty binary. From the Greek Orthodox perspective, sexual intercourse, like menstruation, is a ritually unclean act. In order to receive Holy Communion, for example, men and women alike must have abstained from sexual relations beforehand. However, in this exchange, both Kirios Sterghos and Kiria Paraskevi hold that intercourse, through ejaculation, cleanses a man, just as menstruation from a humoral perspective cleanses a woman.

19. This belief was found widely across Europe into the modern period. For example, in their history of sexual knowledge in Britain between 1650 and 1950, Porter and Hall observe: "Enlightenment hydraulic physiology could see regular genital discharges as cleansing, requisite for health" (1995, 20).

20. In her study of rural Crete, Marlene Arnold (1985) found that a similar list of *mirodhika* herbs (as well as plantain and nettles) was used to bring down the menses.

21. Carole Browner's germinal work (especially Browner 1980, 1985) on the ethnomedical understandings that inform Colombian women's management of early pregnancy allowed me to recognize at an early stage of my own fieldwork the very similar system found on Rhodes.

22. Arnold (1985) reports the emmenagogic use of onion skins for rural Crete also.

23. Rue was also used as an abortifacient and emmenogogue in rural Crete, where it was called *apigano* (Arnold 1985).

24. For a review of the pharmacological effects of many of the emmenagogues and abortifacients mentioned in this chapter, see Browner and Ortiz de Montellano 1986; Etkin 1988; Jochle 1974; Riddle 1997; Siedlecky 2001; and Van de Walle and Renne 2001.

25. Papachristodoulou (1996), in his study of Rhodian place names, alternatively derives the name from *tsambiki*, a kind of ship whose characteristic shape roughly evokes the outline of the hill where the icon was found. This etymology was not shared by the women I interviewed.

26. See Dubisch 1995a (230–40) and Hirschon 1989 (152) for detailed discussions of the differences between Orthodox and Catholic understandings and representations of the Madonna.

27. Marcia Inhorn (1994, 228) makes this point in her study of Egyptian women's visits to shrines specializing in infertility. Like Rhodian supplicants to the Panaghia Tsambika, these women explained their practices in religious terms, "although the nature of the healing rituals taking place within [the shrines] would be described as quite profane by orthodox Muslims."

Chapter 4

1. Reminiscing about his childhood on the island of Ikaros, the novelist Theologhos Malachias described the position of the mammi who lived in his village: "She was the first to be invited to weddings. . . . Besides, there wasn't a bride or groom in our village whose navel had not been cut by the mammi. And of course, without fail she would be present for the baptism [of their child], whose navel the mammi Arghiri would also have cut" (quoted in Rigatos 1992, 32, my translation). Pregnancy, birth, and the postpartum period have received scant attention in the ethnography of rural Greece. Campbell's (1964, 154) description of the postpartum period among the Sarakatsani is a notable, if all too brief, exception. Chryssanthopoulou's (1984) comprehensive analysis of folkloric materials is an invaluable guide to beliefs and

practices elsewhere in Greece. Her study, along with Arnold's (1985) for rural Crete, reveals that while Rhodian practices differ in some details, the similarities with other regions are far more numerous.

2. Among the Sephardic Jews of Rhodes, the foul odor of rue performed the same function (Lévy and Lévy Zumwalt 2002, 98–99).

3. The un-Christian apotropaic number five may derive from the protective power of the Muslim *hamsa* or hand (Lévy and Lévy Zumwalt 2002, 96).

4. I have borrowed the term "ethos of care" from Anne Becker (1995) who coined it to gloss the norm of communal concern for the physical well-being for others in Fiji, as expressed primarily through nurturing and food exchange.

5. The Hippocratic author who described this technique further specified that the birthing woman be held by the arms and legs by four female assistants and given at least ten firm shakes; sometimes, she would also be shaken by the shoulders (Blundell 1995, 111). Jacques Gelis has written one of the few detailed histories of childbirth in early modern Europe. His work reveals a plethora of similarities between ethno-obstetrical practices in Rhodes and those found elsewhere in Europe before medicalization. In the French regions of Saintonge and Poitou, for example, a woman whose labor was progressing too slowly would be treated by a "sack man" who was summoned to shake her just as he would a sack of grain he was filling (1991, 144).

6. Soranus himself cites the earlier work of Demetrius the Herophilean, now lost, when describing the practice of internal podalic version (Temkin 1991, xliii). Early modern European midwifery manuals also drew heavily on Galen, Hippocrates, and Avicenna, but Soranus's text was especially influential. These manuals comprised a conventional genre of publication with similar format, organization, and content that remained relatively unchanged over several centuries (McTavish 2005, 25). Like some of the Greek iatrosophia texts of the same period, they tended to be small, portable books written in the vernacular.

7. The mammi's technique for promoting dilation that Kiria Sterghoula and Kiria Maria describe closely matches that also advocated by Soranus for the same purpose: "And with a circular movement of her finger [which has been anointed with olive oil] the midwife should dilate the orifice of the uterus [and] the labia" (Temkin 1991, 75).

8. In a particularly striking parallel to Rhodian ethno-obstetrical practices, midwives in France used the flower known as the Rose of Jericho to sympathetically promote the "opening" of a laboring woman's womb (Gelis 1991, 117). Although a different plant (*Anastatica hierochuntica*) from the germander Rhodians called the Panaghia's flower, like the latter, the Rose of Jericho was said to have been brought back by pilgrims to the Holy Land. Exactly like the Panaghia's flower, the Rose of Jericho was placed in a glass of water and given to the birthing woman to hold. The Seigneur de Bussy of Picardy, who was present during his wife's confinement in 1713, recorded his observation that "this rose, though very dried up, immediately opens out and blossoms into the same shape as the woman's nature" (quoted in ibid., 145).

9. In rural Crete, the birthing woman sat astride two chairs or stools placed next to each other, and the baby dropped in the space between them, to be caught by the midwife, who sat on a stool in front of her (Arnold 1985, 149).

10. My friend Melina, who introduced me to Kiria Maria (her aunt) and who was with us throughout the interview, was visibly taken aback when she heard that husbands

were formerly present at births if their wives wanted them there. She even asked her own follow-up questions on this point, to confirm what she'd heard. Today, having one's husband present in the delivery room is coded as a distinctively "modern" practice (see Chapters 5 and 6).

11. Recent demographic studies of midwifery in early modern England have begun to revise earlier historical scholarship that routinely portrayed midwives as ignorant, illiterate, and often lethal to their clients. Pollack (1990), for example, found that some 80–85 percent of infants in the seventeenth century did survive for at least a few years and that a woman's cumulative risk of dying in childbirth was less than 10 percent. In his groundbreaking historical study of maternal mortality in Elizabethan England, Roger Schofield (1986) calculates a maternal death rate of 9.3 deaths per 1,000, or a little under 1 percent. Maternal deaths in childbirth were always higher in urban than in rural areas, reaching about 24 per 1,000 in London in the 1590s.

12. In Inner Mani, the placenta was inspected to predict the gender of the next child (Seremetakis 1991, 70).

13. Elsewhere in Greece, the stump was burned with a candle (Chryssanthopoulou 1984, 48).

14. Rigatos (1992, 33) writes that it could take place on the third day or "when the cord fell off."

15. These meanings and practices do not appear to have been confined to Greece. In rural France into the nineteenth century, salt had connotations and ritual uses almost identical to those found in Greece. In Limousin and Perigord, for instance, the newborn was rubbed with salt. In Provence, a packet of salt was placed on the child or wrapped in its swaddling cloths to protect against the evil eye (Gelis 1991, 195). When Provençal villagers visited the newborn, they always brought gifts of small coins and salt so the child would grow to be "wise as salt" (190). And salt was widely used in rituals of exorcism elsewhere in Europe as well (195).

16. Elsewhere in Greece, the word *pentaria* is said to refer to the five times the cloth is wound around the infant's body (Chryssanthopoulou 1984, 66). Soranus specified that the swaddling cloth be "three as well as four fingers in width" (Temkin 1991, 85).

17. Some women told me that in the past, newborns were born with their eyes closed and didn't open them for forty days. Nowadays, they observed, children are much more active and alert from the moment they are born. Commenting on this difference and attributing it to the infant care practices enumerated here (in particular to swaddling), one woman in her sixties remarked to me, "*Kale, ta sklavoname ta pedhia tote!* Goodness, we tormented our children back then!"

18. This is undoubtedly the source of the word *loğusa* that is also used in Turkey to refer to a woman during the forty-day postpartum period (see Delaney 1991, 68ff.).

19. Delaney (1991, 68) reports a similar saying for rural Turkey: "The tomb of the loğusa is open for forty days."

20. On the neighboring island of Halki, the dried cord was bound to a cross-shaped biscuit and hung from the baby's cradle. Later on, it was cut into portions and sewn into little phylactery bundles, called *haimali*, which were worn around the neck by all the family's children as protection against the evil eye and other harm. Elsewhere in Greece, the dried cord was kept on the *iconostasi*, the little shelf that held the family's icons and other holy objects (Hondrou 1984, 10; see also Chryssanthopoulou 1984, 49).

21. This brew, which is reported for many other regions of Greece as well, was also locally known as the *zoumi* (juice or broth) or the *tsai* (tea) *tis lekhonas*, and the *thermomelo*, "warm honey" drink. In France and England, infusions similar to the lekhona's tea, made of cinnamon, nutmeg, and other aromatic and aperient, or opening, ingredients, were prepared to promote the flow of the lochia and speed up the cleansing of "bad blood" (Gelis 1991, 178; Hobby 1999, 163).

22. French women were also given a ritual postpartum meal of broth made from a rooster (a capon, to be precise), often selected months in advance for the occasion (Gelis 1991, 180).

23. Among the minor rituals, for example, the first Saturday after the birth was the day set aside for baking special biscuits, *koulouria*, for the baby. Shaped like a cross, this special *koulouri* was tucked in the baby's cradle. In some Rhodian villages, another cruciform *koulouri* was hung from the archway that divided the house into its two sections. After the child had grown a bit, the *koulouri* was fed to a black dog to remove and destroy any evil that might have been drawn to the child.

24. In patrilineal Inner Mani, boy infants are placed in a flour sifter and only girls are placed in a trough. According to Seremetakis (1991, 71), the trough symbolizes the grave and the coffin, and she interprets the practice of placing girls in the trough as "symbolic infanticide" of the less desirable female infant. In matrifocal Rhodes, both infants were placed in a trough. Infants of both sexes were showered with similar life-enhancing symbols and invocations, although the objects placed beside them in the trough were differentiated by the gendered roles they would assume or aspire to in the future.

25. The blessings invoked during the seven days ritual were fairly formulaic, as in this couplet from the neighboring island of Halki (Skandhalidhi 1965, 178, my translation):

> [Come Fates of fate, and bring the child its share
> Of gold and silver and silks!]

> Elate, Moires ton moiron, na moirasete to pei
> Khrousa ke arghira ke malematenia!

26. The Fates have been represented as occupying an ambiguous conceptual territory between good and evil, the saints and the xotika. Because God ultimately determines all aspects of human affairs, the Fates could be seen as messengers from God (Stewart 1991, 160–61). At the same time, the Moires decided the infant's fate on the spot, and might be capriciously swayed to generosity or cruelty by seemingly minor events (Krikos-Davis 1982, 117). Parents therefore tried to placate them with offerings of honey and other tasty tidbits and, to avoid irritating them, removing from their path any obstacle that might make them trip or stumble. Though the Fates never disclosed their allotments, parents often attempted to divine their will (Campbell 1964, 330). But ultimately, once the child's fate was written by the Fates, it could not be undone. "Ineluctible fate is woven around men by chthonic powers, a fate which, good or bad, is 'written and cannot be unwritten'" (du Boulay 1974, 51–52, 82; see also Campbell 1964, 329).

Chapter 5

1. David Sutton (1998b, 135) also observed of the nearby island of Kalymnos that "the latest child care innovations of T. Berry Brazelton or Penelope Leach are disseminated on Kalymnos no later than they are in Chicago."

2. For a discussion of the meanings of "Europe" in the 1980s in Spain, see Douglass 1992. By the 1990s, a consensus had emerged in which "Spain" confidently encompassed "Europe."

3. This anecdote vividly exemplifies Christina Vlahoutsikou's (1997, 291) astute observation that for this generation, the "defining constituent" of a woman'sidentity as wife and mother is "full correspondence between what she wants for herself and what she wants for her household."

4. This kind of reaction was not confined to ethnomedical beliefs. Another summer, I attended a celebration of St. John's Eve sponsored by the local branch of the Likeon Ellinidhon, the Greek Women's Lyceum, a national women's social organization founded in 1911. Comprised in large part of the town's elite women, the Likeon is devoted to the revival and preservation of Greek folk culture (Bakalaki 1994, 88–89). The program that night included a reenactment of the ritual once performed on St. John's Eve by young women to predict whom they would marry. The narrator, a soignée woman in a dark blue suit who appeared to be in her forties, explained to the audience that in the past, maidens dropped articles of their jewelry into a jar of water, covered the jar with a red cloth, and silently retrieved them the next day in order to divine the name of their future husband. As she described this ritual, many people in the audience, which was composed mainly of mothers and other relatives of the young people performing that night, began to laugh. Taken aback, the narrator looked up from her notes, paused for a moment, and then ad libbed to the audience, "Yes, yes, our society has come a long way since then."

5. Similar pedagogical goals informed women's education at this time in the United States and elsewhere in Europe (Apple 1987; Cole 2000). Bakalaki (1994) provides a detailed analysis of the influence of "European" examples on the prescriptive literature advocating both for and against women's education among nineteenth-century Greek intellectuals.

6. Strictly speaking, the Church does not condone belief in the evil eye and in particular disapproves the spells used to remove it. However, as many Rhodians pointed out to me as support for their continued belief in the practice, the Church "believes in the [evil] eye" (as Veikou [1998] also found among young people in Northern Greece). That is, in fact, the case: despite its official disapproval of popular practices, the Church has devised its own special prayers and rituals for removing the ill effects of the evil eye. More to the point, the logic of these rituals is consistent with popular understandings and practices, so their adoption appears to serve "mainly to safeguard ecclesiastical authority" (Stewart 1991, 235). It is not accidental, then, that while belief in the xotika and in spells of all kinds have practically disappeared, "spells for the evil eye are perhaps the only truly current and widespread form of spell" still practiced (232).

7. On its part, *What to Expect* has undoubtedly become the best-selling and most widely used guide in North America and possibly the world. More than ten million copies have been sold since it was first published in 1984, and it has been translated into more than twenty languages, including, as of 1998, Greek (Oaks 2001, 28).

8. I have translated all quotations from *Birth in Love* from Greek to English myself.

9. See Paxson 2004 for a lucid analysis of the deployment of these key terms in the discourse of Greek family-planning experts.

10. In the early 1990s, Bakalaki (1994, 102) wrote that "in Greece, knowledge about 'Europe' is certainly a source of prestige, especially for men, who like to flaunt their experiences abroad or their awareness of foreign politics." The rhetoric employed in *Birth Is Love* suggests that today women increasingly share this disposition.

11. As Seremetakis (1994, 5) has put it: "Sensory semantics in Greek culture, among others, contain regional epistemologies, in-built theories."

12. See Panopoulos (2003) for a description of the significance of sound and hearing to cultural constructions of the social order on the island of Naxos.

13. I also heard pediatricians at the hospital advise women during postnatal checkups to stay indoors in order to avoid exposing themselves and their infants to microbes.

14. In his compilation of Dodecanese ethnomedical knowledge and practices surrounding birth, the Rhodian teacher Kiriakou Hondrou (1984, 1) concludes his preface with the literally bold contrast between then (*tote*) and now (*tora*):

   > Tote: infants were born using practical means, and with uncertainty as to whether they would survive . . . because many died along with their mothers.

   > Tora: they are born in clinics, private or public, under medical supervision and it is certain that if a child is born, it will live.

15. In 2006, child mortality, that is, deaths among children aged one to five years, was 5 per 1,000 in Greece, but 8 per 1,000 in the United States (for U.S. data, *www.childinfo.org/eddb/mat_mortal/database.htm*; for Greek data, *www.who.int*). For that year, too, average life expectancy at birth was 78.7 years in Greece, 77.4 years in the United States (*www.census.gov/cgi-bin/ipc/idbagg*).

16. Dr. F., who had practiced obstetrics for many years in a large U.S. city before returning to Greece, observed that in his experience, Greek women tended to have fewer problems with pregnancy and birth than his American patients. He attributed their advantage primarily to nonmedical factors. Most importantly, in his opinion, pregnancy among young teenagers and unmarried women was almost nonexistent in Rhodes and very rare throughout Greece (abortion being the usual route taken when these women found themselves pregnant). Intriguingly, Dr. F. also observed that Greek women had a much lower incidence of pre-eclampsia than the women he had cared for in the United States. Overall, he felt that his Greek patients had better levels of health and nutrition.

17. U.S. data from *www.childinfo.org/eddb/mat_mortal/database.htm*; Greek data from *www.who.org*.

18. See Davis-Floyd 2003 (xi) for a comprehensive list of resources that track the voluminous evidence that "standard obstetrical procedures do more harm than good."

19. Aleka Sikaki-Douka, the author of *Birth Is Love*, estimated that in 2002 some forty to fifty home births occurred throughout Greece, most of them in Athens (personal communication).

20. The caesarean section is major abdominal surgery. For the woman, its risks include damage to the uterine blood vessels and to the urinary bladder, infected wounds, anesthesia accidents, and accidentally extended uterine incisions. Risks to babies include depressed Apgar scores, a higher chance of respiratory distress, shortened

length of gestation, and, in a mother's subsequent pregnancies, higher perinatal mortality (J. Miller 1988).

21. While doing research for this book in Athens, I spent a considerable amount of time in the waiting rooms of the prenatal care departments of a large public hospital. On most days, ethnic Greek women waiting for their level II ultrasounds were outnumbered by Roma women in colorful skirts, Albanians, and other immigrants. Still, by 2000 a pattern of stratified reproduction (Ginsburg and Rapp 1995) appears to have emerged in which immigrant women, and Roma in particular, were not undergoing the same panoply of interventions as ethnic Greek women (Mossialos et al. 2005).

22. A recent comparative study of maternity care in nine European countries confirms the continued validity of these trends (Alran et al. 2002).

23. By comparison, during this same period, rates of caesareans in Australia, Denmark, and Finland declined (Stephenson et al. 1993, 49).

24. The decoupling of anesthesia from what is otherwise a fairly standard global package of obstetrical interventions appears to be characteristic of many areas in which birth has recently been medicalized (De Mello e Souza 1994; Donner 2004; Van Hollen 2003).

25. At the time of my hospital study, all of the obstetricians were men.

26. In her fascinating ethnography of medicalized birth in South India, Van Hollen (2003) found that among the reasons poor women valued and expected to be given oxytocin to augment labor was the cultural association between women's valor and power and their ability to withstand pain.

27. The term is from Braidotti 1994; see Reiser 1978 and Bynum and Porter 1993 for historical treatments of the ascendant role of vision in medicine; for ultrasound in particular, see Yoxen 1987.

28. Reflecting this hierarchy of value, Seremetakis (1991, 87) reports that in Inner Mani the death of a young man elicited the most public lamentations, the death of "the deformed or an infant," the most private.

29. The military junta that ruled Greece between 1968 and 1974 passed a law that made premarital screening for the hereditary blood disorders and some other diseases mandatory. This highly unpopular law was widely resisted for its effect on the marriage prospects of those who were discovered to be carriers. The law was rescinded in 1980 (Velogiannis-Moutsopoulos and Bartsocas 1989, 224).

30. Depleted uranium, so-called because it is depleted of its contents of the isotope U-238, is 40 percent less radioactive than regular uranium, but it is still highly dangerous and must be handled with the full high-level radiation precautions (Parsons 2001, 23). All kinds of anomalies that summer were being attributed to radioactive fallout. One rainy day in July, for example, a Rhodian taxi driver commented that even the weather patterns had changed (rain is almost unheard of in the summer) because of the "plutonium the Americans are dropping in Kosovo."

31. The images produced by the scanner in use when I did my hospital study were of fairly poor resolution, and their lack of clarity may have affected the number of anomalies detected. The new hospital policy of requiring level II scans in the fifth month of pregnancy has probably increased the rate of detection. Evangelia's experience reveals some of the unintended negative consequences of this new policy.

32. At one point in our interview, both her husband and her mother-in-law dropped by to visit Fani in the hospital. When her husband urged her to nurse the baby, despite her opinion, shared by her mother-in-law, that giving it chamomile tea was more

appropriate at that moment, her mother-in-law began to complain about her son's interference. In her day, she pointedly remarked, men were like "guests in their own houses" and didn't meddle in a mother's business.

33. The relationship between electronic fetal monitoring and increased performance of caesarean sections is well established; see Davis-Floyd 1992 (279) for a summary of this research.

34. Mossialos et al. (2005, 292) attribute the similarity in the rates of caesareans in public and private hospitals in Athens to convenience and to the fact that because of their complexity, informal payments to public hospital doctors are higher for caesareans than for vaginal births.

35. Ernestine Friedl was the first ethnographer to discuss this process for rural Greece. See also Argyrou (1996, 130) and Stewart (1991, 134) for additional discussion of the concept of "lagging emulation."

Chapter 6

1. I have borrowed the chapter title from Jaggar 1994.

2. While the medical professionals I interviewed were knowledgeable about the pill and the IUD, information about other methods of medical contraception did not appear to be very extensive, as Skilogianis (2001, 222) also found to be the case in Athens.

3. In this regard, the situation in the United States may not be so very different. One married friend who wanted to remain childless told me that she could not convince her doctor to perform a tubal ligation and was forced to find another who would.

4. Substantial differences in men's and women's desired number of children persist into the present: in a recent national survey, 34.5 percent of women with one child did not want to have another, in contrast to 18 percent of men (Symeonidou 2002, 40). However, as I discuss in the next section, although men may express a desire for larger families, they are acutely aware of, and often emotionally stressed by, the economic demands of additional children.

5. Joanna Skilogianis (2001) also found that Athenian couples routinely made abortion decisions jointly. One young woman I interviewed, whose decision to abort was made jointly with her husband, criticized her mother for having had an abortion some years earlier without telling her father.

6. In Athens, Skilogianis (2001) also found that older women were more likely to rely on medical contraception.

7. For a thorough critique of this position, see Paxson 2004.

8. As is the practice in Italy (Gordon and Paci 1997). As a further precaution, doctors may conceal a cancer diagnosis on a patient's chart by using only the English abbreviation, CA.

9. A 2001 national survey found that one-third of Greek women had used the pill at some point in their lives. The majority quit after less than a year because of side effects and concerns over their health. When asked to describe the ideal form of contraception, 75 percent responded that they wanted a method with "no harmful side effects" (Tountas et al. 2004, 193). Anxiety about the harmful health consequences and side effects of the pill are also common cross-culturally, as the comparative studies in Petchesky and Judd 1998 attest.

10. This practice is not confined to Greek women. A 1989 national survey of sex educators in the United States found that less than a quarter knew that women did

not need to stop taking the pill periodically "to give the body a rest" (L. Potter 2001, 146). While this practice may have been reasonable with the older high-dose pill, with the low-dose pills that had replaced them by that time, it was more likely to result in pregnancy.

11. Skilogianis (2001) reports a similar pattern among Athenian women.

12. The binary inside/outside and the ways in which it was linked to the preservation of health and fertility both suggest continuity with preexisting understandings and idiomatic ways of expressing concern over social and bodily order and disorder. However, there was nothing in women's narratives to suggest that their use is associated with older humoral understandings of the body. In particular, there was no conceptual link between the binary opposition of inside/outside and its entailments and those associated with the open/closed opposition so central to the humoral model as described in Chapter 3. There is, however, one significant continuity: however different the conceptual mechanisms underlying the two binaries, both draw on culturally familiar idioms to express and underscore the moral obligation that women have to ensure and protect the health of their bodies in general, and their fertility in particular. This moral imperative remains steady, even if the meanings of the cultural idioms through which it is expressed have shifted.

13. Symeonidou et al. (2000, 86) and Skilogianis (2001) also found this to be the case in their studies of Athenian women, belying the view held by some commentators that Greek women regard abortion as trivial or as a natural method of birth control.

14. I have adapted this section heading from Sant Cassia with Bada (1992).

15. Argyrou (1996, 31) refers to the use of poppy seed tea in rural Cyprus. My grandmother had mentioned to me that it was used by village women around her native Kalamata when they went to work in the fields.

16. For descriptions, see M. Doumanis 1983; Dubisch 1986; du Boulay 1974, 1983; Friedl 1970; Hirschon 1989; Salamone and Stanton 1986.

17. As Bakalaki (1994, 89) has pointed out, the distinctive features of elite nineteenth-century gender discourses and those described by many ethnographers of Greece after the 1960s "present certain striking commonalities in the values, ideas, stereotypes and attitudes that have not been sufficiently noticed." In Greece, as in Europe and North America, women as an aggregate attracted the attention of nineteenth-century reformers concerned with the production of a healthy and educated population. Experts in education, law, and medicine played pivotal roles in devaluing and replacing older "mother-centered" practices of child rearing with a new "child-centered" discourse of the family (Aries 1962; Donzelot 1979; Korasidou 2002). Doctors and other experts scrutinized maternal practices such as nursing and swaddling, chastised women for not maintaining hygienic standards in the home, and repeatedly exhorted mothers to follow modern practices with respect to their children's clothing, bodily care, and cleanliness (Korasidou 2002).

18. Such high rates of homeownership are not peculiar to Rhodes. Greece, along with Ireland, has the highest rate of homeownership in the EU—81 percent in 1995 (Symeonidou 2002, 9).

19. David Sutton (1998a, 100) makes the point that dowry on the neighboring island of Kalymnos has become "naturalized" insofar as it is now considered to be a necessity. However, he attributes this naturalization at least in part to the fact that on Kalymnos, young women may be the main source of funds for their own dwellings, bypassing the hierarchical intergenerational structures of dowry practice in the past.

This was not the case on Rhodes, at least not among native-born Rhodians, for whom "self-endowment" was not common.

20. Filipinas are preferred as domestic workers in Italy, too, where, according to Salazar Parrenas (2001), they tend to be viewed as "status symbols."

21. I have borrowed these terms from Sharon Hays's (1996) study of intensive mothering in the United States for their resonance with many aspects of contemporary mothering in Rhodes.

22. Organization for Economic Cooperation and Development report cited in "Greece Is Largest Student Exporter," *Kathimerini* (English edition), February 12, 2006.

23. The tight conceptual linkage between consumption, especially of technological gadgets, and children is drawn upon to strident rhetorical effect by the conservative New Democracy politician Fani Palli-Petralia, when she asserts in her book *The Birthless Nation*: "Should Greeks' number of children have been even half of the number of computers and cell phones they have, this book would have had no reason for being written" (quoted in Athanasiou 2001, 357).

24. On another occasion, a young married woman, raised in Australia but now living in Rhodes Town, bilingually and pungently remarked to me of her experience as a working mother with two toddlers: "Whoever said *ine eftikhia ta pedhia* was full of shit."

25. It is a common rhetorical strategy, rooted in a long history of antagonism, to favorably contrast Greek Orthodox practices regarding contraception and abortion, as well as other topics, such as divorce, with those of Roman Catholicism. However, there is some ethnographic evidence that, on the ground, Roman Catholic practices may also be pragmatically flexible. As Schneider and Schneider (1991, 888) report for the town of Villamura, Sicily, Catholic parish priests there were not particularly concerned with the issue of contraception, "in contrast to the public voices of the Church."

26. Paxson (2004) and Skilogianis (2001) found that Athenian women also frequently deployed a discourse of greater/lesser evil or sin when explaining their decisions to abort. Paxson (2004, 61) makes the further observation that this form of reasoning may implicitly draw on the Greek Orthodox understanding of *ikonomia*, a notion that "allows the Church to turn away from a smaller wrongdoing (sin) in the interests of facilitating a larger good."

27. In her analysis of Athenian women's abortion narratives, Halkias (2004, 253) discusses the symbolic significance of shoes as a morally tinged justification "for the generation of Greeks who grew up in poor villages during the occupation of Greece by the Nazis and who, very often, did not have shoes to wear."

28. In an interview I saw on television, for example, a transportation worker justified his union's decision to strike by patting his ample belly and declaring to the reporter, "*Piname*, we are hungry."

29. As Petchesky (1998, 305) found in her recent cross-national study of reproductive decision making, women across the globe tend to remain "in dialogue with religion" at the same time they flexibly adapt theology to their own pragmatic ends.

References Cited

Agrafiotis, Dimosthenis, and Mandi, Panagiota. 1997. "Greece." *The International Encyclopedia of Sexuality*. New York: Continuum Press.

Alpu, O., and Fidan, H. 2006. "On the Use of Contraceptive Methods among Married Women in Turkey." *European Journal of Reproductive Health Care* 11(3): 228–36.

Alran, Severine; Sibony, Olivier; Oury, Jean-François; Luton, Dominique; and Blot, Philippe. 2002. "Differences in Management and Results in Term-Delivery in Nine European Referral Hospitals: Descriptive Study." *European Journal of Obstetrics and Gynecology* 103:4–13.

Anagnost, Ann. 1995. "A Surfeit of Bodies: Population and the Rationality of the State in Post-Mao China." In *Conceiving the New World Order*, Faye D. Ginsburg and Rayna Rapp, eds., 22–41. Berkeley: University of California Press.

Angel, Marc. 1998. *The Jews of Rhodes: The History of a Sephardic Community*. *New York*: Sepher-Hermon Press and the Union of Sephardic Congregations.

Appadurai, Arjun. 1986. "Theory in Anthropology: Center and Periphery." *Comparative Studies in Society and History* 28(2): 356–74.

———. 1996. *Modernity at Large: Cultural Dimensions of Globalization*. Minneapolis: University of Minnesota Press.

Apple, Rima. 1987. *Mothers and Medicine: A Social History of Infant Feeding, 1890–1950*. London and Madison: University of Wisconsin Press.

———. 1995. "Constructing Mothers: Scientific Motherhood in the Nineteenth and Twentieth Centuries." *Social History of Medicine* 8(2): 161–78.

Argyrou, Vassos. 1996. *Tradition and Modernity in the Mediterranean: The Wedding as Symbolic Struggle*. Cambridge: Cambridge University Press.

Aries, Philippe. 1962. *Centuries of Childhood*. London: Jonathan Cape.

Armstrong, David. 1983. *The Political Anatomy of the Body*. Cambridge: Cambridge University Press.

Arney, William Ray. 1982. *Power and the Profession of Obstetrics*. Chicago: University of Chicago Press.

Arnold, Marlene S. 1985. "Childbirth among Rural Greek Women in Crete: Use of Popular, Folk, and Cosmopolitan Medical Systems." Ph.D. diss., University of Pennsylvania.

Athanasiou, Athena. 2001. "Nostalgic Futures, Contentious Technologies: Reckoning Time and Population in Greece." Ph.D. diss., New School University.

Avdela, Efi. 2000. "The Teaching of History in Greece." *Journal of Modern Greek Studies* 18(2): 239–53.

Baer, Hans. 1989. "The American Dominative Medical System as a Reflection of Social Relations in the Larger Society." *Social Science and Medicine* 28(11): 1103–12.

———. 2002. "The Growing Interest of Biomedicine in Complementary and Alternative Medicine: A Critical Perspective." *Medical Anthropology Quarterly* 16(4): 403–5.

Bakalaki, Alexandra. 1994. "Gender-Related Discourses and Representations of Cultural Specificity in Nineteenth-Century and Twentieth-Century Greece." *Journal of Modern Greek Studies* 12(1): 75–111.

———. 1997. "Students, Natives, Colleagues: Encounters in Academia and in the Field." *Cultural Anthropology* 12(4): 502–26.

Bakalaki, Alexandra, and Elegmitou, Eleni. 1987. *I ekpedhefsi "is ta tou ikou" ke ta ghinekia kathikonta* [Pedagogy, "Domestic Matters," and Womanly Duties]. Athens: Historical Archive of Greek Youth.

Barley, Stephen R. 1988. "On Technology, Time, and Social Order: Technically Induced Changes in the Temporal Organization of Radiological Work." In *Making Time: Ethnographies of High-Technology Organizations*, F. Dubinskas, ed., 123–69. Philadelphia: Temple University Press.

Bartsocas, C. S. 1997. "Genetic Services in Greece." *European Journal of Human Genetics* 5 (Supplement 2): 89–92.

Beck, Ulrich. 1992a. *Risk Society: Towards a New Modernity*. London: Sage.

———. 1992b. "From Industrial Society to Risk Society: Questions of Survival, Structure, and Ecological Enlightenment." *Theory, Culture, and Society* 9(1): 97–123.

Becker, Ann. 1995. *Body, Self, and Society: The View from Fiji*. Philadelphia: University of Pennsylvania Press.

Becker, Gaylene. 2000. *The Elusive Embryo: How Women and Men Approach New Reproductive Technologies*. Berkeley: University of California Press.

Beer, Gillian. 1989. "Discourses of the Island." In *Literature and Science as Modes of Expression*, Frederick Amrine, ed., 1–27. Dordrecht, Boston, and London: Kluwer.

Beeson, Diane. 1984. "Technological Rhythms in Pregnancy: The Case of Prenatal Diagnosis by Amniocentesis." In *Cultural Perspectives on Biological Knowledge*, T. Duster and K. Garrett, eds., 145–81. Norwood, N.J.: Ablex.

Berlant, Lauren. 1997. *The Queen of America Goes to Washington City: Essays on Sex and Citizenship*. Durham and London: Duke University Press.

Behague, Dominique. 2002. "Beyond the Simple Economics of Caesarean Section Birthing: Women's Resistance to Social Inequality." *Culture, Medicine, and Psychiatry* 26:473–507.

Benthien, Claudia. 2002. *Skin: On the Cultural Border between Self and the World*. New York: Columbia University Press.

Berg, Marc, and Mol, Annemarie, eds. 1998. *Differences in Medicine: Unraveling Practices, Techniques, and Bodies*. Durham and London: Duke University Press.

Beyene, Yewoubdar. 1989. *From Menarche to Menopause: Reproductive Lives of Peasant Women in Two Cultures*. New York: State University of New York Press.

Bledsoe, Carolyn. 1995. "Marginal Members: Children of Previous Unions in Mende Households in Sierra Leone." In *Situating Fertility: Anthropology and Demographic Inquiry*, Susan Greenhalgh, ed., 130–54. Cambridge: Cambridge University Press.

———. 2002. *Contingent Lives: Fertility, Time, and Aging in West Africa*. Chicago: University of Chicago Press.

Blue, Amy. 1993. "Greek Psychiatry's Transition from the Hospital to the Community." *Medical Anthropology Quarterly* 7(3): 301–18.

Blum, Linda. 1999. *At the Breast: Ideologies of Breastfeeding and Motherhood in the Contemporary United States*. Boston: Beacon Press.

Blum, Richard, and Blum, Eva. 1965. *Health and Healing in Rural Greece*. Stanford, Calif.: Stanford University Press.

Blundell, Sue. 1995. *Women in Ancient Greece*. Cambridge, Mass.: Harvard University Press.

Bordo, Susan. 1993. *Unbearable Weight: Feminism, Western Culture, and the Body*. Berkeley: University of California Press.

Borneman, John, and Fowler, Nick. 1997. "Europeanization." *Annual Review of Anthropology* 26:487–514.

Boubouri, Eleni. 1999. "Rodhos: I Dhiki Mas" [Our Rhodes]. *Athenorama*, May 21–27, 71–78.

Bourdieu, Pierre. 1984. *Distinction: A Social Critique of the Judgment of Taste*. Cambridge, Mass.: Harvard University Press.

Bozaninou, Tania. 1996. "Greeks Work More to Purchase Basic Goods." *Athens News*, November 10.

Braidotti, Rosi. 1994. *Nomadic Subjects: Embodiment and Sexual Difference in Contemporary Feminist Theory*. New York: Columbia University Press.

Breart, G.; Mlika-Cabane, N.; Kaminski, M.; Alexander, S.; Herruzo-Nalda, A.; Mandruzzato, P.; Thornton, J. G.; and Trakas, D. 1992. "Evaluation of Different Policies for the Management of Labour." *Early Human Development* 29:309–12.

Breck, John. 1998. *The Sacred Gift of Life: Orthodox Christianity and Bioethics*. Crestwood, N.Y.: St. Vladimir's Seminary Press.

Browner, Carole. 1980. "The Management of Early Pregnancy: Colombian Folk Concepts of Fertility Control." *Social Science and Medicine* 148:25–32.

———. 1985. "Traditional Techniques for Diagnosis, Treatment, and Control of Pregnancy in Cali, Colombia." In *Women's Medicine: A Cross-Cultural Study of Indigenous Fertility Regulation*, Lucille Newman, ed., 99–123. New Brunswick, N.J.: Rutgers University Press.

Browner, Carole, and Ortiz de Montellano, Bernard. 1986. "Herbal Emmenagogues Used by Women in Colombia and Mexico." In *Plants in Indigenous Medicine and Diet: Biobehavioral Approaches*, Nina Etkin, ed., 32–43. Bedford Hills, N.Y.: Redgrave.

Browner, Carole, and Sargent, Carolyn. 1996. "Anthropology and Studies of Human Reproduction." In *Medical Anthropology: Contemporary Theory and Method*, rev. edition, Carolyn Sargent and Thomas Johnson, eds., 219–34. Westport, Conn., and London: Bergin and Garvey.

Buck, Elizabeth. 1993. *Paradise Remade:The Politics of Culture and History in Hawai'i*. Philadephia: Temple University Press.

Buck-Morss, Susan. 1987. "Semiotic Boundaries and the Politics of Meaning: Modernity on Tour—A Village in Transition." In *New Ways of Knowing: The Sciences, Society, and Reconstructive Knowledge*, M. Raskin and H. J. Bernstein, eds., 200–236. Totowa, N.J.: Rowman and Littlefied.

Bynum, W. F., and Porter, Roy, eds. 1993. *Medicine and the Five Senses*. Cambridge: Cambridge University Press.

Campbell, J. K. 1964. *Honour, Family, and Patronage: A Study of Institutions and Moral Values in a Greek Mountain Community*. Oxford: Clarendon Press.

Caraveli, Anna. 1985. "The Symbolic Village: Community Born in Performance." *Journal of American Folklore* 99(289): 260–86.

———. 1986. "The Bitter Wounding: The Lament as Social Protest in Rural Greece." In *Gender and Power in Rural Greece*, Jill Dubisch, ed., 169–94. Princeton: Princeton University Press.

Carrier, James. 1995. Introduction to *Occidentalism: Images of the West*, James Carrier, ed., 1–32. Oxford: Clarendon Press.

Cassell, Joan, ed. 1987. *Children in the Field: Anthropological Experiences*. Philadelphia: Temple University Press.

Castenada, Terri. 1993. "Preservation and the Cultural Politics of the Past on Historic Galveston Island." Ph.D. diss., Rice University.

Chatterjee, Nilanjana, and Riley, Nancy. 2001. "Planning an Indian Modernity: The Gendered Politics of Fertility Control." *Signs* 26(3): 811–45.

Chouliaras, Yiorgos. 1993. "Greek Culture in the New Europe." In *Greece, the New Europe, and the Changing International Order*, Harry Psomiades and Stavros Thomadakis, eds., 79–122. New York: Pella.

Chryssanthopoulou, Vassiliki. 1984. *An Analysis of Rituals Surrounding Birth in Modern Greece.* Master's thesis, University of Oxford.

Clark, Mari. 1995. "From Shelters to Villas: Changing House and Settlement Form on Methana, 1880–1987." *Modern Greek Studies Yearbook* 10/11:511–36

Clark, Patricia. 2002. "Landscape, Memories, and Medicine: Traditional Healing in Amari, Crete." *Journal of Modern Greek Studies* 20(2): 339–65.

Clogg, Richard, ed. 1999. *The Greek Diaspora in the Twentieth Century.* Houndmills, Basingstoke, and Hampshire: Macmillan in association with St. Anthony's College, Oxford; New York: St. Martin's Press.

———. 2002. *A Concise History of Modern Greece.* 2nd edition. Cambridge: Cambridge University Press

Close, David. 2002. *Greece since 1945: Politics, Economy, and Society.* London, New York: Longman.

Cole, Joshua. 2000. *The Power of Large Numbers: Population, Politics, and Gender in Nineteenth Century France.* Ithaca and London: Cornell University Press.

Collier, Jane. 1997. *From Duty to Desire: Remaking Families in a Spanish Village.* Princeton: Princeton University Press.

Colombotos, John, and Fakiolas, Nikos. 1993. "The Power of Organized Medicine in Greece." In *The Changing Medical Profession: An International Perspective.* F. Hafferty and J. McKinlay, eds., 138–49. New York: Oxford University Press.

Colonas, Vassilis. 2002. *Italian Architecture in the Dodecanese Islands (1912–1943).* Athens: Olkos.

Comaroff, Jean, and Comaroff, John L., eds. 1993. *Modernity and Its Malcontents: Ritual and Power in Postcolonial Africa.* Chicago: University of Chicago Press.

Comninos, Anthony. 1988. "Greece." *International Handbook on Abortion.* Paul Sachdev, ed., 207–15. New York: Greenwood Press.

Condit, Celeste M. 1990. *Decoding Abortion Rhetoric: Communicating Social Change.* Urbana and Chicago: University of Illinois Press.

Corbin, Alain. 1986. *The Foul and the Fragrant: Odor and the French Social Imagination.* Leamington Spa, Hamburg, and New York: Berg.

Costa, Janeen. 1993. "The Periphery of Pleasure or Pain: Consumer Culture in the E.C." In *Cultural Change and the New Europe: Perspectives on the European Community,* Thomas Wilson and M. Estellie Smith, eds., 81–98. Boulder, Colo.: Westview Press.

Cowan, Jane. 1990. *Dance and the Body Politic in Northern Greece.* Princeton: Princeton University Press.

———. 1996. "Being a Feminist in Contemporary Greece: Similarity and Difference Reconsidered." In *Practicing Feminism: Identity, Difference, Power,* Nicki Charles and Felicia Hughes-Freeland, eds., 61–85. London: Routledge.

Cowan, Ruth Schwarz. 1987. "The Consumption Junction: A Proposal for Research Strategies in the Sociology of Technology." In *The Social Construction of Technological Systems: New Directions in the Sociology and History of Technology,* Wiebe Bijker, Thomas Hughes, and Trevor Pinch, eds., 261–80. Cambridge, Mass.: MIT Press.

Craig, Marveen. 1990. "Controversies in Obstetric and Gynecologic Ultrasound." In *Medical Sonography: A Guide to Clinical Practice*. Vol. 1, *Obstetrics and Gynecology*, M. Berman, ed., 551–62. Philadelphia: J. B. Lippincott.

Crary, Jonathan. 1990. *Techniques of the Observer: On Vision and Modernity in the Nineteenth Century*. Cambridge, Mass.: MIT Press.

Cressy, David. 1997. *Birth, Marriage, and Death: Ritual, Religion, and the Life-Cycle in Tudor and Stuart England*. Oxford: Oxford University Press.

Crick, Malcolm. 1989. "Representations of International Tourism in the Social Sciences: Sun, Sex, Sights, Savings, and Servility." *Annual Review of Anthropology* 18:307–44.

Danforth, Loring. 1982. *The Death Rituals of Rural Greece*. Princeton: Princeton University Press.

———. 1989. *Firewalking and Religious Healing: The Anastenaria of Greece and the American Firewalking Movement*. Princeton: Princeton University Press.

Davis-Floyd, Robbie. 1992. *Birth as an American Rite of Passage*. Berkeley: University of California Press.

———. 2003. Preface to the Second Edition. *Birth as an American Rite of Passage*, xi–xl. Berkeley: University of California Press.

Davis-Floyd, Robbie, and Arvidson, P. Sven. 1997. *Intuition: The Inside Story*. New York: Routledge.

Davis-Floyd, Robbie, and Franklin, Sarah. 2005. "On Reproduction." *Sage Encyclopedia of Anthropology*. London, Thousand Oaks, Calif., and New Delhi: Sage Publications.

Davis-Floyd, Robbie, and Sargent, Carolyn. 1997. "Introduction: The Anthropology of Birth." In *Childbirth and Authoritative Knowledge: Cross-Cultural Perspectives*. Robbie Davis-Floyd and Carolyn Sargent, eds., 1–51. Berkeley: University of California Press.

Davis-Floyd, Robbie; Pigg, Stacy Leigh; and Cosminsky, Sheila. 2001. "Introduction: Daughters of Time—The Shifting Identities of Contemporary Midwives." *Medical Anthropology* 20:105–39.

Dean-Jones, Lesley. 1994. *Women's Bodies in Classical Greek Science*. Oxford: Clarendon Press.

de Certeau, Michel. 1984. *The Practice of Everyday Life*. Berkeley: University of California Press.

Declerq, Eugene, and Viisainen, Kirsi. 2001. "The Politics of Numbers: The Promise and Frustration of Cross-National Analysis." In *Birth by Design: Pregnancy, Maternity Care, and Midwifery in North America and Europe*, Raymond DeVries, Cecilia Benoit, Edwin van Teijlingen, and Sirpa Wrede, eds., 267–79. New York: Routledge.

de Grazia, Victoria. 1996. "Nationalizing Women: The Competition between Fascist and Commercial Cultural Models in Mussolini's Italy." In *The Sex of Things: Gender and Consumption in Historical Perspective*, Victoria de Grazia, ed., 337–58. Berkeley: University of California Press.

Delaney, Carol. 1991. *The Seed and the Soil: Gender and Cosmology in Turkish Village Society*. Berkeley: University of California Press.

———. 2000. "Making Babies in a Turkish Village." In *A World of Babies: Imagined Childcare Guides for Seven Societies*, Judy DeLoache and Alma Gottlieb, eds., 117–44. Cambridge: Cambridge University Press.

Delighiani-Kwimsi, B. 1993a. "Ta Stereotipa ghia tous Rolous ton Dhio Filon sta Enkhiridhia tou Dhimotikou Skholiou 'I Ghlosa Mou'" [Stereotypes of Gender Roles in the Primary School Text "My Language"]. In *Ekpedhevsi ke Filo* [Education and Gender], B. Delighiani-Kwimsi and S. Zighou, eds., 147–70. Thessaloniki: Vantias Press.

———. 1993b. "Mia Epitikhimeni Kariera ki enas Kalos Sizighos: Onira ke Prosdhokies Koritsion Efivikis Ilikias" [A Successful Career and a Good Husband: Dreams and

Aims of Adolescent Girls]. In *Ekpedhevsi ke Filo* [Education and Gender], B. Delighiani-Kwimsi and S. Zighou, eds., 311–32. Thessaloniki: Vantias Press.

De Mello e Souza, Cecilia. 1994. "C-Sections as Ideal Births: The Cultural Constructions of Beneficence and Patients' Rights in Brazil." *Cambridge Quarterly of Healthcare Ethics* 3:358–66.

DeVries, Raymond; Benoit, Cecilia; van Teijlingen, Edwin; and Wrede, Sirpa, eds. 2001. *Birth by Design: Pregnancy, Maternity Care, and Midwifery in North America and Europe.* New York: Routledge.

Dhimos Rodhion. 2002. *2000–2006 Proghrama: Kinotikis Anaptiksis ke Kinonikis Frondidhas* [2000–2006 Program: Community Development and Social Welfare]. Unpublished report, Office of the Mayor of Rhodes.

Dimitrakakis, Constantine; Papadogiannakis, John; Sakelaropoulos, Gerasimos; Papazefkos, Vasilis; Voulgaris, Zannis; and Michalas, Stylianos. 2001. "Maternal Mortality in Greece (1980–1996)." *European Journal of Obstetrics and Gynecology* 99(1): 6–13.

Dimitriou-Kotsoni, Sibylla. 1993. "The Aegean Cultural Tradition." *Journal of Mediterranean Studies* 3:62–76.

Dixon G. 1992. "Colostrum Avoidance and Early Infant Feeding in Asian Societies." *Asia Pacific Journal of Clinical Nutrition,* 1:225–29.

Donner, Henrike. 2004. "Labour, Privatisation, and Class: Middle-Class Women's Experience of Changing Hospital Births in Calcutta." In *Reproductive Agency, Medicine, and the State: Cultural Transformations in Childbearing,* Maya Unnithan-Kumar, ed., 113–35. New York and Oxford: Berghahn Books.

Donzelot, Jacques. 1979. *The Policing of Families.* New York: Pantheon.

Douglas, Mary. 1980 [1966]. *Purity and Danger: An Analysis of Concepts of Pollution and Taboo.* London and Boston: Routledge and Kegan Paul.

Douglass, Carrie B. 1992. "'Europe,' 'Spain,' and the Bulls." *Journal of Mediterranean Studies* 2(1): 69–79.

Doumanis, Mariella. 1983. *Mothering in Greece: From Collectivism to Individualism.* London and New York: Academic Press.

Doumanis, Nicholas. 1997. *Myth and Memory in the Mediterranean: Remembering Fascism's Empire.* New York: St. Martin's Press.

———. 1999. "The Greeks in Australia." In *The Greek Diaspora in the Twentieth Century,* Richard Clogg, ed., 58–86. New York: St. Martin's Press.

Dragona, Thalia, and Naziri, Despoina. 1995. *Odhighontas pros tin Patrotita* [Toward Fatherhood]. Athens: Eksatas.

Dubisch, Jill. 1986. "Culture Enters through the Kitchen: Women, Food, and Social Boundaries in Rural Greece." In *Gender and Power in Rural Greece,* Jill Dubisch, ed., 195–214. Princeton: Princeton University Press.

———. 1991. "Gender, Kinship, and Religion: 'Reconstructing' the Anthropology of Greece." In *Contested Identities: Gender and Kinship in Modern Greece,* Peter Loizos and Evthemios Papataxiarchis, eds., 29–46. Princeton: Princeton University Press.

———. 1993. "'Foreign Chickens' and Other Outsiders: Gender and Community in Greece." *American Ethnologist* 20(2): 272–87.

———. 1995a. *In a Different Place: Pilgrimage, Gender, and Politics at a Greek Island Shrine.* Princeton: Princeton University Press.

———. 1995b. "Lovers in the Field: Sex, Dominance, and the Female Anthropologist." In *Taboo: Sex, Identity, and Erotic Subjectivity in Anthropological Fieldwork,* Don Kulick and Margaret Willson, eds, 29–50. London and New York: Routledge.

du Boulay, Juliet. 1974. *Portrait of a Greek Mountain Village.* Oxford: Clarendon Press.

———. 1983. "The Meaning of Dowry: Changing Values in Rural Greece." *Journal of Modern Greek Studies* 1:243–70.

———. 1991. "Cosmos and Gender in Village Greece." In *Contested Identities: Gender and Kinship in Modern Greece*, Peter Loizos and Evthemios Papataxiarchis, eds., 47–78. Princeton: Princeton University Press.

Duden, Barbara. 1991. *The Woman beneath the Skin: A Doctor's Patients in Eighteenth-Century Germany*. Cambridge and London: Harvard University Press.

———. 1993. *Disembodying Women: Perspectives on Pregnancy and the Unborn*. Cambridge, Mass.: Harvard University Press.

Durrell, Lawrence. 1960. *Prospero's Cell and Reflections on a Marine Venus*. New York: E. P. Dutton.

Eccles, Audrey. 1982. *Obstetrics and Gynecology in Tudor and Stuart England*. Kent, Ohio: Kent State University Press

Economopoulos, Demetrios. 1990. *In Rodos the Sun Shines Brighter*. Athens: Graphic Arts.

Eisenberg, Arlene; Murkoff, Heidi; and Hathaway, Sandee. 1991. *What to Expect When You're Expecting*. New York: Workman.

Eisner, Robert. 1991. *Travelers to an Antique Land: The History and Literature of Travel to Greece*. Ann Arbor: University of Michigan Press.

Elias, Norbert. 1982. *The Civilizing Process*. New York: Urizen Books.

Emke-Poulopoulou. 1994. *To Dhimoghrafiko* [The Demographic Problem]. Athens: Eleni.

Enloe, Cynthia. 1989. *Bananas, Beaches, and Bases: Making Feminist Sense of International Politics*. Berkeley and Los Angeles: University of California Press.

Etkin, Nina. 1988. "Ethnopharmacology: Biobehavioral Approaches in the Anthropological Study of Indigenous Medicines." *Annual Review of Anthropology* 17:23–42.

Ettore, Elizabeth. 1999. "Prenatal Screening in Europe: A Comparative Study of the Views of Experts in Greece, the Netherlands, and Finland." In *Prenatal Screening in Europe: The Past, the Present, and the Future. Final Report*. In Elizabeth Ettore, et al. Biomedicine and Health Research and Technological Development Programme, Commission of the European Union, unpublished report, EU Contract no. BMH4-CT96-0740.

Evenden, Doreen. 2000. *The Midwives of Seventeenth-Century London*. Cambridge: Cambridge University Press.

Fakinou, Eugenia. 1991. *Astradeni*. Athens: Kendros.

Farmer, Beverly. 1995. *The House in the Light*. Queensland: University of Queensland Press.

Faubion, James. 1993. *Modern Greek Lessons: A Primer in Historical Constructivism*. Princeton: Princeton University Press.

Featherstone, Kevin. 1998. "'Europeanization' and the Centre-Periphery: The Case of Greece in the 1990s." *South European Society and Politics* 3(1): 23–39.

Feher, Michel, with Naddaff, Ramona, and Tazi, Nadia, eds. 1989. *Fragments for a History of the Human Body*. 3 vols. New York: Zone.

Filli, Savva. 2000. *I Rizes Mas* [Our Roots]. Rhodes: Tekhne Publications.

Fischer, Michael. 1986. "Ethnicity and the Post-Modern Arts of Memory." In *Writing Culture: The Poetics and Politics of Ethnography*, George Marcus and James Clifford, eds., 194–233. Berkeley: University of California Press.

Fisher, Sue, and Davis, Kathy. 1993. *Negotiating at the Margins: The Gendered Discourses of Power and Resistance*. New Brunswick, N.J.: Rutgers University Press.

Fiske, John. 1987. *Television Culture*. New York: Routledge.

Flandrin, Jean Louis. 1979. *Families in Former Times: Kinship, Household, and Sexuality*. New York: Cambridge University Press.

Foster, George. 1994. *Hippocrates' Latin American Legacy: Humoral Medicine in the New World*. Amsterdam: Gordon and Breach.

Foucault, Michel. 1978 [1990]. *History of Sexuality: An Introduction*. New York: Vintage.

———. 1982. "The Subject and Power." In *Michel Foucault: Beyond Structuralism and Hermeneutics*, H. L. Dreyfuss and Paul Rabinow, eds., 20–226. Chicago: University of Chicago Press.

———. 1991. "Governmentality." In *The Foucault Effect*, G. Burchell, C. Gordon, and P. Miller, eds. 87–104. Brighton: Harvester Wheatshaft.

Frangoudaki, Anna. 2003. "Greek Education in the Twentieth Century: A Long Process Towards a Democratic European Society." In *Greece in the Twentieth Century*, Theodore A. Couloumbis, Theodore Kariotis, and Fotini Bellou, eds., 198–216. London and Portland, Ore.: Frank Cass.

Friedl, Ernestine. 1964. "Lagging Emulation in the Post-Peasant Society." *American Anthropologist* 66:569–86.

———. 1970. *Vasilika: A Village in Modern Greece*. New York: Holt, Rinehart and Winston.

Fuchs, Victor. 1968. "The Growing Demand for Medical Care." *New England Journal of Medicine* 279:190–95.

Fuller, Mia. 2007. *Moderns Abroad: Architecture, Cities, and Italian Imperialism*. London and New York: Routledge.

Gaines, Atwood, and Robbie Davis-Floyd. 2004. "Biomedicine." *Encyclopedia of Medical Anthropology*. Vol. 1, *Health and Illness in the World's Cultures*, Carol Ember and Melvin Ember, eds., 95–109. New York: Kluwer Academic/Plenum.

Galani Moutafi, Vasiliki. 1993. "From Agriculture to Tourism: Property, Labor, Gender, and Kinship in a Greek Island Village (Part One)." *Journal of Modern Greek Studies*: 11:241–70.

———. 1994. "From Agriculture to Tourism: Property, Labor, Gender, and Kinship in a Greek Island Village (Part Two)." *Journal of Modern Greek Studies* 12:113–31.

Gallant, Thomas 2001. *Modern Greece*. London: Arnold.

Gefou-Madianou, Dimitra. 1992. "Exclusion and Unity, Retsina and Sweet Wine: Commensality and Gender in a Greek Agrotown." In *Alcohol, Gender, and Culture*, Dimitra Gefou-Madianou, ed., 108–36. New York: Routledge.

———. 1999. "Cultural Polyphony and Identity Formation: Negotiating Tradition in Attica." *American Ethnologist* 26(2): 412–39.

Gelis, Jacques. 1991. *History of Childbirth: Fertility, Pregnancy, and Birth in Early Modern Europe*. Boston: Northeastern University Press.

Georges, Eugenia. 1996. "Fetal Ultrasound Imaging and the Production of Authoritative Knowledge in Greece." *Medical Anthropology Quarterly* (ns) 10(2): 157–175.

Georges, Eugenia, and Mitchell, Lisa. 2000. "Baby Talk: Rhetorical Constructions of Women and the Fetus in Greek and Canadian Pregnancy Guidebooks." In *Writing and Speaking the Body: Feminist and Rhetorical Studies of Reproductive Sciences and Technologies*, Mary Lay and Helen Longino, eds., 184–206. Madison: University of Wisconsin Press.

Giannuli, Dimitra. 1998. "'Repeated Disaappointment': The Rockefeller Foundation and the Reform of the Greek Public Health System, 1929–1940." *Bulletin of the History of Medicine* 72:47–72.

Giddens, Anthony. 1991. *Modernity and Self-Identity: Self and Society in the Late Modern Age*. Stanford: Stanford University Press.

Ginsburg, Faye D., and Rapp, Rayna. 1991. "The Politics of Reproduction." *Annual Review of Anthropology* 20:311–43.

———. 1995. "Introduction: Conceiving the New World Order." In *Conceiving the New World*

Order: The Global Politics of Reproduction, Faye Ginsburg and Rayna Rapp, eds., 1–17. Berkeley: University of California Press.

Goddard, Victoria; Llobera, Josep; and Shore, Chris. 1994. *The Anthropology of Europe: Identity and Boundaries in Conflict*. Oxford and Providence, R.I.: Berg.

Goffman, Irving. 1986. *Stigma: Notes on the Management of Spoiled Identity*. Englewood Cliffs, N.J.: Prentice-Hall.

Good, Byron, and DelVecchio Good, Mary-Jo. 1992. "The Comparative Study of Greco-Islamic Medicine: The Integration of Medical Knowledge into Local Symbolic Systems." In *Paths to Asian Medical Knowledge*, Charles Leslie and AllanYoung, eds., 257–71. Berkeley: University of California Press.

Gordon, Deborah. 1988. "Tenacious Assumptions in Western Medicine." In *Biomedicine Examined*, Margaret Lock and Deborah Gordon, eds., 19–46. Dordrecht, Netherlands: Kluwer Academic.

Gordon, Deborah, and Paci, Eugenio. 1997. "Disclosure Practices and Cultural Narratives: Understanding Concealment and Silence around Cancer in Tuscany, Italy." *Social Science and Medicine* 44(10): 1433–52.

Gottlieb, Alma. 2002. "Afterword: Blood Mysteries—Beyond Menstruation as Pollution." *Ethnology* 41(4): 381–89.

Gourgouris, Stathis. 1992. "Nationalism and Oneirocentrism: Of Modern Hellenes in Europe." *Diaspora* 2:43–71.

———. 1996. *Dream Nation: Enlightenment, Colonization, and the Institution of Modern Greece*. Stanford, Calif.: Stanford University Press.

"Greece Is Largest Student Exporter." *Kathimerini* (English edition), February 12, 2006.

Green, Monica. 1985. "The Transmission of Ancient Theories of Female Physiology and Disease through the Early Middle Ages." Ph.D. diss., Princeton University.

———. 1999. Review of John Riddle, *Eve's Herbs: A History of Contraception and Abortion in the West*. *Bulletin of the History of Medicine* 73(2): 308–11.

Greene, Molly. 2000. *A Shared World: Christians and Muslims in the Early Modern Mediterranean*. Princeton: Princeton University Press.

Greenhalgh, Susan. 1995. "Anthropology Theorizes Reproduction: Integrating Practice, Political Economy, and Feminist Perspectives." In *Situating Fertility: Anthropology and Demographic Inquiry*, Susan Greenhalgh, ed., 3–28. Cambridge: Cambridge University Press.

Gunther, Robert. 1934. *The Greek Herbal of Dioscorides*. Oxford: Oxford University Press.

Hahn, Robert, and Gaines, Atwood, eds. 1985. *Physicians of Western Medicine: Anthropological Approaches to Theory and Practice*. Dordrecht, Netherlands: Reidel.

Hahn, Robert, and Kleinman, Arthur. 1983. "Biomedical Practice and Anthropological Theory." *Annual Review of Anthropology* 12:305–33.

Halkias, Alexandra. 1998. "Give Birth for Greece! Abortion and Nation in Letters to the Editor of the Mainstream Greek Press." *Journal of Modern Greek Studies* 16:111–38.

———. 2004. *The Empty Cradle of Democracy: Sex, Abortion, and Nationalism in Modern Greece*. Durham and London: Duke University Press.

Handman, Marie-Elizabet. 1983. *La violence et la ruse. Hommes et femmes dans un village Grec*. La Calade, Aix-en-Provence: Edisud.

Harakas, Stanley. 1996. "Dynamic Elements of Marriage in the Orthodox Church." In *Personhood: Orthodox Christianity and the Connection between Body, Mind, and Soul*, John Chirban, ed., 121–36. Westport, Conn., and London: Bergin and Garvey.

Hart, Laurie. 1992. *Time, Religion, and Social Experience in Rural Greece*. Lanham, Md.: Rowman and Littlefield.

Hays, Sharon. 1996. *The Cultural Contradictions of Motherhood*. New Haven: Yale University Press.

Henshaw, Stanley. 1990. "Induced Abortion: A World Review." *Family Planning Perspectives* 22(2): 76–89.

Herzfeld, Michael. 1980. "The Dowry in Greece: Terminological Usage and Historical Reconstruction." *Ethnohistory* 27:225–41.

———. 1982a. *Ours Once More: Folklore, Ideology, and the Making of Modern Greece*. Austin: University of Texas Press.

———. 1982b. "When Exceptions Define the Rules: Greek Baptismal Names and the Negotiation of Identity." *Journal of Anthropological Research* 38:288–302.

———. 1985. *The Poetics of Manhood: Contest and Identity in a Cretan Mountain Village*. Princeton: Princeton University Press.

———. 1986a. "Within and Without: The Category of 'Female' in the Ethnography of Modern Greece." In *Gender and Power in Rural Greece*, Jill Dubisch, ed., 215–33. Princeton: Princeton University Press.

———. 1986b. "Closure as Cure: Tropes in the Exploration of Bodily and Social Disorder." *Current Anthropology* 27(2): 107–20.

———. 1987. *Anthropology through the Looking-Glass: Critical Ethnography in the Margins of Europe*. Cambridge: Cambridge University Press.

———. 1991. *A Place in History: Social and Monumental Time in a Cretan Town*. Princeton: Princeton University Press.

———. 1992. *The Social Production of Indifference: Exploring the Symbolic Roots of Western Bureaucracy*. Oxford: Berg.

———. 1995. "Hellenism and Occidentalism: The Permutations of Performance in Greek Bourgeois Identity." In *Occidentalism: Images of the West*, James Carrier, ed., 218–33. Oxford: Clarendon Press.

———. 1997. *Cultural Intimacy: Social Poetics in the Nation-State*. New York and London: Routledge.

Hionidou, Violetta. 1995. "The Demographic System of a Mediterranean Island: Mykonos, Greece, 1859–1959." *International Journal of Population Geography* 1(2): 125–46.

Hirsch, Jennifer, and Nathanson, Constance. 2001. "Some Traditional Methods Are More Modern Than Others: Rhythm, Withdrawal, and the Changing Meanings of Sexual Intimacy in Mexican Companionate Marriage." *Culture, Health, and Sexuality* 3(4): 413–28.

Hirschon, Renée. 1978. "Open Body/Closed Space: The Transformation of Female Sexuality." In *Defining Females: The Nature of Women in Society*, Shirley Ardener, ed., 66–88. New York: John Wiley and Sons.

———. 1989. *Heirs of the Greek Catastrophe: The Social Life of Asia Minor Refugees in Piraeus*. Oxford: Clarendon Press.

Hoban, Thomas. 1997. "Consumer Acceptance of Biotechnology: An International Perspective." *Nature Biotechnology* 15:232–34.

Hobby, Elaine, ed. 1999. *The Midwives Book; Or the Whole Art of Midwifery Discovered*, by Jane Sharp (1671). New York and Oxford: Oxford University Press.

Hohlweg, Armin. 1995. "Dhiadhosi ke Epidhrasi tis Vizantinis Iatrikis stous meta tin Alosi Khronous" [The Spread and Influence of Byzantine Medicine in the Years after the Fall]. In *Iatrika Vizantina Khiroghrafa* [Byzantine Medical Manuscripts], Thanasis Diamandopoulos, ed., 31–55. Athens: Domos.

Hondrou, Kiriakou. 1984. *H Mana ke to Pedhi mesa apo ti Laoghrafia tis Dhodhekanisou* [Mother and Child in the Folklore of the Dodecanese]. Rhodes: Tekhni.

Howes, David. 2005. *The Empire of the Senses: The Sensual Culture Reader*. Oxford and New York: Berg.

Hsu, Kuang-Hung; Liao, Pei-Ju; and Hwang, Chorng-Jer. 2008. Factors Affecting Taiwanese Women's Choice of Cesarean Section. *Social Science and Medicine* 66(1): 201–9.

Inhorn, Marcia. 1994. *Quest for Conception: Gender, Infertility, and Egyptian Medical Traditions*. Philadelphia: University of Pennsylvania Press.

———. 2003. *Local Babies, Global Science: Gender, Religion, and In Vitro Fertilization in Egypt*. New York and London: Routledge.

Ipsen, Carl. 1996. *Dictating Demography: The Problem of Population in Fascist Italy*. Cambridge: Cambridge University Press.

Ivy, Marilyn. 1995. *Discourses of the Vanishing: Modernity, Phantasm, Japan*. Chicago: University of Chicago Press.

Jacquart, Danielle. 1991. "The Introduction of Arabic Medicine into the West: The Question of Etiology." In *Health, Disease, and Healing in Medieval Culture*, Sheila Campbell, Bert Hall, and David Klausner, eds., 186–93. New York: St. Martin's Press.

Jaggar, Alison. 1994. *Living with Contradictions: Controversies in Feminist Ethics*. Boulder, Colo.: Westview Press.

Jenkins, Gwynne. 2001. "Changing Roles and Identities of Midwives in Rural Costa Rica." *Medical Anthropology* 20:409–44.

Jochle, Wolfgang. 1974. "Menses-Inducing Drugs: Their Role in Antique, Medieval, and Renaissance Gynecology and Birth Control." *Contraception* 10(4): 425–39.

Johanson, Richard; Newburn, Mary; and Macfarlane, Alison. 2002. "Has the Medicalisation of Childbirth Gone Too Far?" *British Journal of Medicine* 224:892–95.

Jolly, Margaret. 1998. "Introduction: Colonial and Postcolonial Plots in Histories of Maternities and Modernities." In *Maternities and Modernities: Colonial and Postcolonial Experiences in Asia and the Pacific*, Kaplana Ram and Margaret Jolly, eds., 1–25, Cambridge: Cambridge University Press.

Jones, Elise; Forrest, Jacqueline Darroch; Henshaw, Stanley K.; Silverman, Jane; and Torres, Aida. 1989. *Pregnancy, Contraception, and Family Planning Services in Industrialized Countries*. New Haven: Yale University Press.

Jordan, Brigitte. 1993[1978]. *Birth in Four Cultures: A Cross-Cultural Investigation of Childbirth in Yucatan, Holland, Sweden, and the United States*. 4th edition. Prospect Heights, Ill.: Waveland Press.

Joseph, Brian. 1992. "Intellectual Awareness as a Reflex of Linguistic Dimensions of Power: Evidence from Greek." *Journal of Modern Greek Studies* 10:71–85.

Jouanna, Jacques. 1999. *Hippocrates*. Baltimore and London: Johns Hopkins University Press.

Jusdanis, Gregory. 1992. *Belated Modernity and Aesthetic Culture: Inventing National Literature*. Minneapolis and Oxford: University of Minnesota Press.

———. 2001. *The Necessary Nation*. Princeton and Oxford: Princeton University Press.

Just, Roger. 1989. "Triumph of the Ethnos." In *History and Ethnicity*, Elizabeth Tonkin, Malcolm Chapman, and Maryon McDonald, eds., 71–88. London: Routledge.

———. 2000. *A Greek Island Cosmos: Kinship and Community on Meganisi*. Oxford and Santa Fe: School of American Research Press.

Kanaaneh, Rhoda. 2002. *Birthing the Nation: Strategies of Palestinian Women in Israel*. Berkeley: University of California Press.

Karasoulli, Maria. 1994. *Conference Tourism: Can Rhodes Cope?* Master's thesis, University of Ulster.

Kasimati, Koula; Thanopoulou, Maria; and Tsartas, Paris. 1999. *I Ghinekia Apaskholisi ston*

Touristiko Tomea [Women's Employment in the Tourist Sector]. Athens: Panteion University and the European Union, Office of Equal Opportunity.

Kasperson, Roger. 1966. *The Dodecanese: Diversity and Unity in Island Politics*. Chicago: University of Chicago Press.

Katsoudas, Dimitrios. 1987. "The Media: The State and Broadcasting." In *Political Change in Greece: Before and after the Colonels*, Kevin Featherstone and Dimitrios Katsoudas, eds., 189–213. London and Sydney: Croom Helm.

Kelly, Susan. 2003. "Bioethics and Rural Health: Theorizing Place, Space, and Subjects." *Social Science and Medicine* 56(11): 2277–88.

Kenna, Margaret. 1976. "Houses, Fields, and Graves: Property and Ritual Obligation on a Greek Island." *Ethnology* 15:21–34.

———. 1985. "Icons in Theory and Practice: An Orthodox Christian Example." *History of Religions* 24(4): 345–68.

———. 1992. "Changing Places and Altered Perspectives." In *Anthropology and Autobiography*, Judith Okely and Helen Callaway, eds.,147–62. London and New York: Routledge.

Kirtsoglou, Elisabeth. 2004. *For the Love of Women: Gender, Identity, and Same-Sex Relations in a Greek Provincial Town*. London and New York: Routledge.

Knauft, Bruce. 2002. *Critically Modern: Alernatives, Alterities, Anthropologies*. Bloomington and Indianapolis: Indiana University Press.

Koenig, Barbara. 1988. "The Technological Imperative in Medical Practice: The Social Creation of a 'Routine' Treatment." In *Biomedicine Examined*, Margaret Lock and Deborah Gordon, eds., 465–96. Dordrecht, Netherlands: Kluwer Academic.

Kokosalakis, Nikos. 1987. "Religion and Modernization in 19th Century Greece." *Social Compass* 32(2–3): 223–41.

Koliopoulos, John S., and Veremis, Thanos M. 2002. *Greece: The Modern Sequel: From 1821 to the Present*. New York: New York University Press.

Kooij, Loes; Sandall, Jane; Pechlivani, Fani; Toiviainen, Hanna; Santalahti, Paivi; and Jallinoja, Piia. 1999. "The Development of Prenatal Screening in Europe: The Practice and Professional Opinions of Midwives." In *Prenatal Screening in Europe: The Past, the Present, and the Future*. Final Report. Elizabeth Ettore, et al. Biomedicine and Health Research and Technological Development Programme, Commission of the European Union, unpublished report, EU Contract no. BMH4-CT96–0740.

Korasidou, Maria. 2002. *Otan I Arostia Apili* [When Illness Threatens]. Athens: Ghiorghos Dhardhanos.

Kotsamanis, V. 1988. "I Anaparaghoghi ton Elinon: Mithi ke Praghmatikotita" [Greeks' Reproduction: Myths and Realities]. *Greek Review of Social Science Research* 70:136–90.

Koussis, Maria. 1989. "Tourism and Family in a Rural Cretan Community." *Annals of Tourism Research* 16:318–32.

Krause, Elizabeth. 2001. "'Empty Cradles' and the Quiet Revolution: Demographic Discourse and Cultural Struggles of Gender, Race, and Class in Italy." *Cultural Anthropology* 16(4): 576–611.

Krikos-Davis, Katerina. 1982. "Moira at Birth in Greek Tradition." *Folia Neohellenica* 4: 106–34.

Kuriyama, Shigehisa. 1999. *The Expressiveness of the Body and the Divergence of Greek and Chinese Medicine*. New York: Zone Books.

Laderman, Carol. 1983. *Wives and Midwives: Childbirth and Nutrition in Rural Malaysia*. Berkeley: University of California Press.

Laqueur, Thomas. 1990. *Making Sex: Body and Gender from the Greeks to Freud*. Cambridge, Mass., and London: Harvard University Press.

Lash, Scott, and Urry, John. 1994. *Economies of Signs and Space*. London, Thousand Oaks, Calif., and Delhi: Sage Publications.

Lauren, Michaela; Petrogiannis, Konstantine; Jallinoja, Piia; Adam, Eleni; Tymstra, Tjeerd; and Ettore, Elizabeth. 1999. "Prenatal Diagnosis in Lay Press and Professional Journals in Finland, Greece, and the Netherlands." In *Prenatal Screening in Europe: The Past, the Present, and the Future*. Final Report. In Elizabeth Ettore, et al. Biomedicine and Health Research and Technological Development Programme, Commission of the European Union, unpublished report, EU Contract no. BMH4-CT96–0740.

Layne, Linda. 2003. *Motherhood Lost: A Feminist Account of Pregnancy Loss in America*. New York: Routledge.

Leavitt, Judith. 1986. *Brought to Bed: Childbearing in America 1750–1950*. New York: Oxford University Press.

Lefkarites, Mary. 1992. "The Sociocultural Implications of Modernizing Childbirth among Greek Women on the Island of Rhodes." *Medical Anthropology* 13:385–412.

Leontidou, Lila. 1994. "Gendered Dimensions of Tourism in Greece: Employment, Sub-Cultures, and Restructuring." In *Tourism: A Gender Analysis*, Vivian Kinnaird and Derek Hall, eds., 74–105. Chichester and New York: John Wiley and Sons.

Lévy, Isaac Jack, and Lévy Zumwalt, Rosemary. 2002. *Ritual Medical Lore of Sephardic Women*. Urbana and Chicago: University of Illinois Press.

Lieber, Michael. 1990. "Lamarckian Definitions of Identity on Kapingamarangi and Pohnpei." In *Cultural Identity and Ethnicity in the Pacific*, Jocelyn Linnekin and Lin Poyer, eds., 71–101. Honolulu: University of Hawaii Press.

LiPuma, Edward. 1993. "Culture in a Theory of Practice." In *Bourdieu: Critical Perspectives*, Craig Calhoun, Edward LiPuma, and Moishe Postone, eds., 14–34. Chicago: University of Chicago Press.

Litt, Jacquelyn. 2000. *Medicalized Motherhood: Perspectives from the Lives of African-American and Jewish Women*. New Brunswick, N.J., and London: Rutgers University Press.

Littlewood, Ian. 2001. *Sultry Climates: Travel and Sex*. Cambridge, Mass.: Da Capo Press.

Lo, Joan. 2003. "Patients' Attitudes vs. Physicians' Determinations: Implications for Cesarean Sections." *Social Science and Medicine* 57(1): 91–96.

Lock, Margaret. 1993a. *Encounters with Aging: Mythologies of Menopause in Japan and North America*. Berkeley: University of California Press.

———. 1993b. "Cultivating the Body: Anthropology and Epistemologies of Bodily Practice and Knowledge." *Annual Reviews of Anthropology* 22:133–56.

———. 1997. "Culture, Technology, and the New Death: Deadly Disputes in Japan and North America." *Culture* 17(1–2): 27–42.

———. 2004. "Medicalization." *Encyclopedia of Medical Anthropology*. Vol. 1, *Health and Illness in the World's Cultures*, Carol Ember and Melvin Ember, eds., 116–24. New York: Kluwer Academic/Plenum.

Lock, Margaret, and Gordon, Deborah, eds. 1988. *Biomedicine Examined*. Dordrecht, Netherlands: Kluwer Academic.

Lock, Margaret, and Kaufert, Patricia, eds. 1998. *Pragmatic Women and Body Politics*. Cambridge: Cambridge University Press.

Lock, Margaret, and Scheper-Hughes, Nancy. 1996. "A Critical-Interpretive Approach in Medical Anthropology: Rituals and Routines of Discipline and Dissent." In *Medical Anthropology: Contemporary Theory and Method*, rev. edition, Carolyn Sargent and Thomas Johnson, eds., 41–70. Westport, Conn., and London: Bergin and Garvey.

Loizos, Peter, and Papataxiarchis, Evthymios. 1991a. "Introduction: Gender and Kinship in Marriage and Alternative Contexts." In *Contested Identities: Gender and Kinship in Modern*

Greece, Peter Loizos and Evthymios Papataxiarchis, eds., 3–25. Princeton: Princeton University Press.

———. 1991b. "Gender, Sexuality, and the Person in Greek Culture." In *Contested Identities: Gender and Kinship in Modern Greece*, Peter Loizos and Evthymios Papataxiarchis, eds., 221–34. Princeton: Princeton University Press.

Loukissas, Philippos. 1982. "Tourism's Regional Development Impacts: A Comparative Analysis of the Greek Islands." *Annals of Tourism Research* 9:523–41.

Lupton, Deborah. 1994. *Medicine as Culture: Illness, Disease, and the Body in Western Societies*. London: Sage.

———. 1999. Introduction to *Risk and Sociocultural Theory: New Directions and Perspectives*, Deborah Lupton, ed., 1–11. Cambridge: Cambridge University Press.

Luttrell, Anthony. 1999. *The Hospitaller State on Rhodes and Its Western Provinces, 1306–1462*. Aldershot, Eng., and Brookfield, Vt.: Ashgate Valorium.

Machin, Barrie. 1983. "St. George and the Virgin: Cultural Codes, Religion, and Attitudes to the Body in a Cretan Mountain Village." *Social Analysis* 14:107–26.

Mallaby, Thomas. 2002. "Odds and Ends: Mortality and the Politics of Contingency." *Culture, Medicine, and Psychiatry* 26:283–312.

Manderson, Lenore. 1998. "Shaping Reproduction: Maternity in Early Twentieth-Century Malaya." In *Maternities and Modernities: Colonial and Postcolonial Experiences in Asia and the Pacific*, Kaplana Ram and Margaret Jolly, eds., 26–49. Cambridge: Cambridge University Press.

Marangos, Christos, and Adam, Eleni. 1999. "Proghenitikos ke Prosimptotikos Ghenetikos Elekhos: Apopsis Pedhiatron" [Prenatal and Genetic Screening: Views of Greek Paediatricians]. *Pedhiatriki* 62:490–98.

Margharitidhou, Vasso. 1991. *Aksiologhisi ton Ipiresion Ikogheniakou Proghramatismou stin Eladha* [Evaluation of Family Planning Services in Greece]. Athens: Family Planning Society.

Martin, Emily. 1987. *The Woman in the Body: A Cultural Analysis of Reproduction*. Boston: Beacon Press.

Martinoli, Simona, and Perotti, Eliana. 1999. *Architettura coloniale italiana nel Dodecaneso, 1912–1943*. Turin: Edizioni Fondazione Giovanni Agnelli.

Mavrou, Ariadni; Metaxotou, Catherine; and Trichopoulos, Dimitris. 1998. "Awareness and Use of Prenatal Diagnosis among Greek Women: A National Survey." *Prenatal Diagnosis* 18:349–55.

Mazower, Mark. 1993. *Inside Hitler's Greece: The Experience of Occupation, 1941–44*. New Haven: Yale University Press.

McDonald, Maryon. 1993. "The Construction of Difference: An Anthropological Approach to Stereotypes." In *Inside European Identities: Ethnography in Western Europe*, Sharon Macdonald, ed., 219–36. Providence, R.I.: Berg.

McLaren, Angus. 1990. *A History of Contraception: From Antiquity to the Present*. Oxford and Cambridge, Mass.: Blackwell.

McNeill, William H. 1978. *The Metamorphosis of Greece since World War II*. Chicago: University of Chicago Press.

McTavish, Lianne. 2005. *Childbirth and the Display of Authority in Early Modern France*. Hampshire, Eng., and Burlington, Vt.: Ashgate.

Michas, Takis. 2002. *Unholy Alliance: Greece and Milosevic's Serbia*. College Station: Texas A&M University Press.

Michie, Helena, and Cahn, Naomi. 1997. *Confinements: Fertility and Infertility in Contemporary Culture*. New Brunswick, N.J., and London: Rutgers University Press.

Micozzi, Marc. 2002. "Culture, Anthropology, and the Return of 'Complementary Medicine.'" *Medical Anthropology Quarterly* 16(4): 398–414.

Miller, Daniel. 1987. *Material Culture and Mass Consumption*. London: Basil Blackwell.

———. 1994. *Modernity, An Ethnographic Approach: Dualism and Mass Consumption in Trinidad*. Oxford and New York: Berg.

Miller, J. 1988. "Maternal and Neonatal Morbidity and Mortality in Caesarian Section." *Obstetrics and Gynecology Clinics of North America* 15:629–38.

Miller, Timothy. 1997. *The Birth of the Hospital in the Byzantine Empire*. Baltimore: Johns Hopkins University Press.

Mitchell, Lisa. 2001. *Baby's First Picture: Ultrasound and the Politics of Fetal Subjects*. Toronto: University of Toronto Press.

Moore, Henrietta. 1994. *A Passion for Difference: Essays in Anthropology and Gender*. Oxford: Polity Press.

Mossialos, E.; Allin, S.; Karras, K.; and Davaki, K. 2005. "An Investigation of Caesarean Sections in Three Greek Hospitals." *European Journal of Public Health* 15(3): 288–95.

Moutsatsos, Chrisy. 2001. "Transnational Beauty Culture and Local Bodies: An Ethnographic Account of Consumption and Identity in Urban Greece." Ph.D.diss., University of California, Irvine.

Naziri, Despina. 1988. "La femme Greque et l'avortement: étude clinique du recours répétif à l'avortement." Ph.D. diss., University of Paris.

Nederveen Pierterse, Jan. 2004. *Globalization and Culture: Global Melange*. Lanham, Md.: Rowman and Littlefield.

Nelkin, Dorothy. 2003. "Preface: The Social Meaning of Risk." In *Risk, Culture, and Health Inequality: Shifting Perceptions of Danger and Blame*, Barbara Herr Harthorn and Laury Oaks, eds., vii–xiii. Westport, Conn., and London: Praeger.

Nichter, Mark. 2003. "Harm Reduction: A Core Concern for Medical Anthropology." In *Risk, Culture, and Health Inequality: Shifting Perceptions of Danger and Blame*, Barbara Herr Harthorn and Laury Oaks, eds., 13–33. Westport, Conn., and London: Praeger.

Nilsson, Lennart. 1990. *A Child Is Born*. New York: Delacorte Press.

Norgren, Tiana. 2001. *Abortion before Birth Control: The Politics of Reproduction in Postwar Japan*. Princeton: Princeton University Press.

Nutton, Vivian. 1984. "From Galen to Alexander: Aspects of Medicine and Medical Practice in Late Antiquity." *Dunbarton Oaks Papers* 38:1–14.

Oaks, Laury. 2001. *Smoking and Pregnancy: The Politics of Fetal Protection*. New Brunswick, N.J., and London: Rutgers University Press.

Ohnuki-Tierney, Emiko. 1984. *Illness and Culture in Contemporary Japan: An Anthropological View*. Cambridge: Cambridge University Press.

Ong, Walter. 1982. *Orality and Literacy*. London: Metheun.

Osherson, Samuel, and AmaraSingham, Lorna. 1981. "The Machine Metaphor in Medicine." In *Social Context of Health, Illness, and Patient Care*, Elliot Mishler, ed., 218–49. Cambridge: Cambridge University Press.

Palli-Petralia, Fani. 1997. *I Atekni Khora: Dhimografiki Ekseliksi—Prooptikes* [The Birthless Nation: Demographic Development—Perspectives]. Athens: I. Sidheris.

Panopoulos, Panayotis. 2003. "Animal Bells as Symbols: Sound and Hearing in a Greek Island Village." *Journal of the Royal Anthropological Institute* (ns) 9:639–56.

Panourgia, Neni. 1995. *Fragments of Death, Fables of Identity: An Athenian Anthropography*. Madison: University of Wisconsin Press.

Papachristodoulou, Christos. 1994. *Istoria tis Rodhou: apo tous Proistorikous Khronous eos tin*

Ensomatosi tis Dhodhekanisou, 1948 [History of Rhodes, from Prehistoric Times to the Incorporation of the Dodecanese, 1948]. 2nd edition. Athens: Dhimos Rodhou.

———. 1996. *Toponimia tis Rodhou* [Rhodian Toponyms]. Rhodes: SGT.

Papagaroufali, Eleni. 1990. "Greek Women in Politics: Gender Ideology and Practice in Neighborhood Groups and the Family." Ph.D. diss., Columbia University.

———. 1999. "Donation of Human Organs or Bodies after Death: A Cultural Phenomenology of 'Flesh.'" *Ethos* 27:283–314.

Papagaroufali, Eleni, and Georges, Eugenia. 1993. "Greek Women in the Europe of 1992: Brokers of European Cargoes and the Logic of the West." In *Perilous States: Conversations on Culture, Politics, and Nation*, George Marcus, ed., 235–54. Chicago: University of Chicago Press.

———. 2002. *Dhora Meta Thanaton: Politismikes Embiries* [Gifts After Death: Cultural Experiences]. Athens: Ellinika Grammata.

Papataxiarchis, Evthymios. 1995. "Male Mobility and Matrifocality in the Aegean Basin." In *Brothers and Others: Essays in Honor of John Peristiany*, J. Pitt-Rivers and G. Ravis-Giordani, eds., 219–39. Paris: Ecoles des Hautes Etudes.

Parsons, Robert James. 2001. "The Balkan DU Cover Up." *The Nation*, April 9, 22–24.

Paxson, Heather. 2002. "Rationalizing Sex: Family Planning and the Making of Modern Greek Lovers in Urban Greece." *American Ethnologist* 29(2): 307–34.

———. 2004. *Making Modern Mothers: Ethics and Family Planning in Urban Greece*. Berkeley: University of California Press.

Pechlivani, Fani, and Adam, Eleni. 1999. "Greek Midwives on Prenatal Screening." In *Prenatal Screening in Europe: The Past, the Present, and the Future*. Final Report. Elizabeth Ettore, et al. Biomedicine and Health Research and Technological Development Programme, Commission of the European Union, unpublished report, EU Contract no. BMH4-CT96–0740.

Petchesky, Rosalind. 1987. "Foetal Images: The Power of Visual Culture in the Politics of Reproduction." In *Reproductive Technologies: Gender, Motherhood, and Medicine*, Michelle Stanworth, ed., 57–80. Minneapolis: University of Minnesota Press.

———. 1990. *Abortion and Women's Choice: The State, Sexuality, and Reproductive Freedom*. Rev. edition. Boston: Northeastern University Press.

———. 1998. "Cross-Country Comparisons and Political Visions." In *Negotiating Reproductive Rights: Women's Perspectives across Countries and Cultures*, Rosalind Petchesky and Karen Judd, eds., 295–323. London and New York: Zed Books.

Petchesky, Rosalind, and Karen Judd, eds. 1998. *Negotiating Reproductive Rights: Women's Perspectives across Countries and Cultures*. London and New York: Zed Books.

Petryna, Adriana. 2002. *Life Exposed: Biological Citizens after Chernobyl*. Princeton and Oxford: Princeton University Press.

Pettifer, James. 1996. "Greek Political Culture and Foreign Policy." In *Greece in a Changing Europe: Between European Integration and Balkan Disintegration?* Kevin Featherstone and Kostas Ifantis, eds., 17–23. Manchester and New York: Manchester University Press.

Pfaffenberger, Bryan. 1992. "Social Anthropology of Technology." *Annual Review of Anthropology* 21:491–516.

Philalithis, Anastas. 1986. "The Imperative for a National Health System in Greece in a Social and Historical Context." In *Socialism in Greece*, Z. Tzannatos, ed., 145–73. Brookfield, Vt.: Gower.

Phillips, Lynn, and Ilcan, Suzan. 2007. "Responsible Expertise: Governing the Uncertain Subjects of Biotechnology." *Critique of Anthropology* 27(1): 103–26.

Placas, Aimee. 2001. "Who Puts the Romance in Romance Tourism?" Typescript. Author files.

Pollack, Linda. 1990. "Embarking on a Rough Passage: The Experience of Pregnancy in Early Modern Society." In *Women as Mothers in Pre-Industrial England: Essays in Memory of Dorothy McLaren*, Valerie Fildes, ed., 39–67. New York and London: Routledge.

Porter, Roy. 1997. *The Greatest Benefit to Mankind: A Medical History of Humanity from Antiquity to the Present*. London: HarperCollins.

Porter, Roy, and Hall, Lesley. 1995. *The Facts of Life: The Creation of Sexual Knowledge in Britain, 1650–1950*. New Haven and London: Yale University Press.

Potter, Joseph. 1999. "The Persistence of Outmoded Contraceptive Regimes." *Population and Development Review* 25:703–40.

Potter, Linda. 2001. "Menstrual Regulation and the Pill." In *Regulating Menstruation: Beliefs, Practices, Interpretations*, Etienne Van de Walle and Elisha P. Renne, eds., 141–54. Chicago and London: University of Chicago Press.

Probyn, Elspeth. 1991. "The Body Which Is Not One: Speaking an Embodied Self." *Hypatia* 6(3): 111–24.

Rabinow, Paul. 1989. *French Modern: Norms and Forms of the Social Environment*. Cambridge, Mass.: MIT Press.

Ram, Kaplana, and Jolly, Margaret. 1998. *Maternities and Modernities: Colonial and Postcolonial Experiences in Asia and the Pacific*. Cambridge: Cambridge University Press.

Rapp, Rayna. 1994. "Commentary on AAA Panel 'Reproducing Reproduction.'" *Anthropology Newsletter*, November, p. 34.

———. 1999. *Testing Women, Testing the Fetus: The Social Impact of Amniocentesis in America*. New York and London: Routledge.

Reiser, Stanley. 1978. *Medicine in the Reign of Technology*. Cambridge: Cambridge University Press.

Rhodes, Lorna. 1996. "Studying Biomedicine as a Cultural System." In *Medical Anthropology: Contemporary Theory and Method*, rev. edition, Carolyn Sargent and Thomas Johnson, eds., 165–80. Westport, Conn., and London: Bergin and Garvey.

Riddle, John. 1985. *Dioscorides on Pharmacy and Medicine*. Austin: University of Texas Press.

———. 1997. *Eve's Herbs: A History of Contraception and Abortion in the West*. Cambridge, Mass.: Harvard University Press.

Rigatos, Gherasimos. 1992. *I Ighia tou Pedhiou sti Laiki Mas Paradhosi* [The Health of the Child in Our Folk Tradition]. Athens: Dodoni.

———. 1999. *I Arkhea Iatriki sti Laiki Mas Paradhosi* [Ancient Medicine in Our Folk Tradition]. Athens: BHTA.

Riley-Smith, Jonathan. 1999. *Hospitallers: The History of the Order of St. John*. London: Hambledon Press.

Rodd, Rennell. 1892. *The Customs and Lore of Modern Greece*. London: D. Stott.

Roessel, David. 2002. *In Byron's Shadow: Modern Greece in the English and American Imagination*. Oxford and New York: Oxford University Press.

Rollisson, Sharon. 2000. "Official Tourist Figures." *Rodos News*.

Romanucci-Ross, Lola. 1969. "The Hierarchy of Resort in Curative Practices: The Admiralty Islands, Melanesia." *Journal of Health and Social Behavior* 10:201–9.

Rose, Nikolas. 2007. The *Politics of Life Itself: Biomedicine, Power, and Subjectivity in the Twenty-First Century*. Princeton: Princeton University Press.

Rosenthal, Elizabeth. 2006. "Biotech Food Tears Rifts in Europe." *New York Times*, June 6.

Ross, Ellen. 1993. *Love and Toil: Motherhood in Outcast London, 1870–1918*. New York and Oxford: Oxford University Press.

Rothman, Barbara Katz. 1986. *The Tentative Pregnancy*. New York: Viking Press.

Ruiz Jimenez, Antonia Maria. 2004. "Representations of Europe and the Nation: How Do Spaniards See Themselves as Nationals and Europeans?" *Jean Monnet/Robert Schuman Paper Series* 4(13).

Saetnan, Ann. 2000. "Women's Involvement with Reproductive Medicine: Introducing Shared Concepts." In *Bodies of Technology: Women's Involvement with Reproductive Medicine*, Ann Saetnan, Nelly Oudshoorn, and Marta Kirejcyk, eds., 1–30. Columbus: Ohio State University Press.

Said, Edward. 1978. *Orientalism*. New York: Pantheon.

Saka, Erkan. 2003. "Rhodian Turks: Collective Memory and Life Histories in the Making of a Community." Typescript. Author files.

Sakala, Carol. 1993. "Medically Unnecessary Caesarean Section Births: Introduction to a Symposium." *Social Science and Medicine* 37(10): 1177–98.

Salamone, S. D., and Stanton, J. B. 1986. "Women's Roles and House Form and Decoration in Eressos, Greece." In *Gender and Power in Rural Greece*, Jill Dubisch, ed., 97–120. Princeton: Princeton University Press.

Salazar Parrenas, Rhacel. 2001. *Servants of Globalization: Women, Migration, and Domestic Work*. Stanford: Stanford University Press.

Sant Cassia, Paul, with Bada, Constantina. 1992. *The Making of the Modern Greek Family: Marriage and Exchange in Nineteenth Century Athens*. Cambridge: Cambridge University Press.

Savaronakis, N. 1991. *Nisiotikes Kinonies sto Egheo* [Island Communities of the Aegean]. Rhodes: Trohalia.

Sawicki, Jana. 1991. *Disciplining Foucault: Feminism, Power, and the Body*. New York and London: Routledge.

Scarborough, John. 1984. "Introduction: Symposium on Byzantine Medicine." *Dunbarton Oaks Papers* 38:ix–xvi.

Schneider, Jane, and Schneider, Peter. 1991. "Sex and Respectability in an Age of Fertility Decline: A Sicilian Case Study." *Social Science and Medicine* 33:885–95.

Schofield, Roger. 1986. "Did Mothers Really Die? Three Centuries of Maternal Mortality in 'The World We Have Lost.'" In *The World We Have Gained: Histories of Population and Social Structure*, Lloyd Bonfield, Richard M. Smith, and Keith Wrightson, eds., 231–60. Oxford: Oxford University Press.

Seremetakis, C. Nadia. 1991. *The Last Word: Women, Death, and Divination in Inner Mani*. Chicago: University of Chicago Press.

———. 1994. *The Senses Still: Perception and Memory as Material Culture in Modernity*. Chicago: University of Chicago Press.

Sherwin, Susan. 1994. "Abortion through a Feminist Lens." In *Living with Contradictions: Controversies in Feminist Ethics*, Alison Jaggar, ed., 314–24. Boulder, Colo.: Westview Press.

Siampos, George. 1975. "Law and Fertility in Greece." In *Law and Fertility in Europe: A Study of Legislation Directly or Indirectly Affecting Fertility in Europe*, Maurics Kirk, Massimo Livi-Bacci, and Egon Szabady, eds., 337–64. Liege: International Union for the Scientific Study of Population.

Siedlecky, Stefania. 2001. "Pharmacological Properties of Emmenagogues: A Biomedical View." In *Regulating Menstruation: Beliefs, Practices, Interpretations*, Etienne van de Walle, and Elisha P. Renne, eds., 93–112. Chicago and London: University of Chicago Press.

Sikaki-Douka, Aleka. N.d. *O Toketos Ine Aghapi*. [Birth Is Love.] 4th edition. Athens: By author.

Skalkidis, Y.; Petridou, E.; Papathoma, E.; Revinthi, K.; Tong, D.; and Trichopoulos, D. 1996. "Are Operative Deliveries in Greece Socially Conditioned?" *International Journal of Qualitative Health Care* 8(2): 159–65.

Skandhalidhi, Michail. 1965. *Khalki tis Dodhekanisou* [Halki of the Dodecanese]. Athens: By author.

Skilogianis, Joanna. 2001. "Great Expectations vs. State Expectations: Fertility Limitation among Women in Urban Greece." Ph.D. diss., Case Western Reserve University.

Smith, Lindsay. 2002. "Romantic Holidays and Cross-Cultural Marriages: Negotiating Gender, International Power and Prestige, and Erotic Desire." Typescript. Author files.

Sobo, Elisa. 1993. *One Blood: The Jamaican Body*. Albany: State University of New York Press.

Sonderkamp, Joseph. 1984. "Theophanes Nonnus: Medicine in the Circle of Constantine Porphyrogenitus." *Dunbarton Oaks Papers* 38:28–41.

Sontag, Susan. 1989. *On Photography*. New York: Farrar, Straus and Giroux.

Stacey, Jackie. 2001. "The Global Within: Consuming Nature, Embodying Health." In *Global Nature, Global Culture*, Sarah Franklin, Celia Lury, and Jackie Stacey, eds., 97–145. London, Thousand Oaks, Calif., and New Delhi: Sage Publications.

Stamiris, Eleni. 1986. "The Women's Movement in Greece." *New Left Review* 158:98–112.

Stephens, Sharon. 1995. "Introduction: Children and the Politics of Culture in 'Late Capitalism.'" In *Children and the Politics of Culture*, Sharon Stephens, ed., 3–48. Princeton: Princeton University Press.

Stephenson, P. A.; Bakoula, C.; Hemminki, E.; Knudsen, L.; Levasseur, M.; Schenker, J.; Stembera, Z.; Tiba, J.; Verbrugge, H. P.; and Zupan, J. 1993. "Patterns of Use of Obstetrical Interventions in 12 Countries." *Paediatric and Perinatal Epidemiology* 7(1): 45–54.

Stewart, Charles. 1991. *Demons and the Devil: Moral Imagination in Modern Greek Culture*. Princeton: Princeton University Press.

———. 1997. "Fields in Dreams: Anxiety, Experience, and the Limits of Social Constructionism in Modern Greek Dream Narratives." *American Ethnologist* 24(4): 877–94.

Stillwagon, Eileen. 1998. *Stunted Lives, Stagnant Economies: Poverty, Disease, and Underdevelopment*. New Brunswick, N.J., and London: Rutgers University Press.

Stoller, Paul. 1997. *Sensuous Scholarship*. Philadelphia: University of Pennsylvania Press.

Strong, P. M. 1984. "Viewpoint: The Academic Encirclement of Medicine?" *Sociology of Health and Illness* 6:339–58.

Sutton, David. 1998a. *Memories Cast in Stone: The Relevance of the Past in Everyday Life*. Oxford and New York: Berg.

———. 1998b. "'He's Too Cold!' Children and the Limits of Culture on a Greek Island." *Anthropology and Humanism*, Special Issue 23(2): 127–38.

Sutton, David, and Fernandez, Renate, eds. 1998. "In the Field and at Home: Families and Anthropology." *Anthropology and Humanism*, Special Issue 23(2).

Sutton, Susan Buck. 1986. "Family and Work: New Patterns for Village Women in Athens." *Journal of Modern Greek Studies* 4(1): 33–49.

———. 1999. "Fleeting Villages, Moving Households: Greek Housing Strategies in Historical Perspective." In *House Life: Space, Place, and Family in Europe*, Donna Birdwell-Pheasant and Denise Lawrence-Zuniga, eds., 73–103. Oxford and New York: Berg.

———, ed. 2000. *Contingent Countryside: Settlement, Economy, and Land Use in the Southern Argolid since 1700*. Stanford: Stanford University Press.

Symeonidou, Haris. 2002. *Fertility and Family Surveys in Countries of the ECE Region: Standard Country Report: Greece*. New York and Geneva: United Nations.

Symeonidou, Haris; Kavouriaris, Evthimios; Kandhilorou, Eleni; Maghdhalinos, Mikhalis; Mitsopoulos, Ghiorghos; Tsakhalidhis, Ghianis; and Vezirghiani, Katerina. 2000. *Epithimito ke Praghmatiko Meghethos Ikoghenias: Gheghonota tou Kiklou Zois—Mia Dhiakhroniki Prosengisi: 1983–1997* [Desired and Actual Family Size: Events of the Life Cycle—A Diachronic Approach: 1983–1997]. Athens: EKKE.

Taussig, Michael. 1992. *The Nervous System*. New York: Routledge.

Temkin, Oswei. 1962. "Byzantine Medicine: Tradition and Empiricism." *Dunbarton Oaks Papers* 16: 97–115.

———. 1991. *Soranus' Gynecology*. Baltimore and London: Johns Hopkins University Press.

Thompson, Lana. 1999. *The Wandering Womb: A Cultural History of Outrageous Beliefs about Women*. Amherst, N.Y.: Prometheus Books.

Tountas, Yannis; Dimitraki, Christine; Antoniou, Anna; Boulamatsis, Dimitris; and Creatsas, George. 2004. "Attitudes and Behavior towards Contraception among Greek Women during Reproductive Age: A Country-wide Survey." *European Journal of Obstetrics and Gynecology and Reproductive Biology* 116:190–95.

Traina, Cristina; Georges, Eugenia; Inhorn, Marcia; Kahn, Susan; and Ryan, Maura. 2008. "Compatible Contradictions: Religion and the Naturalization of Assisted Reproduction." In *Altering Nature: Religion, Biotechnology and Public Policy*, E. Andrew Lustig, Baruch Brody, and Gerald P. McKenny, eds. Cambridge: Cambridge University Press.

Trakas, Deanna. 1981. "Favism and G6PD Deficiency in Rhodes, Greece: The Interaction of Environment, Inheritance and Culture." Ph.D. diss., Michigan State University.

Traweek, Sharon. 1993. "An Introduction to Cultural and Social Studies of Sciences and Technologies." *Culture, Medicine and Psychiatry* 17:3–25.

Tribe, Laurence. 1990. *Abortion: Clash of Absolutes*. New York: W. W. Norton.

Trouillot, Michel-Rolph. 2002. "The Otherwise Modern: Caribbean Lessons from the Savage Slot." In *Critically Modern: Alternatives, Alterities, Anthropologies*, Bruce Knauft, ed., 220–37. Bloomington and Indianapolis: University of Indiana Press.

Tselikas, Agamenon. 1995. "Ta Elinika Iatrosofia: Mia Perifronimeni Katighoria Khiroghrafon" [Greek Iatrosophia: An Ignored Category of Manuscripts]. In *Iatrika Vizantina Khiroghrafa* [Byzantine Medical Manuscripts], Thanasis Diamandopoulos, ed., 57–69. Athens: Domos.

Tsirpanlis, Zacharias. 1991. *I Rodhos ke i Noties Sporadhes sta Khronia ton Ioaniton Ipoton* [Rhodes and the Southern Sporades in the Years of the Knights of St. John]. Rhodes: n.p.

Tsoukalas, Constantine. 1976. "Some Aspects of 'Over Education' in Modern Greece." In *Regional Variation in Modern Greece and Cyprus: Toward a Perspective on the Ethnography of Greece*, Muriel Dimen and Ernestine Friedl, eds., 419–28. New York: Annals of the New York Academy of Sciences.

———. 1991. "'Enlightened' Concepts in the 'Dark': Power and Freedom, Politics and Society." *Journal of Modern Greek Studies* 9:1–22.

Tulloch, John, and Lupton, Deborah. 2003. *Risk and Everyday Life*. London, Thousand Oaks, Calif., and New Delhi: Sage Publications.

Turner, Bryan. 1995. *Medical Power and Social Knowledge*. 2nd edition. London and Thousand Oaks, Calif.: Sage Publications.

Turner, Victor. 1979. "Betwixt and Between: The Liminal Period in Rites of Passage." In *Reader in Comparative Religion*, W. Lessa and E. Z. Vogt, eds., 234–42. 4th edition. New York: Harper and Row.

Tymstra, Tjeerd. 1989. "The Imperative Character of Medical Technology and the Meaning of 'Anticipated Regret.'" *International Journal of Technology Assessment in Health Care* 5:207–13.

Tziovas, Dimitris. 1989. "Residual Orality and Belated Textuality in Greek Literature and Culture." *Journal of Modern Greek Studies* 7:321–35.

Tzoumaka-Bakoula, C. 1990. "Frondidha kata ton Toketo" [Care during Childbirth]. In *Perighenitiki Frondidha stin Eladha* [Perinatal Care in Greece], E. Valassi Adam, S. Nakou, and D. Trakas, eds., 85–88. Athens: Institute of Child Health.

United Nations Development Program. 2001. *Human Development Report.* New York: Oxford University Press.

Urla, Jacqueline. 1993. "Cultural Politics in an Age of Statistics: Numbers, Nations, and the Making of Basque Identity." *American Ethnologist* 20(4): 818–43.

Valaoras, Vasilios; Polychronopolou, Antonia; and Trichopoulos, Dimitri. 1965. "Control of Family Size in Greece." *Population Studies* 8(3): 265–78.

Van de Walle, Etienne, and Renne, Elisha P., eds. 2001. *Regulating Menstruation: Beliefs, Practices, Interpretations.* Chicago and London: University of Chicago Press.

Van Hollen, Cecilia. 2003. *Birth on the Threshold: Childbirth and Modernity in South India.* Berkeley: University of California Press.

Varon, Laura. 1999. *The Juderia: A Holocaust Survivor's Tribute to the Jewish Community of Rhodes.* Westport, Conn.: Praeger.

Veikou, Christina. 1998. *To Kako Mati: I Kinoniki Kataskevi tis Optikis Epikinonias* [The Evil Eye: The Social Construction of Visual Communication]. Athens: Ellinika Grammata.

Velalidhis, A.; Voughioukas, A.; Kalapanidhas, K.; and Kanakis, N. 1983. *I Ghlosa Mou* [My Language]. Athens: Ministry of National and Religious Education, Pedagogical Institute.

Velogiannis-Moutsopoulos, L., and Bartsocas, C. S. 1989. "Medical Genetics in Greece." In *Human Genetics: A Cross-Cultural Perspective*, D. Wertz and J. Fletcher, eds., 209–34. Heidelberg: Springer.

Vergotis, Ghiorghos. 1997. *H Ekpedhefsi sto Kino tis Rodhou kata tin Italokratia* [Public Education in Rhodes during the Italian Occupation]. Rhodes: Ekdhosi DIKE MME.

Vernier, Bernard. 1984. "Putting Kin and Kinship to Good Use: The Circulation of Goods, Labour, and Names on Karpathos (Greece)." In *Interest and Emotion: Essays on the Study of Family and Kinship*, Hans Medick and David W. Sabean, eds., 28–76. Cambridge: Cambridge University Press.

Vlahoutsikou, Christina. 1997. "Mothers-in-law and Daughters-in-law: Politicizing Confrontations." *Journal of Modern Greek Studies* 15:283–302.

Vratsalis, Antonis. 1990. *Niokhoritika* [New Village Stories]. Rhodes: Tekhni.

Ware, Vron. 1997. Purity and Danger: Race, Gender, and Tales of Sex Tourism. In *Back to Reality? Social Experience and Cultural Studies*, Angela McRobbie, ed., 133–51. Manchester and New York: Manchester University Press.

Wertz, Richard, and Wertz, Dorothy. 1989. *Lying-In: A History of Childbirth in America.* Rev. edition. New Haven: Yale University Press.

Whitaker, Elizabeth. 2000. *Measuring Mama's Milk: Fascism and the Medicalization of Maternity in Italy.* Ann Arbor: University of Michigan Press.

Williams, Raymond. 1961. *The Long Revolution.* London: Penguin.

———. 1973. *The Country and the City.* New York: Oxford University Press.

———. 1980. "Base and Superstructure in Marxist Critical Theory." In *Problems in Materialism and Culture: Selected Essays.* London: Verso.

Williams, Simon. 1997. "Modern Medicine and the 'Uncertain Body': From Corporality to Hyperreality?" *Social Science and Medicine* 45(7): 1041–49.

Wilson, Adrian. 1995. *The Making of Man-Midwifery: Childbirth in England, 1660–1770*. Cambridge, Mass.: Harvard University Press.

Worsley, Peter. 1982. "Non-Western Medical Systems." *Annual Review of Anthropology* 11: 315–48.

Yanagisako, Sylvia, and Delaney, Carol. 1995. "Naturalizing Power." In *Naturalizing Power: Essays in Feminist Cultural Analysis*, Sylvia Yanagisako and Carol Delaney, eds., 1–22. London: Routledge.

Young, Alan. 1982. "The Anthropologies of Illness and Sickness." *Annual Review of Anthropology* 11:257–85.

Yoxen, Edward. 1987. "Seeing with Sound: A Study of the Development of Medical Images." In *The Social Construction of Technological Systems*, W. Bijker, T. Hughes, and T. Pinch, eds., 281–303. Cambridge, Mass.: MIT Press.

Ze'evi, Dror. 2006. *Producing Desire: Changing Sexual Discourse in the Ottoman Middle East, 1500–1900*. Berkeley: University of California Press.

Zighdis, Ioannis. 1993. *I Alaghi Nootropias Aparetiti ghia tin Epiviosi tis Eladhas stin Enomeni Evropi* [The Necessary Change in Mentality for Greece's Survival in the European Union]. Athens: P.I.D. Kleovolos o Lindios.

Zinovieff, Sofka. 1991. "Hunters and Hunted: Kamaki and the Ambiguities of Sexual Predation in a Greek Town." In *Contested Identities: Gender and Kinship in Modern Greece*, Peter Loizos and Evthymios Papataxiarchis, eds., 203–20. Princeton: Princeton University Press.

Index

Page numbers in bold indicate illustrations

Browner, Carole, 20, 107, 109, 283n21
Byron, 50
Byzantine Empire
    Dodecanese islands under, 30, 31
    gynecology of, 84, 90, 282n14
    medical practices of, 27, 83–84, 85, 86, 87,
        97, 272

caesarean section
    anesthesia for, 193, 199
    due date as factor in, 215
    medically unnecessary, 191, 219, 276–77
    rate, 11, 186, 191, 216, 290nn33–34
    women's attitudes concerning, 193, 197,
        198, 199–200
Campbell, J. K., 152
cancer, 209, 242, 243, 290n8
Caraveli, Anna, 118, 122
chamomile tea, 144, 214, 289n32
Chernobyl, 9–10, 209
childbirth
    classes, 157, 188–89, 200
    difficult, procedures for, 132–33, 136–37
    female bodily transformations through,
        71–72, 73
    medicalization of, 10, 193, 195, 289n24
    menstrual problems alleviated through, 73,
        88–89
    menstruation compared to, 103, 150
    as pathological process, 190–91
    persons present at, 136–37, 143, 178–79,
        191, 284–85n10
    position for giving birth, 135–36, 190–91
    risks, potential of, 198, 208
    rituals associated with, 134–38, 141–42,
        143, 157, 158
    ultrasound imaging impact on, 20, 157
childcare practices
    changes in, 255, 291n17
    child mortality blamed on irrational, 224
    mother-centered vs. child-centered, 255,
        291n17
    mother's work impact on, 80–81, 255
    for women in workforce, 260–61, 265
child mortality, 4–5, 74–75, 185, 224, 288n15
children, 70–71, 123, 246, 261–62
Chryssanthopoulou, Vassiliki, 142, 149, 150
cinnamon, 106, 109, 147, 148, 181
cloves, 106, 147, 148
coitus interruptus (withdrawal)
    birth rate, impact on, 223
    cultural aspects of, 245–46
    men's sacrifice in, 245, 246, 253

sexual politics of, 252–54
    use of, 11, 234, 235, 240, 241
    women's attitudes concerning, 245–46,
        250, 251–52
cold (illness), 102–4, 143–44
Collier, Jane, 158
colostrum, avoidance, 144
conception, 97–99, 282n15
condoms
    cultural aspects of, 246, 251
    use of, 11, 223, 234, 235, 241, 244
    women's attitudes concerning, 251
consumption, 255, 257, 259, 264–65, 292n23
contraception. *See also contraceptive method; e.g.,*
        IUD (intra-uterine device)
    access to, 230–33, 244
    vs. "being careful" (terms), 234
    doctor attitudes concerning, 231–32
    generational differences in use of, 239–40
    global variations on, 233–34
    Greek Orthodox Church position on, 227,
        234, 246–47, 251
    men's attitudes concerning, 22–23, 253–54
    men's role in, 245, 246, 252, 254
    nonmedical, 11, 234–35, 245
    use rate for, 11, 13, 230, 234, 239–40
    women's attitudes concerning, 201, 242–45,
        246–47, 248–52, 291n12
contraceptives, oral. *See* birth control pill
cross-cultural marriages, 51, 59, 280n6
cumin, 106

daughters
    houses provided to, 77, 82, 111, 237,
        258–60
    role of, 78–79
    value placed on, 77–78
Davis-Floyd, Robbie, 186, 288n18, 290n33
death, symbolism and practices associated with,
        128–29, 165
De Certeau, Michel, 69
Delaney, Carol, 97, 285n19
demographic problem, 224, 225
demons, 124, 142, 146
devil
    lekhona protection against, 149, 150, 151,
        152
    pregnant women as target of, 123–24
    salt's role in repelling, 14, 142, 145
Dioscorides of Anazarbos, 106, 107
disabilities, stigmatization of, 207–8
distinction, 163, 164
doctor-patient relationships, 217–18, 219

doctors
- abortion, attitudes concerning, 232
- abortions performed by, 110, 228, 230, 235
- gifts to, 217, 218, 219
- midwives compared to, 133, 139–40, 182
- private vs. public sector, 202, 217, 219
- sterilization, attitudes concerning, 232–33, 290n3
- ultrasounds performed by, 204–5, 215–17, 218

Doumanis, Mariella, 80, 281n9
Doumanis, Nicholas, 35, 38, 54, 55
dowry, 76, 77, 82, 258–60, 291n19
dreams, 112–13, 120
Dubisch, Jill, 49, 104–5, 115, 197
du Boulay, Juliet, 92
Duden, Barbara, 173, 180–81
duogenetic theory of procreation, 97, 98
Durrell, Lawrence, 42, 50–51, 280n5

education, 3, 61, 162, 164–65, 255
Eleftherios, St., 114, 120, 126, 141
emmenagogues, 107, 108–10, 148, 282nn22–24
enemas, 18, 186, 190, 197, 200–201
epidurals, 193
episiotomies, 17–18, 190, 199
ethnogynecology
- definition of, 27
- Galenic medicine influence on, 91, 273
- pre-Hippocratic, 84
- women's autonomy and, 274
ethno-obstetrics
- attitudes, contemporary concerning, 158, 168–69
- decline in, 162, 168
- midwifery practices, 91, 156
- women's autonomy and, 274
"ethos of care" (term), 128–29, 181, 238, 284n4
Europe
- ambivalence toward, 57–58
- early modern, childbirth in, 132, 284n5
- early modern, medicine in, 274
Europeanization, 16, 61, 158, 256–57
European Union
- birth practices in, 193, 222
- Greece as member of, 16–17, 22, 226, 256
evidence-based medicine, 17, 186, 222
evil eye
- Orthodox Church position on, 172, 287n6
- pregnant women vulnerable to, 124–25, 129
- protection against, 126, 142, 149, 150, 208, 285n15

young generation's attitudes concerning, 172, 287n6
Evtokia (organization), 188–89, 220

Fakinou, Eugenia, 64, 280n11
Family Law (1983), 46, 258
family planning, 229–30, 231, 235, 245
family size, 226–27, 236–38, 240–41, 254
Fates (Moires), three, 77–78, 154, 155, 156, 286nn25–26
fatherhood
- cultural ideologies of, 74
- men's views on, 22–23
- in prewar period, 71, 79
- transformations in, 20, 254, 264–65, 266
Faubion, James, 201
feeding practices, 104–5, 224
feminism, 8, 166, 188, 220, 229, 270
fertility
- contraception impact on, 241, 243, 244, 247, 251, 276
- declining, concern over, 4
- herbal medicines promoting, 35, 108
- safeguarding as women's duty, 247, 291n12
fetal monitoring, electronic, 186, 190, 216, 290n33
fetal ultrasound imaging. *See* ultrasounds, fetal
fetus, 176, 198, 203, 207, 211, 212, 213, 214, 215
Fischer, Michael, 25
folklor (term), 158–59, 167
food
- cold, classification of, 103–4
- cravings, 123
- sharing, 127–28, 129, 157, 181
- smelling by pregnant women, 127–28, 181
Forty Saints, 127
Foster, George, 20
fosterage, prewar practices involving, 73, 83
Foucault, Michel, 4, 111, 215
Freud, Sigmund, 72, 90, 281n5

Galani Moutafi, Vasilki, 40–41
Galen
- Aristotle compared to, 97, 98
- humoral medicine codified by, 2, 148
- influence and legacy of, 84–85, 90, 272, 273, 282n14
- menstruation, views concerning, 88
- midwifery influenced by, 133, 284n6
- one-sex model of, 98
- sexual intercourse, views concerning, 99–100

millets, 33, 34, 59

mirodhika, 105–6

miscarriage, 111, 124, 127

Mitchell, Lisa, 175

modernity
    belated, 14–15, 17, 18, 220
    biomedical technologies as signifiers of,
        224
    discourses on, 275
    gender and, 13, 177–78

monogenetic theory of procreation, 97–98

motherhood
    contemporary understanding of, 20, 254,
        256, 257, 261–62, 263–64, 265,
        270–71
    education as preparation for, 169
    medical science and, 5
    in prewar period, 71, 74, 79–82, 174

mothers. See also *lekhona* (mother of newborn)
    cultural understanding, shift in, 197, 233
    obligations toward, 82
    responsibilities, 174, 270–71
    women's identity as, 164, 287n3
    in workforce, 260–61, 265, 292n24

Moutsatsos, Chrisy, 257

naming customs, 71, 117, 118

National Health Service (ESY) (Greece), 189,
    191, 217, 218, 228–29, 232

national identity
    education's role in promoting, 171
    forces shaping, 14–15, 16, 57
    Italian occupation impact on, 52–53
    nootropia and, 57
    obstetrics and gynecology linked to, 14

natural childbirth, 24, 188, 197–98, 219

Naziri, Despoina, 265

neraids (*(a)neraes*), 124, 151, 153

newborn infants
    care of, 141–45, 146–47, 181, 285n15
    rituals of incorporation, 146, 154–56
    vulnerability of, 150–51, 153

Nilsson, Lennart, 175

obstetrical interventions and technologies
    global circulation of, 11, 192, 218–19, 221
    nonmedical factors in use of, 220, 221
    overview of, 189, 190–93
    ritual dimensions of, 186–87, 204–5
    women's attitudes concerning, 200–201,
        223

obstetricians, 187–88, 190, 219, 233

obstetrics
    cross-cultural variations in, 12–13, 185–86

lack of opposition to current model of,
    219–20
United States influence on, 186–87

Occidentalism, 179

olfaction, 181–82

one-sex model, 98, 99, 274, 282n16

Ong, Walter, 180

openness, role in pregnancy and birth, 71–72,
    89, 123, 133, 134, 150, 284n8

orgasm, 99, 282n16

Oribasius, 84

Ottoman Empire
    Greek independence from, 2, 16
    medicine of, 84, 86–87, 98, 272, 273, 274
    occupation of Rhodes (1522–1912), 31,
        32–34, 170

oxytocin (pitocin), 190, 192, 196, 197, 198, 201,
    215, 289n26

pain medications, 193. *See also* anesthesia

pain of childbirth
    managing, 193–94
    procedures increasing, 193, 196, 197, 198
    women's attitudes concerning, 197–98, 199,
        200, 289n26

Panaghia (Mother of God)
    manifestations of, 112–13, 114, 119, 120
    mothers' association with, 81
    procreation and fertility, association with,
        113, 126
    vows made to, 114, 117, 118, 119

Panaghia Tsambika, shrine of, 35, 114–15,
    116–17, 118, 283n27

Papachristodoulou, Christos, 32, 34

Patmos island, 45

Paul of Aegina, 84–85, 86

Paxson, Heather, 197, 231, 251, 254, 288n9,
    290n7, 292n26

perineum
    cutting (*see* episiotomies)
    massaging with olive oil during childbirth,
        133, 134
    tearing, preventing, 133, 134, 136, 186

personhood
    children as means to, 70–71
    of fetuses, 268, 270
    of infants and children, 75–76, 109, 149
    marriage as vehicle for, 70

pessaries (vaginal suppositories), 89, 106, 248

Petchesky, Rosalind, 234, 270, 271, 292n29

Petryna, Adriana, 9–10

phylacteries, 126

pilgrimages to shrines. *See* shrines,
    pilgrimages to

pitocin. *See* oxytocin

placenta, 140–41, 285n12

plethora, 88

politics of numbers, 13

postpartum period

    customs and rituals during, 145–46, 149–56, 286n23

    deritualization of, 184–85

    managing dangers of, 27, 103, 210

    maternal care during, 145–49

    maternal seclusion during, 146, 148, 150–51, 152, 153, 184, 185, 273, 288n13

    midwife assistance during, 122, 130, 140–43, 187, 273

Potter, Joseph, 244–45

Pragmateia (Paul of Aegina), 84–85

pregnancy

    ambiguity of, 109–10, 111

    anxiety associated with, 207, 208–10, 212–13

    bodily transformations through, 71–72, 73

    collective responsibility for, 128–29

    early, 20, 107, 109, 283n21

    generational differences in experience of, 208, 210, 212

    guides on, 157–58, 173–79, 189, 200, 206, 223–24, 287–88nn7–10

    humoral model of, 70

    information, media role in, 195

    protective behaviors during, 27, 126, 129, 209

    saints associated with, 126, 127

    ultrasound imaging impact on, 20, 210–15

prenatal care. *See also* midwives and midwifery

    doctor visits, 190

    information, media role in, 195, 230

    technology role in, 190, 194, 276

    universal access to, 191–92

private clinics, 201–2, 204

pronatalism, 226, 227, 230, 237–38

pubic shaves, 18, 186, 190, 197, 200–201

redressive ritual, 220–21, 222

religious healing

    for infertility, 113, 114, 116–17, 118–20, 121, 155, 283n27

    popularity, continuing of, 188

reproduction, medicalization of. *See* medicalization: of reproduction

reproductive decision making, 20, 261, 271, 292n29

Rhodes General Hospital, 23, 190, **202, 203,** 222

rhythm method of birth control, 234, 235

Righatos, Gherasimos, 190

risk, discourse of, 8–9, 208, 210, 241, 254, 276

rue, 108, 110–11, 235, 283n23

rural-to-urban migration, impact of, 164

saints

    specialties associated with, 114, 126–27

    vows made to, 114, 117, 118, 119

Sakala, Carol, 191, 219

Salerno, medical school at, 85–86

salting ritual, 141–42, 145, 154, 155, 273, 285n15

Sant Cassia with Bada, 267

Sarantisma ritual, 149–50

semen, 99, 100, 105

Sephardic Jews, 32–33, 38, 125, 284n2

Serermatakis, C. Nadia, 128, 129

seven days, ritual of, 154–55

sexual desire, male vs. female, 100–101

sexual intercourse

    and conception, 250

    female bodily transformations through, 71–72, 73

    fertility enhancement, role in, 107

    girls' education concerning, 94–96

    male cleansing, role in, 99–100, 101, 283n18

    men's sacrifice in, 245, 246, 253

    oldest generation's experience of, 98–99

    during postpartum period, 148–49, 152

    womb openness due to, 103, 107

shaking or tossing, 73, 101, 132–33, 169, 284n5

Sharp, Jane, 90, 98, 99, 282n15, 282n16

Shirley Valentine, 51, 58, 280n5, 280n8

shrines, pilgrimages to, 114, 116–17, 118, 119, 172, 283n27

Sikaki-Douka, Aleka, 157–58, 174–79, 187, 191, 197, 209, 288n19, 288nn8–10

sin, 92, 107, 109, 125, 251, 266–71

Skilogianis, Joanna, 231, 236, 290n5

social mobility, 20, 163, 259

Society for the Unborn Child, 268

Soranus of Ephesus

    humoral medicine, approach compared to, 2

    infant swaddling, recommendations for, 143, 285n16

    influence and legacy of, 84, 90, 91, 272, 273, 282n14, 284n6

    works of, 133, 142, 144

Spain, 16, 18, 58, 158, 287n2

sterility, 105

sterilization
    female, 234, 250
    legalization of, 229, 232–33
    male, 234
Stewart, Charles, 76, 112, 164–65
stress, 252, 261, 262, 264, 265
Sutton, David, 158, 258, 259, 287n1, 291n19
Sutton, Susan, 20, 279n3
Symeonidou, Haris, 66, 239, 281n13
Symi island, 36, 64, 280n11

tabou (term) 158–59, 167, 199
tea, postpartum, 147–48, 149, 286n21
technological imperative, 220
technological interventions, 7–8, 18, 186,
    195–96, 224
technology
    as birthing place selection factor, 201
    dependence on, 207
    risks and unintended consequences of, 247
    symbolic dimensions, 17, 189, 220, 275
    women's reliance on, 186–87
Temkin, Oswei, 97
thalassemia, 74, 194, 207–8, 268
Theodorakis, Nikolaos, 87, 273
thermantika, 106
Three Fates (Moires), 77–78, 154, 155, 156,
    286nn25–26
tourism
    class and gender assumptions about, 48
    economic benefits of, 42–43
    under Italian occupation, 36, 37–39
    local attitudes toward, 46–52
    seasonal patterns of, 44–46
    women's involvement in, 40–41
Truman Doctrine, 190
tubal ligations, 232, 233, 290n3
Turkey
    birth rate compared to Greece, 225
    mothers of newborns in, 145, 146,
        285nn18–19
    newborn care in, 144
Turks on Rhodes, 32, 34, 38, 118

ultrasounds, fetal
    detection of anomaly through, 10, 194, 209,
        210, 289n31
    doctors' attitudes concerning, 204, 207,
        215–17, 218
    frequency of, 190, 202–3

    impact of, 20, 157, 203–4, 209–10
    overuse of, 17–18, 207, 216
    women's attitudes concerning, 24, 205–7,
        210–15, 216
umbilical cord, 133, 140–41, 146–47, 285n20
undernatality, attitudes concerning, 224–27,
    230
United States
    biomedical model of, 190
    child mortality rate in, 185, 288n15
    evidence-based medicine in, 222
    Greek biomedicine influenced by, 189–90,
        219, 222
    Greek immigration to, 59, 60, 280n9
    obstetrics in, 186–87, 188, 192
urbanization, 20, 63–66, 165, 280n11
uterus, 98, 102. *See also* womb

vacuum extraction, 191, 193
vaginal birth, 199, 218, 277, 290n34
vaginal suppositories (pessaries), 89, 106, 248
vasectomies, 232, 233
virginity, 93, 94, 95, 96
vision, 180, 181, 204, 211, 212. *See also*
    ultrasounds, fetal
Vlahoutsikou, Christina, 164, 287n3

weaning practices, 144–45
What to Expect When You're Expecting, 157, 174,
    287n7
Williams, Raymond, 64
withdrawal. *See* coitus interruptus
womb
    cold, 102, 103–4, 105, 107, 109, 145, 148
    humoral medicine approach to, 89–90
    open/closed, 103–5, 106, 107, 134, 149,
        235, 284n8
    postpartum period, care during, 141, 145,
        147, 149
    smell, sense of, 89–90, 106, 168, 181
    vulnerability, causes of, 103–4
    wandering, 89–90, 102
women's movement. *See* feminism

xotika, 124, 150, 152–53, 164, 165, 167, 172,
    287n6

Zighdis, Ioannis, 54, 56–57
Zinovieff, Sofka, 48

www.ingramcontent.com/pod-product-compliance
Lightning Source LLC
Chambersburg PA
CBHW080412270326
41929CB00018B/2995